Clinical Ophthalmology

A synopsis

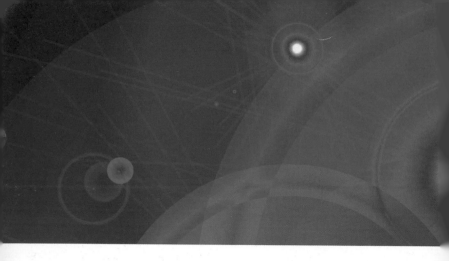

For Elsevier:
Commissioning Editor: **Russell Gabbedy**
Development Editor: **Louise Cook**
Editorial Assistant: **Poppy Garraway**
Project Manager: **Frances Affleck**
Design: **Stewart Larking**
Marketing Manager(s) (UK/USA): **John Canelon/Bill Veltre**

SECOND EDITION

Clinical
Ophthalmology
A synopsis

Jack J Kanski
MD, MS, FRCS, FRCOphth
Honorary Consultant Ophthalmic Surgeon
Prince Charles Eye Unit
King Edward VII Hospital
Windsor, UK

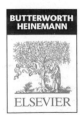

BUTTERWORTH
HEINEMANN

ELSEVIER

BUTTERWORTH
HEINEMANN
ELSEVIER

First published 2009
First edition published 2004

The right of Jack J Kanski to be identified as author of this work has been
asserted by him in accordance with the Copyright, Designs and Patents Act
1988.

ISBN: 978-0-7020-3135-9

International Student Edition ISBN: 978-0-8089-24241

British Library Cataloguing in Publication Data
Kanski, Jack J.
    Clinical ophthalmology : a synopsis. – 2nd ed.
    1. Ophthalmology
    I. Title
    617.7

Library of Congress Cataloging in Publication Data
A catalog record for this book is available from the Library of Congress

ELSEVIER your source for books,
journals and multimedia
in the health sciences

www.elsevierhealth.com

Working together to grow
libraries in developing countries
www.elsevier.com | www.bookaid.org | www.sabre.org

 ELSEVIER BOOK AID International Sabre Foundation

The
publisher's
policy is to use
**paper manufactured
from sustainable forests**

Printed in China
Last digit is the print number: 9 8 7 6 5 4 3 2 1

Contents

15 Ocular Tumours and Related Conditions 271

16 Retinal Vascular Disease 303

20 Strabismus 393

21 Neuro-ophthalmology 407

22 Drug-induced Disorders 437

Preface

Five years have elapsed since the last edition of this book. This edition has undergone major modifications. The text has been expanded and is more detailed, and many new illustrations have been incorporated. It is, however, still the intention of the author for this book to act as a companion to 'Clinical Ophthalmology, 6th Edition' and should be of particular value as a revision guide to those preparing for examinations, as well as the busy clinician requiring a quick reference to a particular diagnostic or therapeutic problem.

Jack J Kanski
2009

Acknowledgements

I am extremely grateful to the following colleagues and medical photographic departments for supplying me with additional material:

Abu El-Asrar L 14.90; **Albert DM, Jakobiec FA** *Principles and Practice of Ophthalmology*, **WB Saunders, 1994** 21.17a-c; **Armstrong D** 6.46; **Barabino S** 8.48; **Barry C** 3.37, 4.99, 8.14, 11.13, 13.26, 14.44, 14.66, 15.51, 15.66, 15.73, 15.84, 15.97, 16.18, 16.27, 16.57, 16.66, 17.12, 17.17, 17.25, 17.27, 17.32, 17.36, 17.37, 17.44, 17.49, 17.50, 18.2, 18.8, 18.60, 19.32, 21.12; **Baruchoff S** 3.17; **Bashshur Z** 14.50; **Bates R** 3.5, 3.20, 4.54, 4.72, 8.36, 9.38, 9.52, 9.58, 15.3, 15.23, 15.33; **Bolton A** 17.10, 17.31, 18.53; **Bonini S** 9.42; **Bouloux P-M** *Clinical Medicine Assessment Questions in Colour*, **Wolfe, 1993** 24.83; **Chisholm L** 3.35; **Curi A** 14.53; **Curtis R** 9.19, 9.21, 12.37, 13.20, 15.13, 15.29, 15.36, 15.38, 15.40, 23.9, 24.24; **Damato B** 15.19, 15.47, 15.48, 15.53, 15.57, 15.58, 15.83, 15.85, 15.91, 15.92, 15.93, 15.94, 15.95, 15.101, 16.61; **Delva S** 4.42; **Desai A** 2.20, 24.67; **Eye Academy** 10.10; **Emond RT, Welsby PD, Rowland HA** *Colour Atlas of Infectious Diseases*, **Mosby, 2003** 24.28, 24.32, 24.39; **ffytche T** 24.33, 24.68, 24.77; **Fogla R** 3.18, 8.49, 8.54, 9.60, 9.62, 9.64, 10.1, 11.19, 24.38; **Forbes CD, Jackson WF** *Color Atlas and Text of Clinical Medicine*, **Mosby, 2003** 24.22, 24.34; **Garcia C de A** 14.57, 14.58, 14.61; **Garner A** 4.38, 6.52, 15.42, 15.43, 15.69; **Gass JDM** *Stereoscopic Atlas of Macular Diseases: Diagnosis and Treatment*, **Mosby, 1997** 14.23, 14.84, 15.57, 16.54, 17.23, 17.48, 18.41, 22.9; **Gilbert C** 24.37; **Gili P** 13.2, 13.7, 14.69, 14.77, 15.7, 15.81, 16.51, 17.9, 17.35, 17.45, 17.48, 18.18, 18.19, 21.1, 21.6, 22.11; **Govan J** 18.37, 18.38; **Hamza M** 15.50; **Harry J** 4.34, 15.68; **Harry J, Misson G** *Clinical Ophthalmic Pathology*, **Butterworth-Heinemann, 2001** 15.67, 15.70; **Hayreh Singh S** 16.31, 21.7; **Horton L** 3.11, 4.17, 4.26, 4.30, 4.66; **Hoyng C** 18.50, 18.51; **Isaacs T** 18.39; **Jager M** 2.13, 4.16, 4.32, 8.12, 8.53, 9.1, 9.31, 9.32, 11.1; **Kerr-Muir M** 9.50; **Krachmer JH, Mannis MJ, Holland EJ** *Cornea*, **Mosby, 2005** 4.28, 4.45, 5.15, 5.16, 8.48, 9.15, 9.24, 9.25, 9.86, 10.6, 10.7, 15.14, 24.76; **Kumar Puri S** 4.67, 13.34; **Leyland M** 10.8; **Leys A** 15.102; **Lightman S** 14.45; **Lisch W** 9.96; **MacKeen L** 13.14, 13.16; **Manoj B** 21.32, 21.44; **Marsh R** 16.38, 16.40; **Martinkova R** 13.45; **Merin L** 12.8, 12.11, 13.24, 14.89, 15.35, 16.17, 17.28, 17.33, 18.55, 22.10; **Mermoud A** 13.68; **Messmer E** 18.48; **Meyer D** 3.11; **Milewski S** 12.16, 14.85, 14.86, 15.100, 16.32, 17.23, 18.17, 23.15; **Mir A** *Atlas of Clinical Diagnosis*, **Saunders, 2003** 21.17d, 24.20, 24.35, 24.36, 24.44, 24.56, 24.59, 24.84; **Moore A** 18.28; **Moorfields Eye Hospital** 14.70, 14.76, 16.23, 17.21, 18.5, 18.26, 18.27, 18.31, 18.36, 18.40, 18.58, 18.61, 24.63; **Morse P** 14.18, 15.87, 18.32, 18.33, 18.34; **Mroczkowska H** 3.8; **Nerad JA, Carter KD, Alford MA** *Oculoplastic and reconstructive surgery*, in *Rapid Diagnosis in Ophthalmology*, **Mosby, 2008** 4.40, 24.4; **Nischal K** 2.9, 6.10, 6.38, 9.82, 12.34, 13.52, 15.79, 16.38, 21.25, 24.47, 24.64, 24.86, 24.87; **Parluekar M** 3.7, 20.12, 20.18, 24.90; **Pavesio C** 14.10, 14.32, 14.43, 14.47, 14.79; **Pearson A** 4.12, 4.14, 4.28, 4.50, 4.78, 4.86, 4.88, 4.90, 4.100, 5.1, 5.2, 5.3, 5.7, 5.13, 5.14, 5.15, 6.7, 6.23, 6.24, 6.25, 6.31, 6.32, 6.45, 6.46, 6.49, 6.54, 8.7, 23.2, 23.6, 23.7; **Pe'er J** 15.78; **Prost M** 14.83;

Raik N 4.22; **Raina U** 14.38, 24.27, 24.50, 24.89; **Ridgway A** 9.73, 9.76, 9.77; **Rogers N** 3.4, 9.15, 9.63, 12.30, 13.36, 21.20, 24.91; **Rose G** 6.43; **Saine P** 16.33, 16.88, 17.46, 18.1, 21.4, 21.11; **Salmon J** 13.9, 13.51, 13.64; **Schepens CL, Hartnett ME, Hirose T** *Schepens Retinal Detachment and Allied Diseases,* Butterworth-Heinemann, 2000 19.12; **Schuman JS, Christopoulos V, Dhaliwal DK, Kahook MY, Noecker RJ Lens and glaucoma,** in *Rapid Diagnosis in Ophthalmology,* Mosby, 2008 3.18, 3.21, 12.33, 12.38, 13.13; **Shun Shin A** 23.13; **Sibtain N** 2.19, 24.60; **Singh AD** 15.103; **Singh AD, Damato BE, Pe'er J, Murphree AL, Perry JD** *Clinical Ophthalmic Oncology,* Saunders, 2007 4.35 4.39; **Sloper J** 2.11; **Talks J** 18.46; **Tanner V** 19.29; **Taylor D** 6.59; **Taylor D, Hoyt CS** *Pediatric Ophthalmology and Strabismus,* Elsevier, 2005 3.50; **Thomas D** 21.23, 21.43; **Trobe JD** Neuro-ophthalmology, in *Rapid Diagnosis in Ophthalmology,* Mosby, 2008 21.7; **Tuft S** 4.50, 4.60, 4.61, 7.1, 7.6, 7.7, 8.6, 8.11, 8.16, 8.17, 8.22, 8.25, 8.26, 8.27, 8.29, 8.31, 8.33, 8.34, 8.35, 8.36, 8.39, 8.43, 8.44, 8.47, 8.51, 8.55, 9.4, 9.5, 9.24, 9.27, 9.28, 9.29, 9.30, 9.33, 9.34, 9.41, 9.45, 9.46, 9.88, 10.3, 10.4, 12.17, 12.18, 24.40; **Visser R** 3.14, 9.61; **Waggoner T** 1.21; **Watson P** 11.6, 11.9, 11.11, 11.12; 11.14, 11.20, 11.22; **Watts P** 16.43; **Wykes W** 16.50; **Wylegala E** 8.41; **Yanguela J** 20.6, 23.4; **Zitelli BL, Davis HW** *Atlas of Pediatric Physical Diagnosis,* Mosby, 2002 6.67, 24.48; **Zografos L** 22.2.

Abbreviations

AAU	acute anterior uveitis
AC/A ratio	accommodative convergence/accommodation ratio
ACTH	adrenocorticotrophic hormone
AD	autosomal dominant
AIDS	acquired immune deficiency syndrome
AION	anterior ischaemic optic neuropathy
AMD	age-related macular degeneration
ANA	antinuclear antibody
APD	afferent pupillary defect
APMPPE	acute posterior placoid pigment epitheliopathy
AR	autosomal recessive
ARC	abnormal retinal correspondence
ARN	acute retinal necrosis
BDR	background diabetic retinopathy
BDUMP	bilateral diffuse uveal melanocytic proliferation
BRAO	branch retinal artery occlusion
BRVO	branch retinal vein occlusion
BSV	binocular single vision
cANCA	antineutrophilic cytoplasmic antibody
CAU	chronic anterior uveitis
CHED	congenital hereditary endothelial dystrophy
CHRPE	congenital hypertrophy of retinal pigment epithelium
CMO	cystoid macular oedema
CMV	cytomegalovirus
CNS	central nervous system
CNV	choroidal neovascularization
CPEO	chronic progressive external ophthalmoplegia
CPSD	corrected pattern standard deviation
CRAO	central retinal artery occlusion
CRV	central retinal vein
CRVO	central retinal vein occlusion
CSF	cerebrospinal fluid
CSR	central serous retinopathy
CSMO	clinically significant macular oedema
CT	computed tomography
CV	colour vision
DA	dark adaptation
DCR	dacryocystorhinostomy
DR	diabetic retinopathy
DVD	dissociated vertical deviation
ECCE	extracapsular cataract extraction
EKC	epidemic keratoconjunctivitis
ELISA	enzyme-linked immunosorbent assay

EOG	electro-oculogram
ERG	electroretinogram
ESR	eryrthrocyte sedimentation rate
FA	fluorescein angiography
FAP	familial adenomatous polyposis
FAZ	foveal avascular zone
5-FU	5-fluorouracil
GCA	giant cell arteritis
GPC	giant papillary conjunctivitis
HAART	highly active antiretroviral therapy
HIV	human immunodeficiency virus
HSV-1	herpes simplex virus type 1
HSV-2	herpes simplex virus type 2
HZO	herpes zoster ophthalmicus
ICG	indocyanine green (angiography)
Ig	immunoglobulin
INOP	internuclear ophthalmoplegia
IOL	intraocular lens
IOP	intraocular pressure
IRMA	intraretinal microvascular abnormality
ISNT	inferior, superior, nasal and temporal
JFRT	juxtafoveolar retinal telangiectasia
JIA	juvenile idiopathic arthritis
KCS	keratoconjunctivitis sicca
KP	keratic precipitate
LASEK	laser *in situ* keratectomy
LASIK	laser *in situ* keratomileusis
MD	mean deviation
MEWDS	multiple evanescent white dot syndrome
MLF	medial longitudinal fasciculus
MPS	mucopolysaccharidosis
MRA	magnetic resonance angiography
MR	magnetic resonance imaging
MS	multiple sclerosis
MU	mega units
NF 1	neurofibromatosis 1
NF 2	neurofibromatosis 2
NFL	retinal nerve fibre layer
NSAID	non-steroidal anti-inflammatory drug
NVD	new vessels at disc
NVE	new vessels elsewhere
OCT	optical coherence tomography
OKN	optokinetic nystagmus
PACG	primary angle-closure glaucoma
PAM	primary acquired melanosis
PAS	peripheral anterior synechiae

PCF	pharyngoconjunctival fever
PCR	polymerase chain reaction
PDR	proliferative diabetic retinopathy
PED	pigment epithelial detachment
PEX	pseudoexfoliative material
PIC	punctate inner choroidopathy
PMMA	polymethylmethacrylate
POAG	primary open-angle glaucoma
POHS	presumed ocular histoplasmosis syndrome
PORN	progressive outer retinal necrosis
PPDR	preproliferative diabetic retinopathy
PPRF	pontine paramedian reticular formation
PRK	photorefractive keratectomy
PRP	panretinal laser photocoagulation
PSD	pattern standard deviation
PVD	posterior vitreous detachment
PVR	proliferative vitreoretinopathy
RD	retinal detachment
RP	retinitis pigmentosa
RPE	retinal pigment epithelium
SF	short-term fluctuation
SLK	superior limbic keratoconjunctivitis
SRF	subretinal fluid
TB	tuberculosis
TGF	transforming growth factor
TINU	tubulointerstitial nephritis and uveitis
TTT	transpupillary thermotherapy
US	ultrasonography
VA	visual acuity
VEP	visual evoked potential
VF	visual field
VZV	varicella zoster virus
X-L	X-linked
X-LD	X-linked dominant
X-LR	X-linked recessive

Chapter 1

Ocular Examination Techniques

Slit-lamp biomicroscopy of the anterior segment

1. **Direct illumination** – diffuse light is used to detect gross abnormalities and a narrow slit-beam provides a cross-section of the cornea (*Fig. 1.1a*).
2. **Scleral scatter** – detects subtle stromal lesions (*Fig. 1.1b*).
3. **Retroillumination** – detects fine epithelial and endothelial changes (*Fig. 1.1c*).

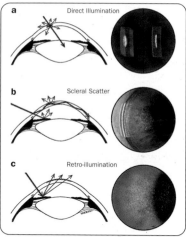

Fig. 1.1 Slit-lamp biomicroscopy of the anterior segment

Fundus examination

Slit-lamp biomicroscopy

1. **Indirect biomicroscopy** – high power convex lenses obtain a wide field of view (*Fig. 1.2*); image is vertically inverted and laterally reversed.

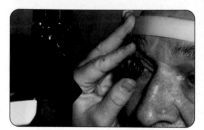

Fig. 1.2 Slit-lamp biomicroscopy of the fundus

2. **Goldmann three-mirror examination** – lens consists of a central part and three mirrors set at different angles (*Fig. 1.3*).
   - Central mirror – affords 30° upright view of the posterior pole.
   - Oblong-shaped – from 30° to the equator.
   - Square-shaped – from equator to the ora serrata.
   - Dome-shaped – for gonioscopy.
   - When viewing the vertical meridian the image is upside-down but not laterally reversed (*Fig. 1.4*).

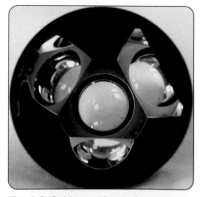

Fig. 1.3 Goldmann three-mirror lens

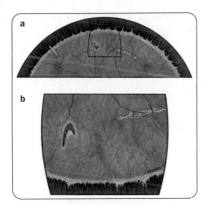

Fig. 1.4 (a) U-tear left of 12 o'clock and an island of lattice degeneration; (b) the same lesion seen with the three-mirror Goldmann lens positioned at 6 o'clock

- When viewing the horizontal meridian the image is laterally reversed.

Indirect ophthalmoscopy

The light emitted from the instrument is transmitted to the fundus through a condensing lens which provides an inverted and laterally reversed image of the fundus (*Fig. 1.5*).

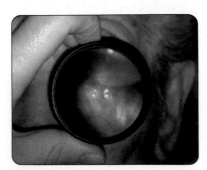

Fig. 1.5 Indirect ophthalmoscopy

Tonometry

1. **Goldmann** – applanation tonometer with a double prism (*Fig. 1.6*).
   - Excess fluorescein – semi-circles are too thick and the radius too small (*Fig. 1.7a*).
   - Insufficient fluorescein – semi-circles are too thin and the radius too large (*Fig. 1.7b*).
   - Appropriate – semi-circles of correct thickness and radius (*Fig. 1.7c*).

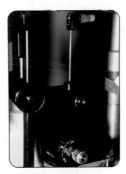

Fig. 1.6 Goldmann tonometer

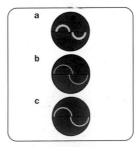

Fig. 1.7 (a) Too much fluorescein; (b) insufficient; (c) correct

2. **Perkins** – hand-held, portable, applanation tonometer (*Fig. 1.8*).
3. **Tono-Pen** – hand-held, portable, contact tonometer (*Fig. 1.9*).
4. **Non-contact tonometers** – central part to the cornea is flattened by a jet of air and the time taken from the onset of the puff to applanation of the cornea is related to the IOP; examples include the non-portable Reichert and the portable Keeler Pulsair (*Fig. 1.10*).

Gonioscopy

Goniolenses

1. **Indirect** – provide a mirror image of the opposite angle and can be used only in conjunction with a slit-lamp.

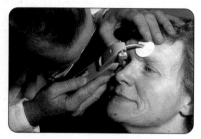

Fig. 1.8 Perkins tonometer

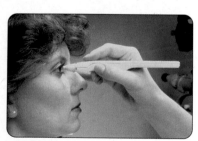

Fig. 1.9 Tono Pen

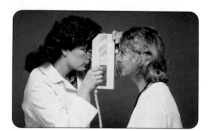

Fig. 1.10 Keeler Pulsair

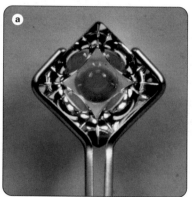

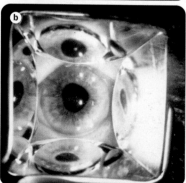

Fig. 1.11 Zeiss lens

a. *Goldmann* (see *Fig. 1.3*) – diagnostic lens that requires a coupling fluid; modifications with one mirror and two mirrors are available for laser trabeculoplasty.

b. *Zeiss* – diagnostic four-mirror lens (*Fig. 1.11a*) that does not require a coupling fluid; simultaneous view of the entire angle (*Fig. 1.11b*); may be used for indentation gonioscopy.

2. **Direct** (gonioprisms) – provide a direct view of the angle.

a. *Koeppe* – diagnostic lens.

b. *Swan–Jacob* – used for goniotomy (*Fig. 1.12*).

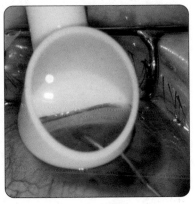

Fig. 1.12 Swan–Jacob lens

Identification of angle structures
(*Fig. 1.13*)

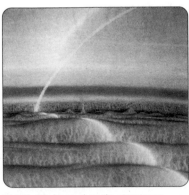

Fig. 1.13 Normal angle structures

1. **Schwalbe line** – demarcates the peripheral termination of Descemet membrane and the anterior limit of the trabeculum.
2. **Trabeculum** – extends from Schwalbe line to the scleral spur.
   - Anterior non-functional part lies adjacent to Schwalbe line.
   - Posterior functional pigmented part is adjacent to the scleral spur.
3. **Scleral spur** – narrow, dense, often shiny, whitish band.
4. **Ciliary body** – band just behind the scleral spur.
5. **Angle recess** – posterior dipping of the iris as it inserts into the ciliary body.
6. **Iris processes** – insert at the level of the scleral spur.

Shaffer grading of angle width

The Shaffer system assigns a numerical grade (4–0) to each angle with associated anatomical description, angle width in degrees and implied clinical interpretation (*Fig. 1.14*).

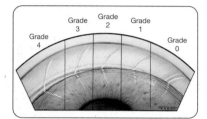

Fig. 1.14 Grading of angle width

- **Grade 4** (35–45°) – ciliary body visualized with ease; closure impossible.
- **Grade 3** (25–35°) – at least the scleral spur identified; closure impossible.
- **Grade 2** (20°) – only the trabeculum identified; closure possible but unlikely.
- **Grade 1** (10°) – only Schwalbe line and perhaps the top of the trabeculum identified; high risk of closure.
- **Slit angle** – no angle structures identified without obvious iridocorneal contact; very high risk of closure.
- **Grade 0** (0°) – inability to identify the apex of the corneal wedge; angle is closed.

Psychophysical tests

Visual acuity

Spatial visual acuity is quantified by the minimum angle of separation (subtended at the nodal point of the eye) between two objects that allow them to be perceived as separate.

1. **Snellen** – testing distance over the distance at which the letter would subtend 5 min of arc vertically (*Fig. 1.15*).

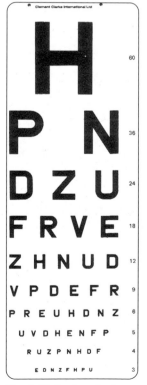

Fig. 1.15 Snellen chart

- At 6 metres a 6/6 letter subtends 5 min of arc and a 6/60 letter 50 min.
- Snellen fraction (i.e. 6/6 = 1; 6/60 = 0.10).

2. Bailey–Lovie – records the minimum angle of resolution (MAR) that relates to the resolution required to resolve the elements of a letter (*Fig. 1.16*).

- 6/6 equates to a MAR of 1 min of arc and 6/12 equates to 2 min.
- LogMAR is the log of the MAR; as letter size changes by 0.1 logMAR units per row and there are five letters in each row, each letter can be assigned a score of 0.02.

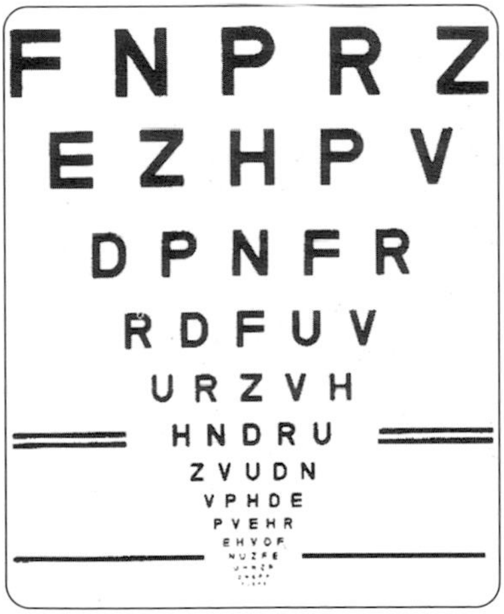

F N P R Z
E Z H P V
D P N F R
R D F U V
U R Z V H
H N D R U
Z V U D N
V P H D E
P V E H R
E H V O F
H U Z F E
U H R F E

Fig. 1.16 Bailey–Lovie chart

Contrast sensitivity

This is a measure of the minimal amount of contrast required to distinguish a test object. The Pelli–Robson contrast sensitivity letter chart (*Fig. 1.17*) is viewed at 1 metre and consists of rows of letters of equal size but with decreasing contrast of 0.15 log units for every group of three letters.

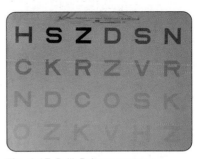

Fig. 1.17 Pelli–Robson contrast sensitivity letter chart

Amsler grid

- Evaluates the 20° of the visual field centred on fixation.
- There are seven charts, of which chart 1 is the most frequently used.
- Grid consists of 400 squares each of which measures 5 mm.
- When viewed at about one-third of a metre, each small square subtends an angle of 1°.
- The subject draws the perceived abnormality such as a scotoma or an area of metamorphopsia on a separate paper grid (*Fig. 1.18*).

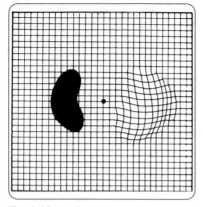

Fig. 1.18 Amsler grid recording

Dark adaptometry

1. **Definition** – phenomenon by which the visual system adapts to decreased illumination.
2. **Indications**
   - Investigation of nyctalopia.
   - Diagnosis of fundus dystrophies.
3. **Goldmann–Weekes adaptometry**
   - Subject is exposed to an intense light that bleaches the photore-ceptors and is then placed in the dark.
   - Flashes of light of gradually increasing intensity are presented.
   - The threshold at which the subject just perceives the light is plotted.
4. **Sensitivity curve** – plot of the light intensity of a minimally perceived spot versus time (*Fig. 1.19*).
   a. *Cone branch* – represents the initial 5–10 minutes of darkness during which cone sensitivity rapidly improves.
   b. *'Rod–cone' break* – in normals occurs after 7–10 minutes when cones achieve their maximum sensitivity and the rods become

perceptibly more sensitive than cones.
   c. *Rod branch* – slower and represents the continuation of improvement of rod sensitivity.

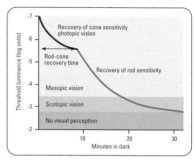

Fig. 1.19 Dark adaptation curve

Colour vision tests

1. **Ishihara** – used mainly to screen for congenital protan and deuteran defects.
   - Consists of a test plate followed by 16 plates each with a matrix of dots arranged to show a central shape or number which the subject is asked to identify (*Fig. 1.20*).
   - A colour deficient person identifies some of the figures.
2. **Hardy–Rand–Rittler** – similar to Ishihara but can detect all three congenital defects (*Fig. 1.21*).
3. **City University** – 10 plates each containing a central colour and four peripheral colours (*Fig. 1.22*); subject selects one of the peripheral colours which most closely matches the central colour.
4. **Farnsworth–Munsell 100-hue** – for both congenital and acquired colour defects; 85 hue caps contained in four separate racks in each of which

the two end caps are fixed while the others are loose so they can be randomized by the examiner (*Fig. 1.23*).

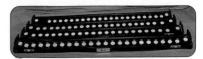

Fig. 1.23 Farnsworth–Munsell 100-hue test

Orthoptic examination

Visual acuity

Testing in preverbal children

1. **Fixation and following** – using bright attention-grabbing targets.
2. **Comparison** – occlusion of one eye, if strongly objected to, indicates poorer acuity in the other eye (*Fig. 1.24*).

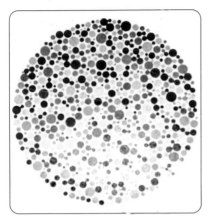

Fig. 1.20 Ishihara test

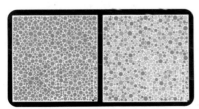

Fig. 1.21 Hardy–Rand–Ritter test

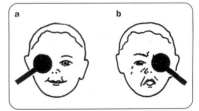

Fig. 1.24 (a) No objection to covering eye with worse acuity; (b) objection to covering better eye

3. **Fixation behaviour** – to establish unilateral preference if a manifest squint is present.
4. **The 10 Δ test** – promotion of diplopia.
5. **Rotation test** – gross qualitative test of the ability of an infant to fixate with both eyes open.

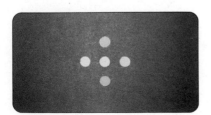

Fig. 1.22 City University test

6. Preferential looking – infants prefer to look at a pattern rather than a homogeneous stimulus; Cardiff (*Fig. 1.25*), Teller or Keeler acuity cards.

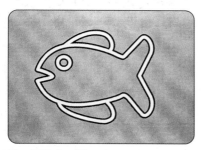

Fig. 1.25 Cardiff acuity card

Testing in verbal children

1. Age 2 years – picture naming test such as the crowded Kay pictures (*Fig. 1.26*).
2. Age 3 years – matching of letter optotypes; Sheridan–Gardiner (*Fig. 1.27*), Keeler logMAR or Sonksen.

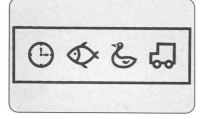

Fig. 1.26 Kay pictures

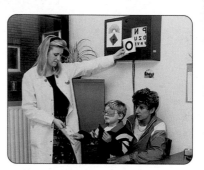

Fig. 1.27 Sheridan–Gardiner test

Tests for stereopsis

Stereopsis is measured in seconds of arc (1° = 60 min of arc; 1 min = 60 sec of arc); normal spatial visual acuity is 1 min and normal stereo-acuity is 60 sec (which equals 1 minute); the lower the value the better the acuity.

1. TNO – requires complementary red–green spectacles (*Fig. 1.28*); disparity is 480–15 sec.
2. Frisby – spectacles not required (*Fig. 1.29*); disparity is 600–15 sec.
3. Lang – spectacles not required (*Fig. 1.30*); disparity is 1200–600 sec.
4. Titmus – requires polarized spectacles (*Fig. 1.31*).
   - Fly – disparity is 3000 sec.
   - Circles – disparity is 800–40 sec.
   - Animals – disparity is 400–100 sec.

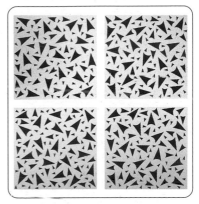

Fig. 1.29 Frisby test

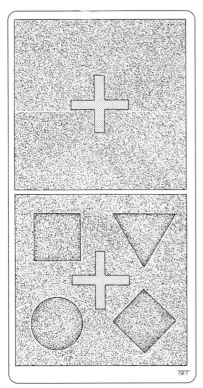

Fig. 1.28 TNO test

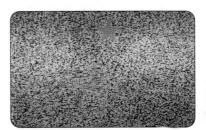

Fig. 1.30 Lang test

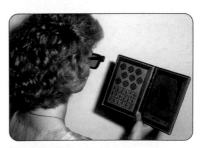

Fig. 1.31 Titmus test

Tests for sensory anomalies

1. **Worth four-dot** – requires red–green spectacles (*Fig. 1.32*).
2. **Bagolini striated glasses** – lenses with fine striations at 45° and 135° convert a point light source into an oblique line perpendicular to that seen by the fellow eye (*Figs 1.33 & 1.34*).
3. **Synoptophore** – compensates for the angle of squint and allows stimuli to be presented to both eyes simultaneously (*Fig. 1.35*); can be used to investigate the potential for binocular function in the presence of a manifest squint (*Fig. 1.36*).

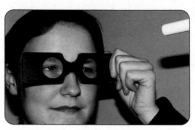

Fig. 1.33 Bagolini glasses

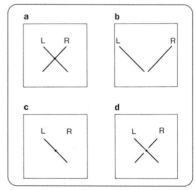

Fig. 1.34 Possible results of Bagolini test. (a) Normal fusion or ARC; (b) diplopia; (c) suppression; (d) small central suppression scotoma

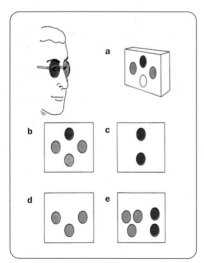

Fig. 1.32 Worth four-dot test. (a) Patient wears a right red lens and a left green lens and views a box with one red light, two green lights, and one white light; (b) normal fusion or ARC; (c) left suppression; (d) right suppression; (e) diplopia

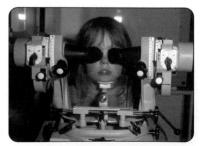

Fig. 1.35 Synoptophore

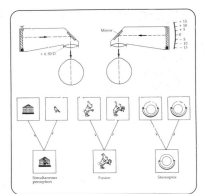

Fig. 1.36 Grades of binocular vision

Cover tests

1. **Cover–uncover test**
   - Cover test for heterotropia (*Fig. 1.37*).
   - Uncover test for heterophoria (*Fig. 1.38*).
2. **Alternate cover test** – reveals the total deviation when fusion is suspended (*Fig. 1.39*); performed after the cover–uncover test.
3. **Prism cover test** – measures the angle of deviation and combines the alternate cover test with prisms.

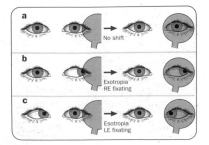

Fig. 1.37 Possible results of the cover test

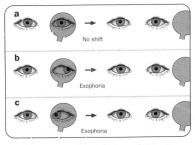

Fig. 1.38 Possible results of the uncover test

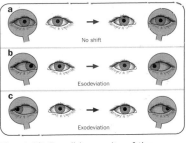

Fig. 1.39 Possible results of the alternate cover test

Measurement of deviation

1. **Hirschberg** – each mm of deviation = 7° (1° ≈ 2 Δ).
2. **Krimsky test** – prisms are placed in front of the fixating eye until the corneal reflexes are symmetrical (*Fig. 1.40*).
3. **Maddox wing** – dissociates the eyes for near fixation (1/3 m) and measures heterophoria; right eye sees only a white vertical arrow and a red horizontal arrow; left eye sees only horizontal and vertical rows of numbers (*Fig. 1.41*).

4. Maddox rod – dissociates the eyes but cannot differentiate heterotropia from heterophoria; fused cylindrical red glass rods convert a white spot of light into a red streak at an angle of 90° with the long axis of the rods (*Fig. 1.42*); amount of dissociation is measured by the superimposition of the two images using prisms.

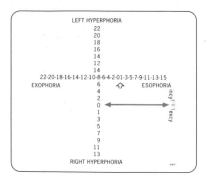

Fig. 1.40 Krimsky test

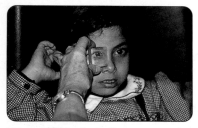

Fig. 1.41 Maddox wing

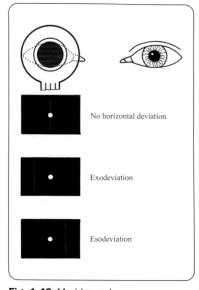

No horizontal deviation

Exodeviation

Esodeviation

Fig. 1.42 Maddox rod

Investigation of diplopia

The Hess test and the Lees screen (*Fig. 1.43*) plot the dissociated ocular position as a function of the extraocular muscles.

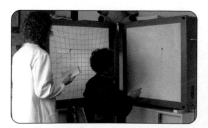

Fig. 1.43 Lees screen

1. Recently acquired right 4th nerve palsy (*Fig. 1.44*).

- Right chart – smaller than the left.
- Right chart – underaction of the superior oblique and overaction of the inferior oblique.
- Left chart – overaction of the inferior rectus and underaction (inhibitional palsy) of the superior rectus.
- Primary deviation FL is R/L 8°.
- Secondary deviation FR is R/L 17°.

2. Right 6th nerve palsy (*Fig. 1.45*).

- Right chart – smaller than the left.
- Right esotropia – note that the fixation spot of the right inner chart is deviated nasally.
- Right chart – marked underaction of the lateral rectus and slight overaction of the medial rectus.
- Left chart – marked overaction of the medial rectus.
- Primary angle FL is +15°.
- Secondary angle FR is +20°.

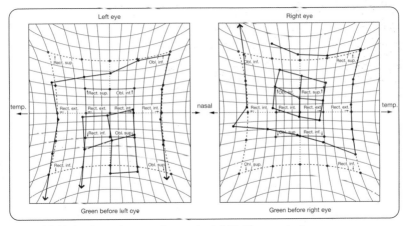

Fig. 1.44 Hess chart of a recently acquired right 4th nerve palsy

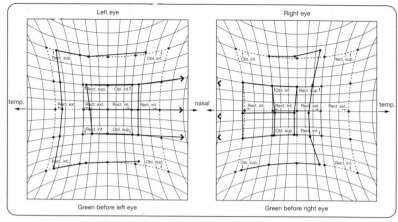

Fig. 1.45 Hess chart of a recently acquired right 6th nerve palsy

Electrophysical tests

Electroretinography

Principles

The electroretinogram (ERG) is the record of an action potential produced by the retina when it is stimulated by light of adequate intensity. The potential between the active electrode and the reference electrode is amplified and displayed (*Fig. 1.46*).

1. **The a-wave** – initial fast negative deflection directly generated by photoreceptors.
2. **The b-wave** – next slower positive deflection with larger amplitude; amplitude of the b-wave is measured from the trough of the a-wave to the peak of the b-wave, and increases with both dark adaptation and increased light stimulus.

Normal ERG

The normal ERG consists of five recordings (*Fig. 1.47*); first three are elicited

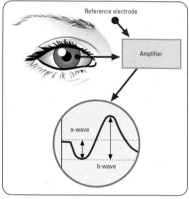

Fig. 1.46 Principles of ERG

after 30 min of dark adaptation (scotopic), and the last two after 10 min of adaptation to moderately bright diffuse illumination (photopic).

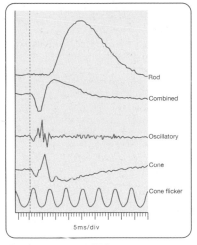

Fig. 1.47 Normal ERG

1. Scotopic ERG
  a. *Rod responses* – elicited with a very dim flash of white light or a blue light resulting in a large b-wave and a small or non-recordable a-wave.
  b. *Combined rod and cone responses* – elicited with a very bright white flash resulting in a prominent a-wave and a b-wave.
  c. *Oscillatory potentials* – elicited by using a bright flash and changing the recording parameters.
2. Photopic ERG
  a. *Cone responses* – elicited with a single bright flash, resulting in an a-wave and a b-wave with small oscillations.

  b. *Cone flicker* – isolates cones by using a flickering light stimulus at a frequency of 30 Hz to which rods cannot respond.

Multifocal ERG

Multifocal ERG is a topographical map of retinal function. The stimulus is scaled for variation in photoreceptor density across the retina. The information can be summarized in the form of a three-dimensional plot which resembles the hill of vision (*Fig. 1.48*). The technique can be used for almost any disorder which affects retinal function.

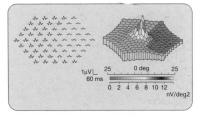

Fig. 1.48 Multifocal ERG

Electro-oculography

1. Principle – measures the standing potential between the electrically positive cornea and the electrically negative back of the eye (*Fig. 1.49*). Diffuse or widespread disease of the RPE is needed to affect the EOG response significantly.

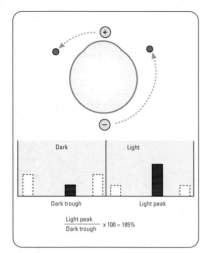

Fig. 1.49 Principles of EOG

2. Technique
- The test is performed in both light- and dark-adapted states.
- Electrodes are attached to the skin near the medial and lateral canthi.
- The patient is asked to look rhythmically from side to side, making excursions of constant amplitude.
- The potential difference between the two electrodes is amplified and recorded.

3. Interpretation – maximal height of the potential in the light (light peak) is divided by the minimal height of the potential in the dark (dark trough); expressed as a ratio (Arden ratio) or as a percentage; normal is over 1.85 or 185%.

Visual evoked potential

1. Principle – recording of electrical activity of the visual cortex created by stimulation of the retina; monitoring of visual function in babies and the investigation of optic neuropathy, particularly when associated with demyelination.

2. Technique – stimulus is either a flash of light or a black-and-white checker-board pattern, which periodically reverses polarity on a screen (*Fig. 1.50*).

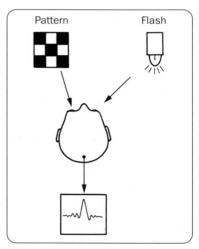

Fig. 1.50 Principles of VEP

3. Interpretation – latency (delay) and amplitude are assessed; in optic neuropathy there is prolongation of latency and decrease in amplitude.

Perimetry

Types of perimetry

1. **Kinetic** – two-dimensional assessment of the boundary of the hill of vision; a moving stimulus of known luminance or intensity is presented from a non-seeing area to a seeing area until it is perceived (*Fig. 1.51a*).
2. **Static** – three-dimensional assessment of the height (differential light sensitivity) of a pre-determined area of the hill of vision; non-moving stimuli of varying luminance are presented in the same position to obtain a vertical boundary of the visual field (*Fig. 1.51b*).
3. **Suprathreshold** – stimuli at luminance levels above normal threshold values are presented in various locations.
4. **Threshold** – plots the threshold luminance value in various locations and compares the results with age-matched 'normal' values.

Humphrey perimetry

Programs

1. **Suprathreshold** – rapid (6 minutes per eye) 88 point screening test using a 3-zone strategy.
2. **Full-threshold strategy** – initially four points are tested to determine threshold levels which are then used as a starting level for neighbouring points and so on until the entire field has been tested; points where the anticipated response is out by 5 dB of that expected are re-tested.
3. **SITA** – standard program shows greater sensitivity than full-threshold for early defects; fast program is quicker but less sensitive.

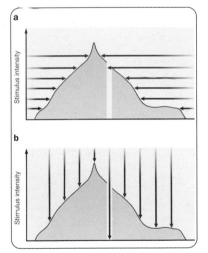

Fig. 1.51 (a) Kinetic perimetry; (b) static perimetry

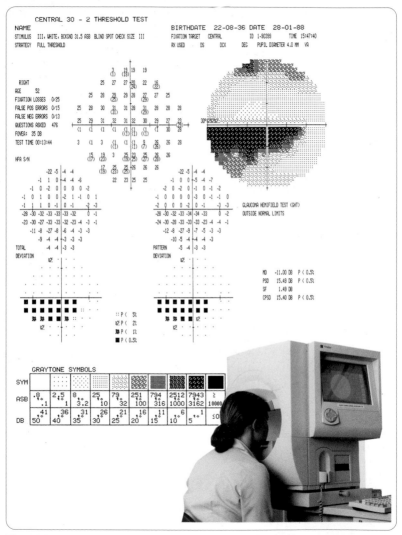

Fig. 1.52 Humphrey perimeter and display

Displays (Fig. 1.52)

1. **Numerical** – gives the threshold (dB) for all points checked; figures in brackets indicate threshold at the same point checked a second time.
2. **Grey scale** – decreasing sensitivity represented by darker tones is the simplest to interpret; scale at the bottom shows corresponding values of the grey tone symbols in abs and dB; each change in grey scale tone is equivalent to 5 dB change in threshold.
3. **Total deviation** – deviation of the patients' result from that of age-matched controls; upper numerical display illustrates the differences in dB and the lower display exhibits these differences as grey symbols.
4. **Pattern deviation** – similar to total deviation except that it is adjusted for any generalized depression in the overall field which might be caused

by other factors such as lens opacities or miosis.

5. **Probability values** (P) – indicate the significance of the defects are shown as <5%, <2%, <1% and <0.5%; the lower the P value the greater its clinical significance and the lesser the likelihood of the defect having occurred 'by chance'.

Reliability indices

1. **Fixation losses** – stimuli are presented in the physiological blind spot; if the patient responds, a fixation loss is recorded; the less the number of losses the more reliable is the test.
2. **False positives** – stimulus is accompanied by a sound; if the sound alone is presented (without an accompanying light stimulus) and the patient responds a false positive is recorded; grey scale printout in 'trigger happy' patients appears abnormally pale (Fig. 1.53).

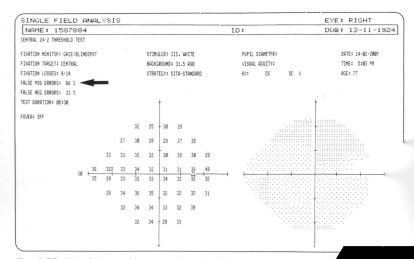

Fig. 1.53 High false-positive score (arrow) with an abnormally pale d

3. False negatives – detected by presenting a stimulus much brighter than threshold at a location where sensitivity has already been recorded; if the patient fails to respond a false negative is recorded; grey scale printout with high false negative responses has a clover leaf shape (*Fig. 1.54*).

Global indices

Global indices summarize the results in a single number and are principally used to monitor progression of glaucomatous damage rather than for initial diagnosis.

1. Mean deviation (MD) (elevation or depression) – measure of the overall field loss.

2. Pattern standard deviation (PSD) – measure of focal loss or variability taking into account any generalized depression in the hill of vision; increased PSD is a more specific indicator of glaucomatous damage than MD.

3. Short-term fluctuation (SF) – indication of the consistency of responses.

4. Corrected pattern standard deviation (CPSD) – measure of variability after correcting for short-term fluctuation (intra-test variability).

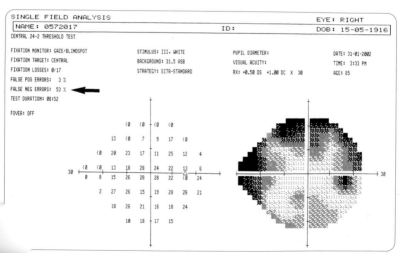

54 High false-negative score (arrow) with a clover leaf-shaped display

Chapter 2

Imaging Techniques

Cornea

Specular microscopy

- Specular microscopy is a study of the changes in different layers of the cornea under magnification which is 100 times greater than slit-lamp biomicroscopy.
- It is principally used to photograph the corneal endothelium and the image is analysed with respect to cellular size, shape, density and distribution.
- The normal endothelial cell is a regular hexagon with a density of about 3000 cells/mm^2 (*Fig. 2.1*); counts below 1000 are associated with a significant risk of endothelial decompensation.

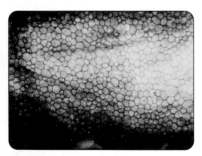

Fig. 2.1 Specular micrograph of normal endothelium

Corneal topography

Corneal topography provides a colour-coded map of the corneal surface; power in dioptres of the steepest and flattest meridia and their axes are calculated and displayed (*Fig. 2.2*).

- Steep curvatures (high dioptres) are coloured orange and red.
- Flat curvatures (low dioptres) are coloured violet and blue.
- Most normal corneas remain within the yellow–green spectrum.
- Absolute scales have fixed end-points and each individual colour represents a specific power interval in dioptres.
- An absolute scale should always be used to facilitate comparison over time and between patients.
- Relative (normalized) scales are not fixed and vary according to the range in dioptres of the individual cornea.

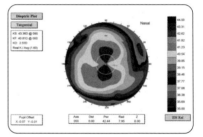

Fig. 2.2 Normal relative scale map shows 3.5 D of with-the-rule astigmatism and a typical bow-tie pattern

Fluorescein angiography

Phases of the angiogram

1. **Red free image** (*Fig. 2.3a*).
2. **Choroidal (pre-arterial)** – patchy choroidal filling.
3. **Arterial** – arterial filling and the continuation of choroidal filling (*Fig. 2.3b*).
4. **Arteriovenous (capillary)** – complete filling of arteries and capillaries with early laminar venous flow (*Fig. 2.3c*).

5. Venous

a. *Early* – complete arterial and capillary filling, with more marked laminar venous flow.

b. *Mid* – almost complete venous filling (*Fig. 2.3d*).

c. *Late* – complete venous filling with reducing concentration of dye in the arteries (*Fig. 2.3e*).

6. Late (elimination) – continuous recirculation, dilution and elimination of the dye; late staining of the disc is a normal finding (*Fig. 2.3f*).

7. Dark appearance of the fovea caused by three phenomena.

- Absence of blood vessels in the foveal avascular zone.
- Blockage of background choroidal fluorescence by increased density of xanthophyll at the fovea.
- Blockage of background choroidal fluorescence by the RPE cells at the fovea, which are larger and contain more melanin than elsewhere.

Causes of abnormal fluorescence

1. Hyperfluorescence

- Transmission (window) defect caused by deficiency of the RPE (e.g. dry AMD – see *Fig. 17.8*).
- Pooling in the subretinal space (e.g. CSR – see *Fig. 17.28*) or sub-RPE space (e.g. PED – see *Fig. 17.11*).
- Leakage from neovascularization in the retina or choroid (e.g. CNV – see *Fig. 17.14*).
- Breakdown of the inner blood–retinal barrier (e.g. CMO – see *Fig. 17.32*).
- Staining due to prolonged retention of dye in tissue (e.g. macular drusen – see *Fig. 17.3b*).

2. Hypofluorescence

- Blockage of normal fluorescence (*Fig. 2.4*).

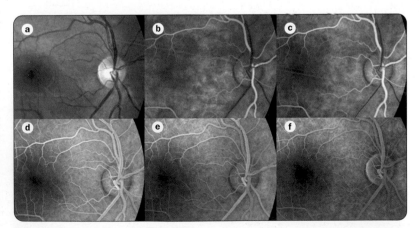

Fig. 2.3 Normal fluorescein angiogram

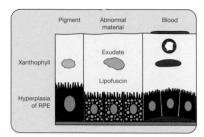

Fig. 2.4 Causes of blocked fluorescence

- Inadequate perfusion due to vascular occlusion or loss of the vascular bed (e.g. severe degenerative myopia – see *Fig. 17.43*).

Indocyanine green angiography

Normal angiogram

1. **Early phase** (within 2–60 sec of injection – *Fig. 2.5a*)

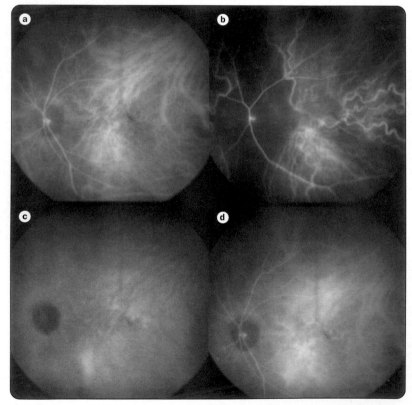

Fig. 2.5 Normal indocyanine green angiogram

- Hypofluorescence of the optic disc and poor perfusion of the watershed zone.
- Prominent filling of choroidal arteries and early filling of choroidal veins.
- Retinal arteries are visible but not veins.

2. Early mid phase (1–3 min – *Fig. 2.5b*)
- Filling of watershed zone.
- Fading of choroidal arteries with increased prominence of choroidal veins.
- Both retinal veins and arteries are visible.

3. Late mid phase (3–15 min – *Fig. 2.5c*)
- Fading of choroidal vascular filling.
- Diffuse hyperfluorescence due to diffusion of dye from the choriocapillaris.
- Retinal vessels are still visible.

4. Late phase (15–30 min – *Fig. 2.5d*)
- Hypofluorescence of choroidal vasculature against a background of hyperfluorescence resulting from staining of extrachoroidal tissue.
- Decreased visibility of retinal vasculature.
- Dye may remain in neovascular tissue after it has left the choroidal and retinal circulations.

Causes of abnormal fluorescence

1. Hyperfluorescence
- RPE 'window' defect.
- Leakage from the retinal or choroidal circulations, or the optic nerve head.
- Abnormal blood vessels.

2. Hypofluorescence
- Blockage of fluorescence by pigment, blood or exudate.
- Obstruction of the circulation.
- Loss of vascular tissue.
- PED (see *Fig. 17.9b*).

Ultrasonography

A-Scan

1. Indications – measurement of anterior chamber depth, lens thickness, and axial length.
2. Display – vertical spikes along a baseline (*Fig. 2.6*) the height of which is proportional to the strength of the echo; the greater the distance to the right, the greater the distance between the source of the sound and the reflecting surface.

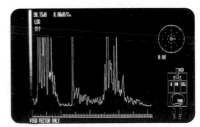

Fig. 2.6 A-scan display

B-Scan

The amount of reflected sound is portrayed as a dot of light; the more sound reflected, the brighter the dot; the frequency of the transducer determines which part of the globe or orbit is examined.

1. Low (2–5 MHz) – for orbital pathology (*Fig. 2.7*).

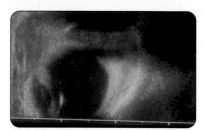

Fig. 2.7 Low frequency ultrasonography shows an anterior orbital capillary haemangioma

2. Moderate (7–10 MHz):
- Detection of RD in eyes with opaque media (*Fig. 2.8*).
- Evaluation of posterior intraocular tumours.
- Detection of calcification (e.g. retinoblastoma and optic disc drusen).

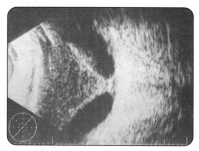

Fig. 2.8 B-scan shows intragel vitreous haemorrhage and total tractional retinal detachment

3. High (30–50 MHz) – for high-definition imaging of the anterior segment, particularly in the evaluation of congenital corneal opacification (*Fig. 2.9*).

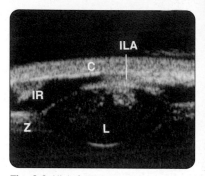

Fig. 2.9 High frequency ultrasonography shows corneal opacification and lenticulocorneal apposition

Optical coherence tomography

1. **Physics** – cross-sectional images are generated by scanning the optical beam in the transverse direction, thus yielding a two-dimensional data set that can be displayed as a false-colour or grey scale image.
2. **Indications**
   - Macular pathology.
   - To monitor progression of disease processes and response to treatment.
   - Analysis of the optic nerve head and retinal nerve fibre layer (NFL) thickness.
3. **Normal appearance** (*Fig. 2.10*)
   - Nerve fibre and plexiform layers – red, yellow or bright-green.
   - Inner and outer nuclear layers – blue or black.
   - Inner and outer plexiform layers – bright-green.

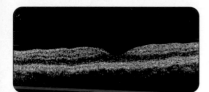

Fig. 2.10 Normal OCT

Imaging in glaucoma

1. **Heidelberg Retinal Tomograph** (HRT) – scanning laser ophthalmoscope that can interpret differences in the profile of the optic nerve head and peripapillary NFL to produce a computerized three-dimensional topographical image (*Fig. 2.11*).

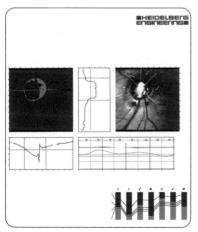

Fig. 2.11 HRT display

2. **GDxVCC analyser** measures the change in polarization caused by the birefringence of NFL axons; degree of polarization is assessed over an area of 1.75 disc diameters concentric to the disc and the profile of the density of the NFL established; the thicker the NFL the greater the polarization (*Fig. 2.12*).

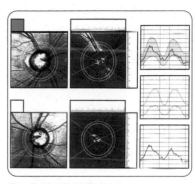

Fig. 2.12 GDxVCC display

3. **STRATUS OCT** images and analyses the NFL, macular thickness, and the optic nerve head (*Fig. 2.13*).

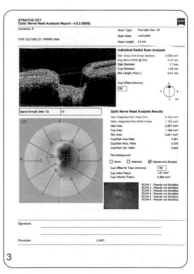

Fig. 2.13 STRATUS OCT

Neuroimaging

Computed tomography

1. Physics – x-ray beams obtain tissue density values from which detailed cross-sectional images are formed by a computer; tissue density is represented by a grey scale, white being maximum density (e.g. bone) and black being minimum density (e.g. air); image may be coronal (*Fig. 2.14*) or axial (*Fig. 2.15*).

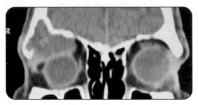

Fig. 2.14 Coronal CT image shows a right orbital tumour

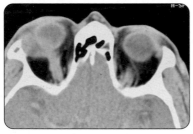

Fig. 2.15 Axial CT image of the same patient

2. Indications
- Orbital disease and trauma.
- Intraocular foreign bodies.
- Detection of intraocular calcification.

- Acute cerebral or subarachnoid haemorrhage.

3. Iodinated contrast material – improves sensitivity and specificity but is not indicated in acute cerebral haemorrhage, bony injury or localization of foreign bodies because it may mask visualization of these high density structures.

Magnetic resonance imaging

Physics

Magnetic resonance imaging (MR) depends on the rearrangement of hydrogen nuclei when a tissue is exposed to a short electromagnetic pulse. When the pulse subsides, the nuclei return to their normal position, re-radiating some of the energy they have absorbed. Exposed tissues produce radiation with characteristic intensity and time patterns. The signals are analysed, computed and displayed as a cross-sectional image which may be: (a) axial, (b) coronal or (c) sagittal.

Imaging sequences

Weighting refers to two methods of measuring the relaxation times of the excited protons after the magnetic field has been switched off. Various body tissues have different relaxation times so that a given tissue may be T1- or T2-weighted (i.e. best visualized on that particular type of image).

1. T1-weighted – best for normal anatomy (*Fig. 2.16*).
- Hypointense (dark) – CSF and vitreous.
- Hyperintense (bright) – fat, blood, and contrast agents.

2. T2-weighted – useful for pathological changes (*Fig. 2.17*).
- Hypointense – fat and contrast agents.
- Hyperintense – CSF and vitreous.
- Blood vessels – black unless occluded.

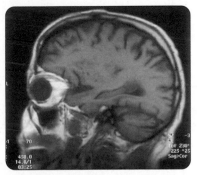

Fig. 2.16 T1-weighted sagittal MR image

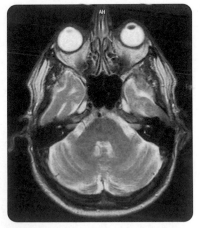

Fig. 2.17 T2-weighted axial MR image

Enhancement

1. Gadolinium – acquires magnetic moment when placed in an electro-magnetic field; only visualized on T1-weighted images, and enhancing lesions such as tumours (*Fig. 2.18*) and areas of inflammation which appear bright.

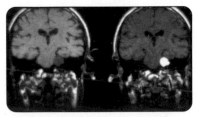

Fig. 2.18 T1-weighted MR images of an acoustic neuroma; (left) without gadolinium; (right) with gadolinium

2. Orbital fat-suppression techniques – the bright signal of orbital fat on conventional T1-weighted imaging obscures other orbital contents; two fat suppression sequences are T1 fat suppression with gadolinium and STIR (Short T1 Inversion Recovery) for detecting intrinsic lesions of the intraorbital part of the optic nerve.

3. FLAIR (fluid attenuation inversion recovery) – suppresses the bright CSF on T2-weighted images to allow better visualization of adjacent pathological tissue such as periventricular plaques of demyelination (see *Fig. 24.60*).

Angiography

1. Magnetic resonance angiography (MRA) – for the carotid and vertebrobasilar circulations (*Fig. 2.19*) to demonstrate stenosis, dissection, occlusion, arteriovenous malformations, and aneurysms; thrombosed aneurysms may be missed and is unreliable in detecting very small lesions.

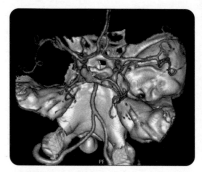

Fig. 2.20 CT angiogram showing a left superior cerebellar artery aneurysm

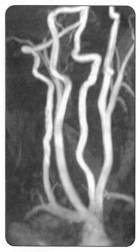

Fig. 2.19 MR angiogram

2. **Magnetic resonance venography** (MRV) – for venous sinus thrombosis.
3. **Computed tomography angiography** (CTA) – for intracranial aneurysms; images of the vessels can be reconstructed in three dimensions (*Fig. 2.20*).
4. **Computed tomography venography** (CTV) – useful when MRA is contraindicated or there are difficulties in distinguishing slow flow from thrombus on MRA; similar to CTA but images are acquired in the venous phase of contrast enhancement (*Fig. 2.21*).

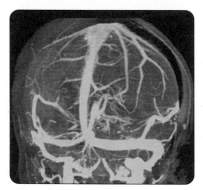

Fig. 2.21 CT venogram

5. **Conventional intra-arterial catheter angiography** – a catheter is passed through the femoral artery into the internal carotid and vertebral arteries in the neck under fluoroscopic guidance; digital subtraction results in images of the contrast-filled vessels without any background structure such as bone (*Fig. 2.22*).

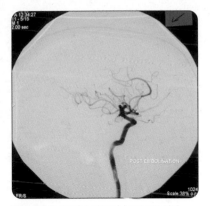

Fig. 2.22 Conventional intra-arterial angiogram with subtraction

Positron emission tomography

Positron emission tomography (PET/CT) uses radioactive glucose that accumulates within malignant cells because of their high rate of metabolism. Following injection the patient is imaged on a whole body scanner to reveal tumours that may have been overlooked by conventional CT or MR. It is a sensitive tool for the detection and staging of hepatic and extra-hepatic metastatic choroidal melanoma.

Chapter 3

Developmental Malformations and Anomalies

Eyelids

Epicanthic folds

1. **Signs** – bilateral vertical folds of skin that extend from the upper or lower lids towards the medial canthi; according to distribution the four types are: palpebralis (*Fig. 3.1* – most common), tarsalis, inversus, and superciliaris.
2. **Treatment** – of small folds is by Y-V plasty; large folds require Mustarde Z-plasty.

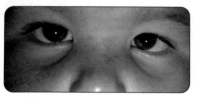

Fig. 3.1 Epicanthic folds (palpebralis)

Telecanthus

1. **Signs** – increased distance between the medial canthi as a result of abnormally long medial canthal tendons (*Fig. 3.2*).

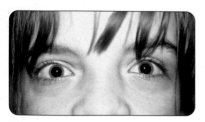

Fig. 3.2 Telecanthus

2. **Associated syndromes** – blepharophimosis, Waardenburg, Möbius, Treacher Collins, Rubinstein–Taybi, and Turner.
3. **Differential diagnosis** – hypertelorism in which there is wide separation of the orbits.

Blepharophimosis syndrome

1. **Inheritance** – AD.
2. **Signs** – ptosis with poor levator function, short horizontal palpebral aperture, telecanthus, epicanthus inversus, lateral ectropion of lower lids, poorly developed nasal bridge, and hypoplasia of the superior orbital rims (*Fig. 3.3*).
3. **Treatment** – correction of epicanthus and telecanthus, and later bilateral frontalis suspension.

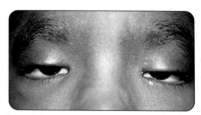

Fig. 3.3 Blepharophimosis syndrome

Epiblepharon

1. **Signs** – extra horizontal fold of skin stretches across the anterior lid margin; lashes are directed vertically, especially medially (*Fig. 3.4*).
2. **Treatment** – Hotz procedure if persistent.
3. **Differential diagnosis** – congenital entropion.

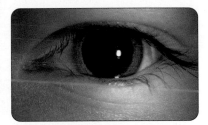

Fig. 3.4 Epiblepharon

Congenital entropion

1. **Pathogenesis** – improper development of the inferior retractor aponeurosis.
2. **Signs** – in-turning of the entire lower eyelid and lashes with absence of the lower lid crease (*Fig. 3.5*).
3. **Treatment** – Hotz procedure urgently.
4. **Differential diagnosis** – epiblepharon.

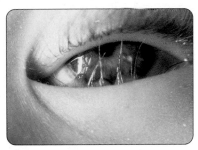

Fig. 3.5 Congenital lower lid entropion

Euryblepharon

1. **Signs** – horizontal enlargement of the palpebral fissure with associated lateral canthal malposition and lateral ectropion (*Fig. 3.6*).

2. **Associations** – lateral displacement of the proximal lacrimal drainage system, a double row of meibomian gland orifices, telecanthus, and strabismus.
3. **Treatment** – lateral canthal tightening or tarsorrhaphy.

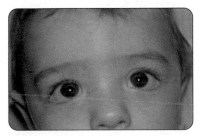

Fig. 3.6 Euryblepharon

Coloboma

1. **Definition** – partial or full-thickness eyelid defect occurring when eyelid development is incomplete.
2. **Pathogenesis** – failure of migration of lid ectoderm to fuse the lid folds, or mechanical forces such as amniotic bands.
3. **Upper lid** – at junction of the middle and inner thirds (*Fig. 3.7*); may be occasionally associated with Goldenhar syndrome.
4. **Lower lid** – at junction of the middle and outer thirds; associated with Treacher Collins syndrome and amniotic band syndrome.
5. **Treatment** – small defects can be closed directly; large defects require skin grafts and rotation flaps.

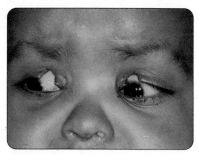

Fig. 3.7 Upper lid colobomas

Microblepharon

Microblepharon is characterized by small eyelids, often associated with anophthalmos (see *Fig. 3.31*).

Ablepharon

1. **Signs** – deficiency of the anterior lamellae of the eyelids.
2. **Treatment** – reconstructive skin grafting.
3. **Systemic anomalies** – ablepharon-macrostomia syndrome characterized by an enlarged fish-like mouth, ear and genital anomalies, and redundant skin (*Fig. 3.8*).

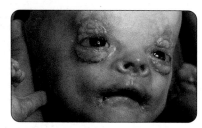

Fig. 3.8 Ablepharon-macrostomia syndrome – following lid reconstruction

Cryptophthalmos

1. **Signs**
   a. *Incomplete* – lids are replaced by layer of skin which is fused with a microphthalmic eye (*Fig. 3.9*).
   b. *Complete* – microphthalmos, rudimentary lids and a small conjunctival sac (*Fig. 3.10*).
2. **Systemic association** – Fraser syndrome.

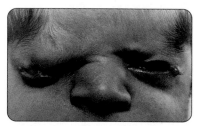

Fig. 3.9 Incomplete cryptophthalmos

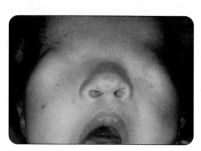

Fig. 3.10 Complete cryptophthalmos

Congenital upper lid eversion

1. **Predispositions** – black infants, Down syndrome, and collodion skin disease (*Fig. 3.11*).
2. **Treatment** – may resolve spontaneously depending on cause or may require surgery.

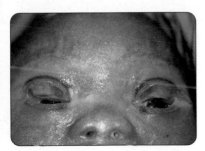

Fig. 3.11 Congenital ectropion in collodion disease

Cornea

Microcornea

1. **Inheritance** – AD.
2. **Signs** – unilateral or bilateral; horizontal corneal diameter is 10 mm or less (*Fig. 3.12*), hypermetropia, shallow anterior chamber but other dimensions are normal.
3. **Ocular associations** – glaucoma, congenital cataract, leukoma, cornea plana, Rieger anomaly, microphakia, and optic nerve hypoplasia.
4. **Syndromic associations** – fetal alcohol, Ehlers–Danlos, Weill–Marchesani, Waardenburg, Nance–Horan, and Cornelia de Lange.

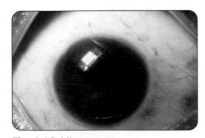

Fig. 3.12 Microcornea

Megalocornea

1. **Inheritance** – X-LR (90%).
2. **Signs** – bilateral; corneal diameter is 13mm or more, very deep anterior chamber (*Fig. 3.13*), high myopia and astigmatism, and pigment dispersion syndrome but normal IOP.
3. **Systemic associations** – Alport syndrome, Marfan syndrome, Ehlers–Danlos syndrome, Down syndrome, osteogenesis imperfecta, progressive facial hemiatrophy, renal carcinoma, and megalocornea–mental retardation syndrome.

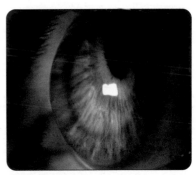

Fig. 3.13 Megalocornea

Cornea plana

1. **Inheritance** – AD is less severe than AR.
2. **Signs** – bilateral; small flat cornea and shallow anterior chamber (*Fig. 3.14*), hypermetropia, and predisposition to angle-closure glaucoma.
3. **Ocular associations** – hazy corneal limbus, early arcus senilis, microcornea, sclerocornea, microphthalmos, and Peters anomaly.

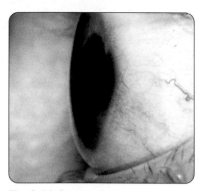

Fig. 3.14 Cornea plana

Sclerocornea

1. **Signs** – usually bilateral; variable opacification and vascularization of the cornea (*Fig. 3.15*).
2. **Associations** – Peters anomaly and cornea plana.

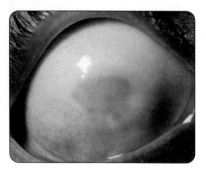

Fig. 3.15 Sclerocornea

Keratectasia

1. **Pathogenesis** – probably intrauterine keratitis and perforation.
2. **Signs** – unilateral; protuberance between the eyelids or an opaque and sometimes vascularized cornea (*Fig. 3.16*).

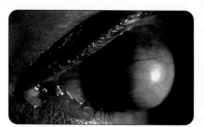

Fig. 3.16 Keratectasia

Posterior keratoconus

1. **Definition** – sporadic, unilateral, non-progressive increase in curvature of the posterior corneal surface.
2. **Classification**
   a. *Generalis* – involves entire cornea.
   b. *Conscriptus* – localized paracentral or central posterior indentation (*Fig. 3.17*).

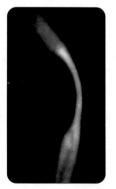

Fig. 3.17 Posterior keratoconus conscriptus

Lens

Anterior lenticonus

1. **Signs** – bilateral; axial projection of the anterior lens surface (*Fig. 3.18*).

2. Systemic association – Alport syndrome in 90% (also retinal flecks; see *Figs 18.37 & 18.38*).

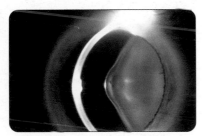

Fig. 3.18 Anterior lenticonus

Posterior lenticonus

1. Inheritance – majority are sporadic and not associated with systemic abnormalities.
2. Signs – usually unilateral; round or conical bulge of the posterior axial zone of the lens with local thinning or absence of the capsule (*Fig. 3.19*).

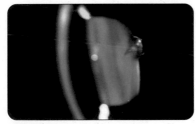

Fig. 3.19 Posterior lenticonus

Lentiglobus

Very rare, usually unilateral, generalized hemispherical deformity of the lens which may be associated with a posterior polar opacity.

Microspherophakia

1. Signs – bilateral; small spherical lens (*Fig. 3.20*).
2. Classification:
   a. Familial (AD) without systemic associations.
   b. With systemic associations – Marfan syndrome, Weill–Marchesani syndrome, hyperlysinaemia, and congenital rubella.
3. Ocular associations – Peters anomaly and familial ectopia lentis et pupillae.
4. Complications – lenticular myopia, subluxation, and total dislocation into the anterior chamber.

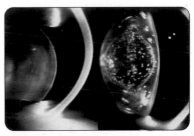

Fig. 3.20 Microspherophakia

Microphakia

1. Sign – bilateral; lens with a smaller than normal diameter.
2. Systemic association – Lowe syndrome.

Coloboma

1. Signs – unilateral or bilateral; notching (segmental agenesis) at the equator (*Fig. 3.21*) with corresponding absence of zonular fibres.
2. Ocular association – occasional coloboma of the iris or fundus.

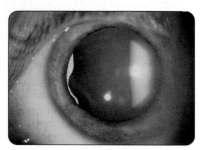

Fig. 3.21 Lens coloboma

Iridocorneal dysgenesis

Posterior embryotoxon

1. **Signs** – thin grey–white, peripheral
   ridge adjacent to the limbus which
   comprises a prominent and anteriorly
   displaced Schwalbe line (*Fig. 3.22*).
2. **Associations**
   a. Axenfeld–Rieger anomaly –
      invariable.
   b. Alagille syndrome – in 95% of
      cases.

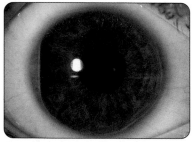

Fig. 3.22 Posterior embryotoxon

Axenfeld–Rieger syndrome

A spectrum of disorders designated by
the following AD eponyms:
1. **Axenfeld anomaly** – posterior
   embryotoxon with attachment of
   peripheral iris strands (*Fig. 3.23*).

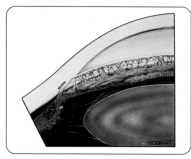

Fig. 3.23 Iris strands in Axenfeld
anomaly

2. **Rieger anomaly** – posterior
   embryotoxon, iris stromal hypoplasia,
   ectropion uveae, corectopia, full
   thickness iris defects (*Fig. 3.24*), and
   broad iris adhesions anterior to
   Schwalbe line (*Fig. 3.25*); glaucoma
   develops in about 50% of cases.

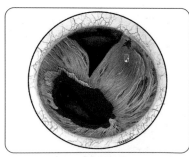

Fig. 3.24 Severe changes in Rieger
anomaly

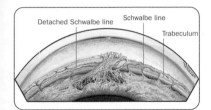

Fig. 3.25 Broad iris adhesions in Rieger anomaly

3. **Rieger syndrome** – comprises Rieger anomaly and the following malformations:
   a. *Dental* – hypodontia and microdontia (*Fig. 3.26*).
   b. *Facial* – maxillary hypoplasia, broad nasal bridge, telecanthus and hypertelorism.
   c. *Other* – redundant paraumbilical skin and hypospadias.

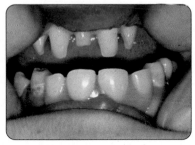

Fig. 3.26 Microdontia and hypodontia in Rieger syndrome

Peters anomaly

1. **Pathogenesis** – defective neural crest cell migration in the 6th to 8th weeks of fetal development, during which time the anterior segment of the eye is formed.

2. **Signs** – usually bilateral.
   • Corneal opacity + posterior corneal defect alone.
   • Above + iridocorneal adhesions (*Fig. 3.27a*).
   • Above + kerato-lenticular contact or cataract (*Fig. 3.27b*).

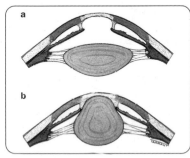

Fig. 3.27 Peters anomaly

3. **Ocular associations** – glaucoma in 50%; occasionally Axenfeld–Rieger syndrome, aniridia, microphthalmos, persistent fetal vasculature, and retinal dysplasia.
4. **Systemic associations** – chromosomal, craniofacial and CNS anomalies, fetal alcohol syndrome, and Peters plus syndrome (short-limbed dwarfism, cleft lip/palate, prominent forehead, and mental handicap).

Aniridia

1. **Pathogenesis** – abnormal neuroectodermal development secondary to a mutation in the PAX6 gene linked to 11p13.

2. Classification

    a. *AN-1* – AD; accounts for 66% of cases.

    b. *AN-2 (Miller syndrome)* – sporadic; accounts for 33% of cases and carries a 30% risk of Wilm tumour before the age of 5 years.

    c. *AN-3 (Gillespie syndrome)* – AR; mental handicap and cerebellar ataxia.

3. Presentation – at birth with nystagmus and photophobia.

4. Aniridia – ranges from minimal to partial and total (*Fig. 3.28*).

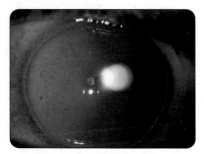

Fig. 3.28 Aniridia

5. Gonioscopy – rudimentary iris tissue that may cause synechial angle closure (*Fig. 3.29*).

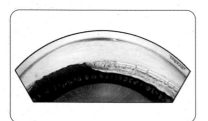

Fig. 3.29 Partial synechial angle closure in aniridia

6. Cornea – epithelial defects, limbal stem cell deficiency and 'conjunctivalization' of the peripheral cornea, and epibulbar dermoids.

7. Lens – cataract, subluxation, congenital aphakia and persistent pupillary membranes.

8. Fundus – foveal hypoplasia, optic nerve hypoplasia, and choroidal coloboma.

9. Glaucoma – 75% of cases.

Globe

Microphthalmos

1. Definition – total axial length (TAL) at least 2 standard deviations below age-similar controls; usually unilateral.

2. Pathogenesis – non-specific growth failure in response to a variety of prenatal insults.

3. Classification

    a. *Simple* – isolated.

    b. *Complex (colobomatous)* – coloboma, usually of the iris (*Fig. 3.30*).

    c. *Microphthalmos with cyst* – orbital cyst communicates with the globe.

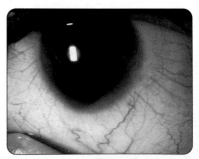

Fig. 3.30 Colobomatous microphthalmos

d. *Posterior* – TAL is reduced in the setting of normal corneal diameter, resulting in high hypermetropia and papillomacular retinal folds.
4. **Differential diagnosis** – nanophthalmos (microphthalmos, microcornea, and tendency to uveal effusions).

Anophthalmos

1. **Pathogenesis** – either a complete failure of budding of the optic vesicle or early developmental arrest.
2. **Simple** – associated with absence of extraocular muscles, short conjunctival sac, and microblepharon (*Fig. 3.31*).
3. **Anophthalmos with cyst (congenital cystic eyeball)** – globe is replaced by a cyst (*Fig. 3.32*).

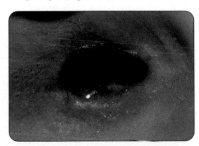

Fig. 3.31 Simple anophthalmos

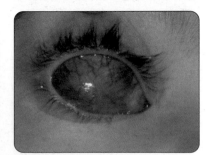

Fig. 3.32 Anophthalmos with cyst (congenital cystic eyeball)

Retina and choroid

Choroidal coloboma

1. **Pathogenesis** – incomplete closure of the embryonic fissure.
2. **Signs** – sharply circumscribed white area in the inferior fundus devoid of blood vessels (*Fig. 3.33*).
3. **Complications** – RD.

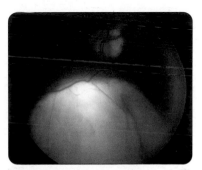

Fig. 3.33 Choroidal coloboma

Myelinated nerve fibres

1. **Signs** – white feathery streaks running within the NFL towards the disc (*Fig. 3.34*).

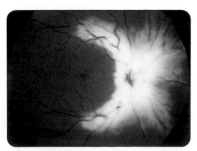

Fig. 3.34 Myelinated nerve fibres

2. **Ocular associations if extensive** – high myopia, anisometropia, macular aplasia, epiretinal membrane, and amblyopia.
3. **Systemic associations** – NF 1, Down syndrome, and Gorlin–Goltz syndrome.

Aicardi syndrome

1. **Inheritance** – X-LD.
2. **Systemic signs** – infantile spasms, CNS and skeletal malformations, and psychomotor retardation with early demise.
3. **Ocular signs** – bilateral, multiple depigmented 'chorioretinal lacunae' clustered around the disc that may be hypoplastic, colobomatous or pigmented (Fig. 3.35).
4. **Ocular associations** – microphthalmos, iris coloboma, persistent pupillary membranes, and cataract.

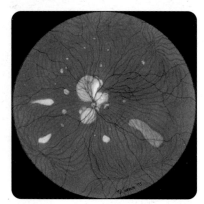

Fig. 3.35 Fundus in Aicardi syndrome

Retinal macrovessel

A unilateral, large, aberrant retinal vessel, usually a vein, in the posterior pole that may cross the horizontal raphe (Fig. 3.36).

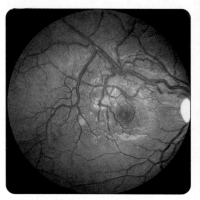

Fig. 3.36 Retinal macrovessel

Arteriovenous communications

Congenital arteriovenous communications can be divided into three types on the basis of severity:

- **Group 1** – anastomosis between a small arteriole and venule with the intervention of an abnormal capillary or arteriolar plexus.
- **Group 2** – direct arteriovenous communications between a branch retinal artery and vein (Fig. 3.37).

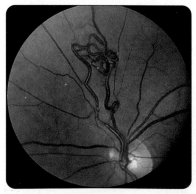

Fig. 3.37 Arteriovenous communication

- **Group 3** – diffuse marked dilatation of the vascular tree with many large calibre anastomosing channels.

Optic nerve

Prepapillary loop

1. **Signs** – vascular loop extending from the disc into the vitreous cavity and then back (*Fig. 3.38*).
2. **Complications** – obstruction in the distribution of the retinal artery supplying the loop occurs in 10% of cases.

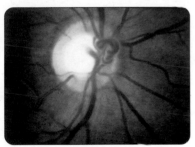

Fig. 3.38 Prepapillary loop

Bergmeister papilla

1. **Pathogenesis** – unilateral anomaly derived from avascular remnants of the hyaloid system.
2. **Signs** – raised glial tissue on the disc surface (*Fig. 3.39*).

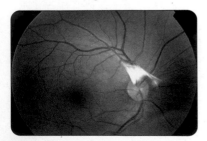

Fig. 3.39 Bergmeister papilla

Tilted disc

1. **Signs** – oval or D-shaped disc, situs inversus, inferonasal chorioretinal thinning, and myopic astigmatic refractive error (*Fig. 3.40*).
2. **Perimetry** – superotemporal defects that do not respect the vertical midline may be present.
3. **Complications** – occasional CNV and sensory macular detachment.

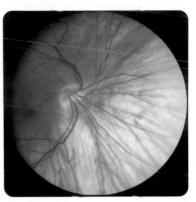

Fig. 3.40 Tilted disc

Optic disc pit

1. **Signs** – large disc contains a round or oval pit usually located temporally (*Fig. 3.41*) but may occasionally be central.
2. **Perimetry** – visual field defects are common and may mimic those due to glaucoma.
3. **Serous macular detachment** – develops in about 45% of eyes with non-central disc pits (median age 30

years); subretinal fluid is thought to be derived from the vitreous and resolves spontaneously in 25% of cases.

4. **Treatment** – persistent detachment may require laser photocoagulation or vitrectomy with air–fluid exchange.

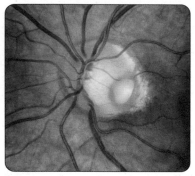

Fig. 3.41 Optic disc pit

Optic disc drusen

1. **Histology** – hyaline-like calcific material within the substance of the optic nerve head.
2. **Signs**
   a. *Buried drusen* – elevated disc with a scalloped margin without a physiological cup; anomalous vascular patterns include early branching, increased number of major retinal vessels and vascular tortuosity (*Fig. 3.42*).
   b. *Exposed drusen* – during the early 'teens drusen usually emerge to the surface of the disc as waxy pearl-like irregularities (*Fig. 3.43*).

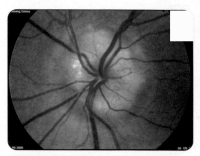

Fig. 3.42 Buried optic disc drusen

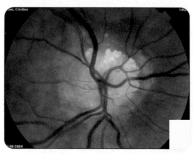

Fig. 3.43 Exposed optic disc drusen

3. **Associations** – RP, angioid streaks, Alagille syndrome, and congenital hamartoma of the retina and RPE.
4. **Complications** – juxtapapillary CNV, disc neovascularization, central retinal arterial and venous occlusion, and progressive but limited loss of visual field are rare.
5. **Imaging**
   a. *FA* – autofluorescence prior to dye injection and then progressive hyperfluorescence due to staining without leakage.
   b. *US* – high acoustic reflectivity.
   c. *CT* – calcification.

Optic disc coloboma

1. **Signs** – discrete, focal, glistening, white, bowl-shaped disc excavation, decentred inferiorly (*Fig. 3.44*).

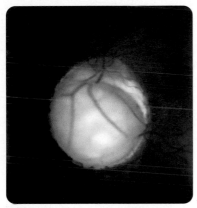

Fig. 3.44 Optic disc coloboma

2. **Ocular associations** – microphthalmos and other colobomas.
3. **Complications** – rarely serous macular detachment and peripapillary CNV.
4. **Systemic associations**
   a. *Chromosomal anomalies* – Patau syndrome (trisomy 13), Edward syndrome (trisomy 18) and Cat-eye syndrome (trisomy 22).
   b. *'CHARGE'* (**C**oloboma, **H**eart defects, choanal **A**tresia, **R**etarded growth and development, **G**enital and **E**ar anomalies).
   c. *Other syndromes* – Meckel–Gruber, Goltz, Walker–Warburg, Goldenhar, Aicardi, Dandy–Walker cyst and linear sebaceous naevus.
   d. *CNS anomalies*.

Morning glory anomaly

1. **Signs**
   - Large disc with a funnel-shaped excavation surrounded by an annulus of chorioretinal disturbance (*Fig. 3.45*).
   - Supernumerary blood vessels emerge radially like the spokes of a wheel.

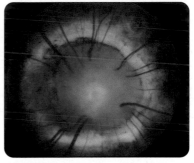

Fig. 3.45 Morning glory anomaly

2. **Complications** – serous RD in 30%; CNV is less common.
3. **Systemic associations** – frontonasal dysplasia, NF 2, PHACE syndrome (posterior fossa brain malformations, facial haemangiomas and cardiovascular anomalies).

Optic nerve hypoplasia

1. **Predispositions** – agents used by the mother during gestation include excess alcohol, LSD, quinine, protamine zinc insulin, steroids, diuretics, cold remedies, and anticonvulsants.
2. **Signs**
   - Small grey disc surrounded by hypopigmentation (double-ring sign – *Fig. 3.46*).
   - Normal calibre retinal vessels that may be tortuous.

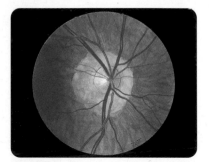

Fig. 3.46 Optic disc hypoplasia

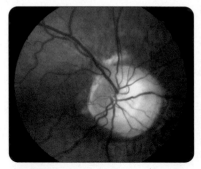

Fig. 3.47 Megalopapilla

3. **Associated signs** – astigmatism, field defects, dyschromatopsia, afferent pupillary defect, foveal hypoplasia, aniridia, microphthalmos, strabismus and nystagmus.
4. **Systemic associations** – de Morsier syndrome (septo-optic dysplasia) in 10%.

Miscellaneous anomalies

1. **Megalopapilla** – horizontal and vertical disc diameters are 2.1 mm or more (*Fig. 3.47*).
2. **Peripapillary staphyloma** – normal disc sits at the base of a deep excavation which is surrounded by chorioretinal atrophy (*Fig. 3.48*).
3. **Optic disc dysplasia** – markedly deformed disc that does not conform to any recognizable category described above (*Fig. 3.49*).
4. **Papillorenal (renal-coloboma) syndrome** – discs are normal in size and may be surrounded by variable pigmentary disturbance; the excavation is central, and the disc appears 'vacant', with replacement of the central retinal vasculature by vessels of cilioretinal origin (*Fig. 3.50*).
5. **Optic nerve aplasia** – absent or rudimentary disc; blood vessels are absent or sparse.

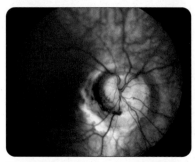

Fig. 3.48 Peripapillary staphyloma

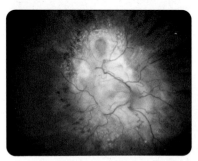

Fig. 3.49 Dysplastic disc

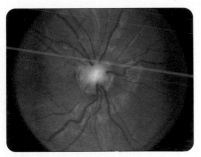

Fig. 3.50 Papillorenal syndrome

Vitreous

Persistent hyaloid artery

1. Signs
- Glial remnants extending from the disc to the lens (Cloquet canal).
- A partly patent artery may contain blood (*Fig. 3.51*) at its point of attachment to the posterior lens capsule and may form a white ('Mittendorf') dot (see *Fig. 12.33*).

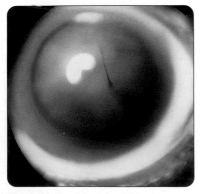

Fig. 3.51 Persistent hyaloid artery partly filled with blood

2. Complications – vitreous haemorrhage is very rare.
3. Ocular associations – posterior vitreous cyst, optic disc coloboma, and optic nerve hypoplasia.

Persistent fetal vasculature

1. Presentation – unilateral leukocoria in a microphthalmic eye (*Fig. 3.52*).

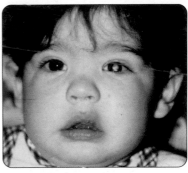

Fig. 3.52 Persistent fetal vasculature involving the left eye

2. Signs
- Retrolental mass into which elongated ciliary processes are inserted.
- Prominent iris blood vessels and shallow anterior chamber.
- With time the mass contracts and pulls the ciliary processes centrally so that they become visible through the pupil.
3. Complications – cataract, elevation of intraocular pressure, and RD.
4. Treatment – vitreoretinal surgery in early cases may salvage some vision.

Vitreoretinal dysplasia

1. **Pathogenesis** – faulty differentiation of the retina and vitreous.
2. **Signs** – retrolental vascularized retrolental mass resulting in leukocoria (*Fig. 3.53*).

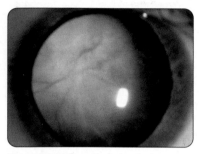

Fig. 3.53 Vitreoretinal dysplasia

3. **Systemic associations** – Norrie disease, incontinentia pigmenti (Bloch–Sulzberger syndrome), and Warburg syndrome.

Vitreous cyst

Rare congenital remnants of the primary hyaloidal system or ciliary body pigment epithelium (*Fig. 3.54*).

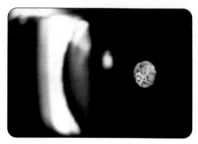

Fig. 3.54 Vitreous cyst

Eyelids

Benign nodules and cysts

Chalazion ('meibomian cyst')

1. **Pathogenesis** – inflammatory reaction induced by leakage of retained sebaceous secretions into stromal tissues.
2. **Histology** – lipogranulomatous inflammatory reaction with epithelioid cells and multinucleated giant cells intermixed with lymphocytes and plasma cells (*Fig. 4.1*).

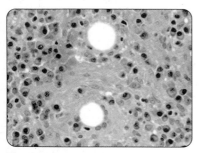

Fig. 4.1 Histology of chalazion

3. **Predispositions** – chronic posterior blepharitis, acne rosacea, and seborrhoeic dermatitis.
4. **Signs** – non-tender, roundish, nodule within the tarsal plate (*Fig. 4.2*).

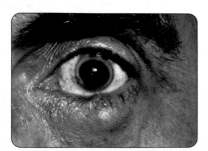

Fig. 4.2 Chalazion

5. **Treatment** – incision and curettage, or injection of triamcinolone diacetate aqueous suspension diluted with lignocaine (or equivalent).
6. **Complications** – polypoidal conjunctival granuloma (*Fig. 4.3*).

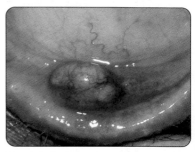

Fig. 4.3 Chalazion granuloma

7. **Differential diagnosis** – external hordeolum (stye), cyst of Zeis, and sebaceous gland carcinoma.

Epidermoid cyst

1. **Pathogenesis** – implantation of surface epidermis during trauma or surgery.
2. **Histology** – keratin-filled cavity within the dermis lined by stratified squamous epithelium.
3. **Signs** – firm, round, mobile lesion (*Fig. 4.4*).
4. **Complications** – rupture may result in a foreign body reaction and secondary infection.
5. **Treatment** – marsupialization or excision.

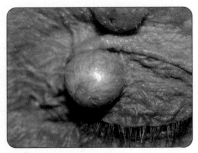

Fig. 4.4 Epidermoid cyst

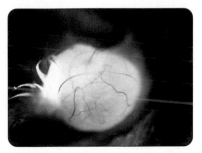

Fig. 4.6 Cyst of Moll

Miscellaneous cysts and nodules

1. Cyst of Zeis – small, non-translucent lesion on the anterior lid margin (*Fig. 4.5*).

3. Eccrine hidrocystoma – similar to a cyst of Moll but located along the medial or lateral aspects of the lid without involving the lid margin itself (*Fig. 4.7*).

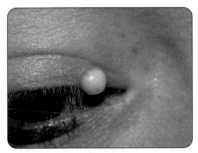

Fig. 4.5 Cyst of Zeis

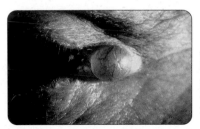

Fig. 4.7 Eccrine hidrocystoma

4. Syringoma – multiple, small papules (*Fig. 4.8*).

2. Cyst of Moll (apocrine hidrocystoma) – translucent fluid-filled lesion on the anterior lid margin (*Fig. 4.6*).

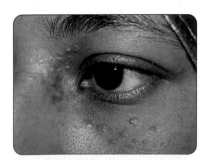

Fig. 4.8 Syringomas

5. Milia – crops of tiny, white, round, superficial cysts (*Fig. 4.9*).

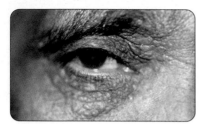

Fig. 4.9 Milia

6. Comedones – tiny papules that occur in patients with acne vulgaris (*Fig. 4.10*).

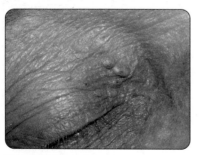

Fig. 4.10 Comedones

Benign tumours

Squamous papilloma

1. Histology – finger-like projections of fibrovascular connective tissue covered by irregular acanthotic and hyperkeratotic squamous epithelium (*Fig. 4.11*).

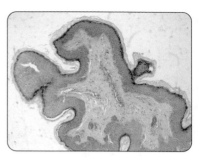

Fig. 4.11 Histology of papilloma

2. Signs are variable:
- Narrow-based pedunculated lesion (skin tag – *Fig. 4.12*).
- Sessile lesion with raspberry-like surface (*Fig. 4.13*).
- Hyperkeratotic filiform lesion similar to a cutaneous horn.

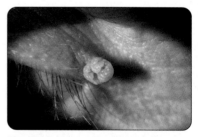

Fig. 4.12 Pedunculated papilloma

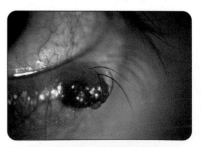

Fig. 4.13 Sessile papilloma

3. **Treatment** – simple excision.
4. **Differential diagnosis** – viral wart, seborrhoeic keratosis, and intra-dermal naevus.

Basal cell papilloma (seborrhoeic keratosis, seborrhoeic wart, senile verruca)

1. **Histology** – expansion of the squamous epithelium of the epidermis by a proliferation of basal cells; acanthotic epidermis may show keratin-filled cystic inclusions which may be either horn cysts or pseudo-horn cysts.
2. **Signs** – greasy, brown plaque with a friable verrucous surface and a 'stuck-on' appearance (*Fig. 4.14*).

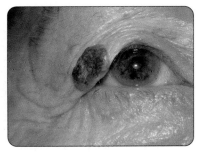

Fig. 4.14 Basal cell papilloma

3. **Treatment** – shave excision of flat lesions and excision of pedunculated lesions.
4. **Differential diagnosis** – pigmented basal cell carcinoma, naevus, and melanoma.

Inverted follicular keratosis (inverted seborrhoeic keratosis, irritated basal cell papilloma, basosquamous acanthoma)

1. **Histology** – resembles seborrhoeic keratosis but also shows zones of squamous cells arranged in whorls (squamous eddies).
2. **Signs** – non-pigmented papilloma-tous lesion on the lid margin that may grow rapidly (*Fig. 4.15*).

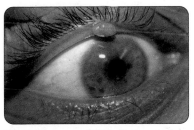

Fig. 4.15 Inverted follicular keratosis

3. **Treatment** – excision.

Actinic (solar, senile) keratosis

1. **Predispositions** – elderly, fair-skinned individuals who have been exposed to excessive sunlight.
2. **Histology** – irregular dysplastic epidermis with hyperkeratosis, parakeratosis, and cutaneous horn formation.
3. **Malignant potential** – into squa-mous cell carcinoma is low.
4. **Signs** – hyperkeratotic plaque with distinct borders with a scaly surface that may become fissured (*Fig. 4.16*).

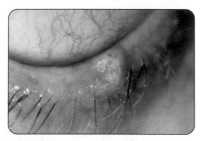

Fig. 4.16 Actinic keratosis

5. Treatment – biopsy followed by excision or cryotherapy.

Keratoacanthoma

1. Histology – irregular thickened epidermis surrounded by acanthotic squamous epithelium; sharp transition from the thickened to normal adjacent epidermis (shoulder formation – *Fig. 4.17*).

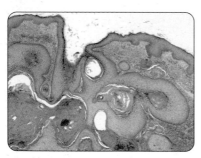

Fig. 4.17 Histology of keratoacanthoma

2. Signs in chronological order:
- Rapidly growing pink lesion, often on the lower lid.
- Stops growing and remains static for 2–3 months and then starts to involute.

- During involution the central part becomes hyperkeratotic and a keratin-filled crater may develop (*Fig. 4.18*).
- Complete involution may take up to a year.

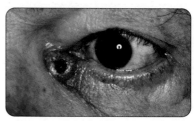

Fig. 4.18 Keratoacanthoma with crater

3. Treatment – excision, radiotherapy, cryotherapy, and topical or intra-lesional 5-fluorouracil.
4. Differential diagnosis – squamous cell carcinoma and basal cell carcinoma.

Acquired melanocytic naevus

1. Histology – naevus cells derived either from epidermal melanocytes (junctional, compound and intradermal naevi) or from dermal melanocytes (blue naevi).
2. Malignant potential – related to the junctional component.
3. Classification
  a. *Junctional*
  - Brown macule or papule in a young individual.
  - Naevus cells – at junction of epidermis and dermis; low malignant potential.
  b. *Compound*
  - Raised papular lesion with variable pigmentation in a middle-aged individual (*Fig. 4.19*).

- Naevus cells – extend from the epidermis into the dermis; low malignant potential.

c. *Dermal*

- Papillomatous non-pigmented lesion in an elderly individual that may be associated with dilated vessels and protruding lashes (*Fig. 4.20*).
- Naevus cells – confined to dermis (*Fig. 4.21*); no malignant potential.

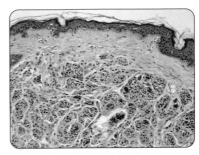

Fig. 4.21 Histology of dermal naevus

4. Treatment – excision for cosmesis or concern about malignancy.

Congenital melanocytic naevus

1. Signs – uniform coloured lesion which may occasionally equally involve the upper and lower lids ('kissing' naevus – *Fig. 4.22*).

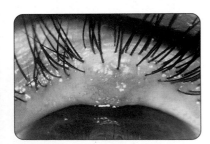

Fig. 4.19 Compound naevus

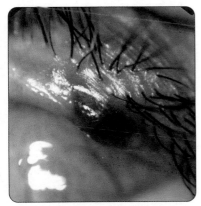

Fig. 4.20 Dermal naevus

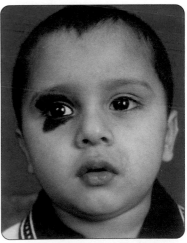

Fig. 4.22 Congenital 'kissing' naevus

2. Treatment – excision and reconstruction with skin grafts.

Capillary haemangioma (strawberry naevus)

1. Histology – proliferation of varying-sized vascular channels within the dermis and subcutaneous tissue.
2. Presentation – shortly after birth.
3. Signs – raised bright red lesion (*Fig. 4.23*) which blanches on pressure and may swell on crying; orbital extension may be present.

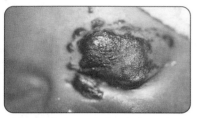

Fig. 4.23 Capillary haemangioma

4. Treatment – observation for regression of small lesions; steroid injection of vision-threatening lesions.

Port-wine stain (naevus flammeus)

1. Histology – dilated blood-filled spaces separated by thin fibrous septae.
2. Signs
  • Congenital, sharply demarcated, pink patch which does not blanch on pressure.
  • Darkens with age and the overlying skin may become hypertrophied and coarse (*Fig. 4.24*).

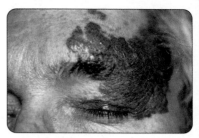

Fig. 4.24 Port-wine stain

3. Systemic associations – Sturge–Weber syndrome in 5% of cases with extensive lesions.
4. Treatment – erbium laser in relatively flat or mildly hypertrophic lesions.

Pyogenic granuloma

1. Pathogenesis – usually antedated by surgery, trauma or infection although some are idiopathic.
2. Histology – granulation tissue composed of wide, thin-walled vascular channels and inflammatory cellular infiltration.
3. Signs – painful, rapidly growing, vascular polypoidal lesion (*Fig. 4.25*).

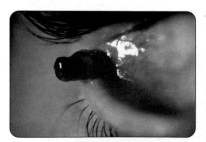

Fig. 4.25 Pyogenic granuloma

4. Treatment – excision.

Xanthelasma

1. Histology – lipid-laden histiocytes within the dermis (*Fig. 4.26*).

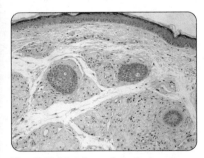

Fig. 4.26 Histology of xanthelasma

2. Signs – usually bilateral, yellowish, subcutaneous plaques at the medial aspects of the eyelids (*Fig. 4.27*).

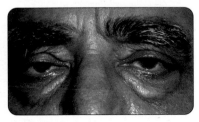

Fig. 4.27 Xanthelasma

3. Systemic association – increased serum cholesterol and low-density lipoprotein, especially in young individuals with corneal arcus.

4. Treatment – excision or laser destruction.

Pilomatricoma (pilomatrixoma, calcifying epithelioma of Malherbe)

1. Histology – irregular epithelial islands exhibiting viable basophilic cells at the periphery and degenerate shadow cells more centrally; calcification is common.

2. Signs – deep, dermal nodule that may be calcified (*Fig. 4.28*).

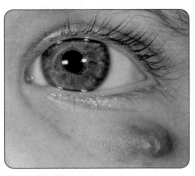

Fig. 4.28 Pilomatricoma

3. Treatment – excision.

Neurofibroma

1. Histology – proliferation of Schwann cells, fibroblasts, and nerve axons.

2. Signs – subcutaneous upper lid lesion giving rise to an S-shaped deformity (*Fig. 4.29*).

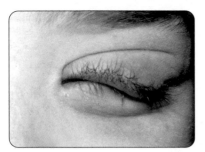

Fig. 4.29 Neurofibroma

3. Systemic association – NF 1.
4. Treatment – excision, if solitary.

Malignant tumours

Basal cell carcinoma (BCC)

1. **Rare predisposing conditions** (see Chapter 24)
   a. *Xeroderma pigmentosum.*
   b. *Gorlin–Goltz syndrome.*
   c. *Muir–Torre syndrome.*
   d. *Bazex syndrome.*
   e. *Linear basal cell carcinoma.*
2. **General features**
   • 90% occur in the head and neck and of these about 10% involve the eyelid.
   • Accounts for 90% of eyelid malignancies.
   • Location in decreasing frequency – lower lid, medial canthus, upper lid, and lateral canthus.
3. **Histology** – downward proliferation of basal cells arising from the epidermis that may exhibit palisading at the periphery of a lobule of cells (*Fig. 4.30*).

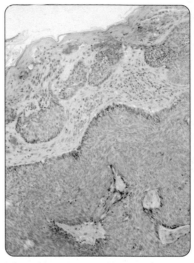

Fig. 4.30 Histology of BCC

4. **Clinical types**
   a. *Nodular* – slow-growing, shiny, firm, pearly nodule with dilated surface vessels (*Fig. 4.31*).
   b. *Noduloulcerative (rodent ulcer)* – central ulceration, pearly raised rolled edges and dilated vessels over its lateral margins (*Fig. 4.32*).
   c. *Sclerosing (morphoeic)* – indurated plaque with loss of lashes (*Fig. 4.33*).

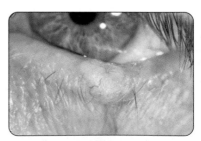

Fig. 4.31 Nodular BCC

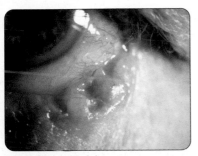

Fig. 4.32 Rodent ulcer

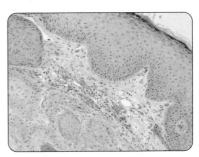

Fig. 4.34 Histology of SCC

3. Clinical types

  a. *Nodular* – hyperkeratotic nodule which may develop crusting erosions and fissures (*Fig. 4.35*).

  b. *Ulcerating* – red base and sharply defined, indurated and everted borders but absence of pearly margins and surface vessels (*Fig. 4.36*).

  c. *Cutaneous horn* – with underlying invasive SCC (*Fig. 4.37*).

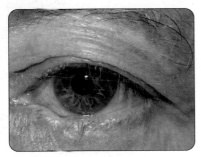

Fig. 4.33 Sclerosing BCC

Squamous cell carcinoma (SCC)

1. General features

- Less common than BCC; more aggressive.
- Accounts for 5–10% of eyelid malignancies.
- May arise de novo or from pre-existing actinic keratosis or carcinoma in-situ.
- Predilection for the lower eyelid.

2. Histology

- Groups of atypical epithelial cells with prominent nuclei and abundant eosinophilic cytoplasm within the dermis (*Fig. 4.34*).
- Keratin 'pearls' and intercellular bridges (desmosomes) in well-differentiated tumours.

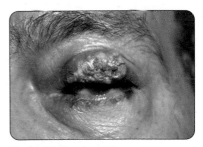

Fig. 4.35 Nodular SCC

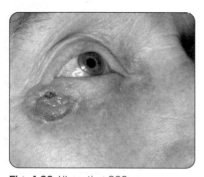

Fig. 4.36 Ulcerating SCC

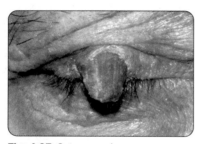

Fig. 4.37 Cutaneous horn

Sebaceous gland carcinoma (SGC)

1. General features

- Aggressive tumour that usually arises from the meibomian glands, and occasionally from the glands of Zeis or sebaceous glands in the caruncle.
- Predisposition for the upper lid.
- In early cases signs of malignancy may be subtle and the tumour may be misdiagnosed as chalazion or chronic blepharitis.

2. Histology – lobules of cells with pale foamy vacuolated cytoplasm and large hyperchromatic nuclei that stain positive (red) for lipid (*Fig. 4.38*).

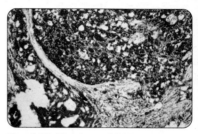

Fig. 4.38 Histology of SGC with oil red stain

3. Clinical types

  a. *Nodular* – discrete, hard, immobile nodule that may exhibit yellow discoloration (*Fig. 4.39*).
  b. *Spreading* – diffuse infiltration of the epidermis (pagetoid spread) causes diffuse thickening of the lid margin and loss of lashes; similar conjunctival infiltration may occur (*Fig. 4.40*).

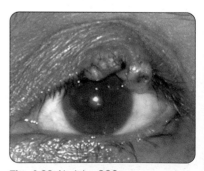

Fig. 4.39 Nodular SGC

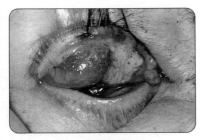

Fig. 4.40 Spreading SGC with conjunctival involvement

4. Systemic association – Muir–Torre syndrome.

Lentigo maligna (melanoma in-situ, Hutchinson freckle)

1. Presentation – sun-damaged skin in elderly individuals.
2. Histology – intraepidermal proliferation of atypical spindle-shaped melanocytes that replace the basal layer of the epidermis; later dermal infiltration and malignant transformation may occur.
3. Signs
- Slow-growing pigmented macule with an irregular border (*Fig. 4.41*).
- Nodular thickening and areas of irregular pigmentation are highly suggestive of malignant transformation (*Fig. 4.42*).

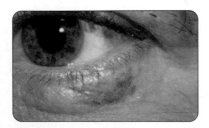

Fig. 4.41 Lentigo maligna

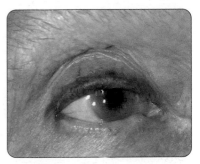

Fig. 4.42 Melanoma arising from lentigo maligna

Melanoma

1. Histology – large atypical melanocytes within the dermis.
2. Clinical types
  a. *Superficial spreading* – plaque with an irregular outline and variable pigmentation (*Fig. 4.43*).
  b. *Nodular* – blue-black nodule (*Fig. 4.44*).

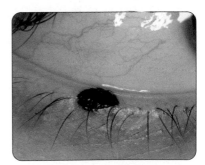

Fig. 4.43 Superficial spreading melanoma

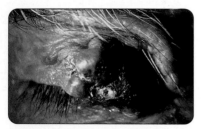

Fig. 4.44 Nodular melanoma

Merkel cell (cutaneous neuroendocrine) carcinoma

1. **Histology** – sheets of cells with scanty cytoplasm, round or oval nuclei and numerous mitotic figures.
2. **Signs** – fast-growing, violaceous, well demarcated nodule with intact overlying skin (*Fig. 4.45*).

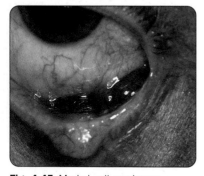

Fig. 4.45 Merkel cell carcinoma

3. **Treatment** – excision and chemotherapy.

Kaposi sarcoma

1. **Histology** – proliferating spindle cells, vascular channels, and inflammatory cells within the dermis.
2. **Predisposition** – AIDS.

3. **Signs** – pink, red-violet to brown lesion which may be mistaken for a haematoma or naevus (*Fig. 4.46*).

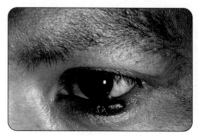

Fig. 4.46 Kaposi sarcoma

4. **Treatment** – radiotherapy.

Treatment options of malignant tumours

1. **Surgical excision** – entire tumour must be removed with preservation of as much of normal tissue as possible.
   a. *Small BCC* – excision with a 4 mm margin of clinically normal tissue.
   b. *Large BCC and aggressive tumours* – radical surgery with frozen section control by either standard methods or Mohs micrographic surgery.
2. **Reconstruction** – depends on the extent of tissue removed.
   a. *Small defects* – direct closure with or without lateral cantholysis (*Fig. 4.47*).
   b. *Moderate defects* – Tenzel semicircular flap (*Fig. 4.48*).
   c. *Large defects* – Mustarde procedure (*Fig. 4.49*) and reconstruction of anterior and posterior lamellae.

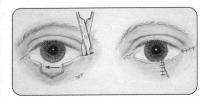

Fig. 4.47 Direct closure of a small defect with lateral cantholysis

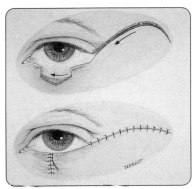

Fig. 4.48 Tenzel flap

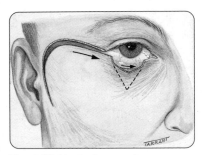

Fig. 4.49 Mustarde procedure

3. **Radiotherapy** – small BCC not involving the medial canthal area, and Kaposi sarcoma.

Disorders of lashes

Trichiasis

1. **Predispositions** – chronic anterior blepharitis, herpes zoster ophthalmicus, and trachoma.
2. **Signs** – posterior misdirection of lashes arising from normal sites of origin (*Fig. 4.50*).

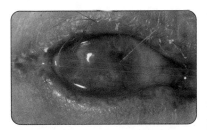

Fig. 4.50 Trichiasis

3. **Complications** – punctate epithelial erosions, corneal ulceration, and pannus formation.
4. **Treatment options** – epilation, electrolysis, cryotherapy (*Fig. 4.51*), argon laser ablation, and full-thickness wedge resection.

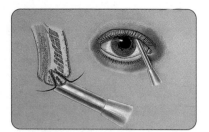

Fig. 4.51 Cryotherapy for trichiasis

5. Differential diagnosis – distichiasis and entropion (pseudo-trichiasis).

Congenital distichiasis

1. **Pathogenesis** – primary epithelial germ cell destined to differentiate into a specialized sebaceous gland develops into a complete pilosebaceous unit.
2. **Inheritance** – AD.
3. **Signs** – partial or complete second row of thin short lashes emerging at or slightly behind the meibomian gland orifices and often pointing posteriorly (*Fig. 4.52*).

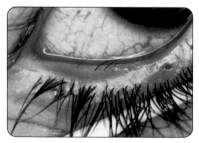

Fig. 4.52 Congenital distichiasis

4. Treatment
 a. *Lower lid* – cryotherapy.
 b. *Upper lid* – lamellar eyelid division and cryotherapy to posterior lamella (*Fig. 4.53*).

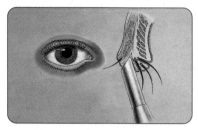

Fig. 4.53 Lamella division and cryotherapy for trichiasis

5. Systemic association – leg lymphoedema (lymphoedema-distichiasis syndrome).

Acquired distichiasis (metaplastic lashes)

1. **Pathogenesis** – metaplasia and dedifferentiation of the meibomian glands to become hair follicles associated with late stage cicatrizing conjunctivitis.
2. **Signs** – non-pigmented lashes originating from meibomian gland orifices (*Fig. 4.54*).
3. **Treatment**
 a. *Mild* – as for trichiasis.
 b. *Severe* – lamellar eyelid division and cryotherapy to the posterior lamella.

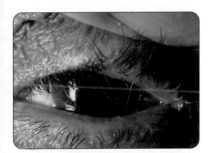

Fig. 4.54 Acquired distichiasis (metaplastic lashes)

Eyelash ptosis

1. **Predispositions** – floppy eyelid syndrome, dermatochalasis with anterior lamellar slip, and long-standing facial palsy.
2. **Signs** – downward sagging of upper lashes (*Fig. 4.55*).

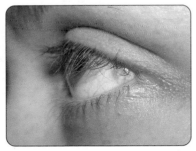

Fig. 4.55 Eyelash ptosis

Trichomegaly

Trichomegaly is excessive eyelash growth (*Fig. 4.56*); causes are listed in *Table 4.1*.

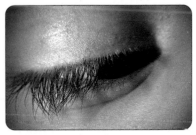

Fig. 4.56 Trichomegaly

Table 4.1 **Causes of trichomegaly**

1. *Acquired*
   • Drug-induced – phenytoin, ciclosporin, and prostaglandin analogues
   • Malnutrition
   • AIDS
   • Porphyria
   • Hypothyroidism
   • Familial
2. *Congenital*
   • Oliver–McFarlane syndrome
   • Cornelia de Lange syndrome
   • Goldstein–Hutt syndrome
   • Hermansky–Pudlak syndrome
   • Oculocutaneous albinism type 1

Madarosis

Madarosis is a decrease in the number of lashes (*Fig. 4.57*); causes are listed in *Table 4.2*.

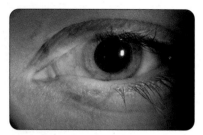

Fig. 4.57 Madarosis following irradiation

Table 4.2 **Causes of madarosis**

1. *Local*
   • Chronic anterior lid margin disease
   • Infiltrating lid tumours
   • Burns
   • Radiotherapy or cryotherapy of lid tumours
 2. *Skin disorders*
   • Generalized alopecia
   • Psoriasis
 3. *Systemic diseases*
   • Myxoedema
   • Systemic lupus erythematosus
   • Acquired syphilis
   • Lepromatous leprosy
 4. *Following removal*
   • Iatrogenic for trichiasis
   • Trichotillomania (psychiatric disorder of hair removal)

Poliosis

Poliosis is a premature localized whitening of hair, which may involve the lashes and eyebrows (*Fig. 4.58*); causes are listed in *Table 4.3*.

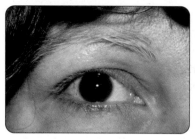

Fig. 4.58 Poliosis of lashes and eyebrows

Table 4.3 **Causes of poliosis**

1. *Ocular*
   • Chronic anterior blepharitis
   • Sympathetic ophthalmitis
   • Idiopathic uveitis
 2. *Systemic*
   • Vogt–Koyanagi–Harada syndrome
   • Waardenburg syndrome
   • Vitiligo
   • Marfan syndrome
   • Tuberous sclerosis

Allergic disorders

Acute allergic oedema

1. **Aetiology** – insect bites, angioedema and urticaria, and occasionally drugs.

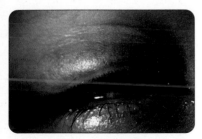

Fig. 4.59 Acute allergic oedema

2. **Signs** – sudden onset of pitting periorbital oedema (*Fig. 4.59*).
3. **Treatment** – systemic antihistamines if severe.

Contact dermatitis

1. **Pathogenesis** – sensitization on initial exposure followed, on further exposure, by an immune reaction mediated by a delayed type IV hypersensitivity response.
2. **Symptoms** – itching and tearing following exposure.
3. **Signs** – lid erythema, scaling, and angular fissuring which may be associated with papillary conjunctivitis (*Fig. 4.60*).

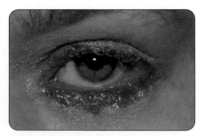

Fig. 4.60 Contact dermatitis

4. **Treatment** – stopping exposure to the allergen, cold compresses and oral antihistamines.

Atopic dermatitis

1. **Signs** – thickening, crusting and vertical fissuring of the lids associated staphylococcal blepharitis and madarosis (*Fig. 4.61*).

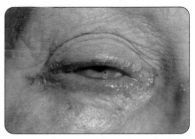

Fig. 4.61 Atopic dermatitis

2. **Treatment** – emollients to hydrate the skin and mild topical steroids.
3. **Associations**
   a. *Ocular* – vernal disease in children, chronic keratoconjunctivitis in adults, keratoconus, early-onset cataract, and RD.
   b. *Systemic* – asthma and hay fever.

Bacterial infections

External hordeolum (stye)

1. **Definition** – acute staphylococcal abscess of a lash follicle and its associated gland of Zeis.
2. **Signs** – tender swelling in the lid margin pointing through the skin often with a lash at its apex (*Fig. 4.62*).

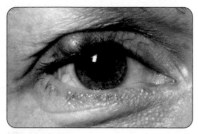

Fig. 4.62 Stye

3. Treatment – topical antibiotics and hot compresses; epilation of the associated lash may hasten resolution.

Impetigo

1. **Definition** – superficial skin infection caused by *S. aureus* or *S. pyogenes*.
2. **Signs** – erythematous macules which develop into thin-walled blisters which on rupturing produce golden-yellow crusts (*Fig. 4.63*).

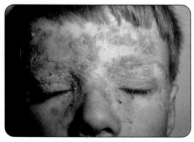

Fig. 4.63 Impetigo

3. Treatment – topical antibiotics and oral flucloxacillin or erythromycin.

Erysipelas (St Anthony fire)

1. **Definition** – acute cellulitis caused by *S. pyogenes* at a site of minor skin trauma.
2. **Signs** – expanding, well-defined, indurated, erythematous, subcutaneous plaque (*Fig. 4.64*).

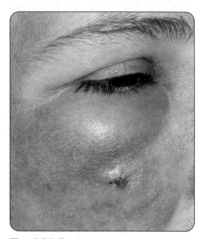

Fig. 4.64 Erysipelas

3. Treatment – oral phenoxymethyl-penicillin.

Necrotizing fasciitis

1. **Definition** – rapidly progressive necrosis involving subcutaneous soft tissues and later the skin; caused by *S. pyogenes* and occasionally *S. aureus*.
2. **Signs** – bullae and black discoloration of skin due to gangrene secondary to underlying thrombosis (*Fig. 4.65*).

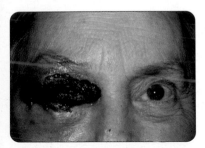

Fig. 4.65 Necrotizing fasciitis

3. **Complications** – ophthalmic artery occlusion and lagophthalmos.
4. **Treatment** – intravenous benzylpenicillin and debridement of necrotic tissue.

Viral infections

Molluscum contagiosum

1. **Pathogenesis** – poxvirus transmitted by contact with infected people and then by autoinoculation.
2. **Histology**
   - Central pit and lobules of hyperplastic epidermis with intracytoplasmic (Henderson–Patterson) inclusion bodies that displace the nuclear remnant to the edge of the cell.
   - Near the surface the bodies are small and eosinophilic and deeper down they are large and basophilic (*Fig. 4.66*).

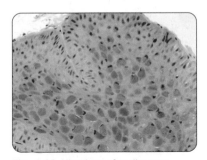

Fig. 4.66 Histology of molluscum contagiosum

3. **Signs** – single or multiple, pale, waxy, umbilicated nodules (*Fig. 4.67*).

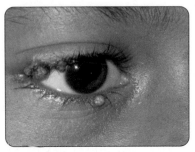

Fig. 4.67 Molluscum contagiosum

4. **Treatment** – excision, or destruction by cauterization, cryotherapy or laser.
5. **Complications** – ipsilateral, chronic, follicular conjunctivitis.
6. **Systemic association** – immunocompromised patients may develop multiple lesions.

Herpes zoster ophthalmicus

1. **Pathogenesis** – reactivation of latent varicella zoster virus (VZV) in the sensory ganglion of the trigeminal nerve causing a vesicular skin reaction.
2. **Presentation** – pain in the distribution of the first division of the trigeminal nerve.
3. **Signs** – maculopapular rash followed by vesicles, pustules to crusting (*Fig. 4.68*).

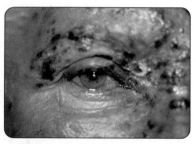

Fig. 4.68 Herpes zoster ophthalmicus

4. **Complications** – conjunctivitis, episcleritis, scleritis, keratitis, uveitis, optic neuritis, extraocular nerve palsies, hemianopia, and encephalitis.
5. **Treatment**
   a. *Systemic*
   - Oral aciclovir 800 mg five times daily for 3–7 days.
   - Alternatives – valaciclovir 1 g t.i.d. or famciclovir 250 mg t.i.d., or 750 mg once daily for 7 days.
   b. *Topical* – aciclovir or penciclovir cream, and a steroid–antibiotic combination.

Herpes simplex

1. **Pathogenesis** – reactivation of herpes simplex virus (HSV) previously dormant in the trigeminal ganglion.
2. **Signs** – crops of small vesicles (*Fig. 4.69*).

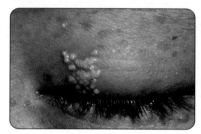

Fig. 4.69 Herpes simplex vesicles

3. **Complications** – transient follicular conjunctivitis and dendritic ulceration are uncommon.
4. **Treatment** – topical or oral aciclovir.

Blepharitis

Chronic anterior marginal blepharitis

1. **Pathogenesis**
   a. *Staphylococcal* – abnormal cell-mediated response to cell wall of *S. aureus*.
   b. *Seborrhoeic* – often associated with generalized seborrhoeic dermatitis.
2. **Signs**
   a. *Staphylococcal*
   - Hard scales, crusting around the bases of the lashes (collarettes), and madarosis (*Fig. 4.70*).
   - Notching (tylosis), trichiasis, and poliosis.

- Secondary tear film instability, papillary conjunctivitis, stye formation, marginal keratitis, and phlyctenulosis.

b. *Seborrhoeic*

- Soft scales located anywhere on the lid margin and lashes (*Fig. 4.71*).
- Greasy anterior lid margins with sticking together of lashes.

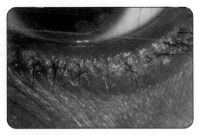

Fig. 4.70 Staphylococcal blepharitis

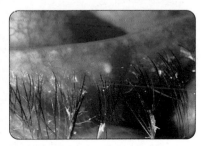

Fig. 4.71 Seborrhoeic blepharitis

3. Treatment

- Lid hygiene with diluted baby shampoo.
- Weak topical steroids for severe papillary conjunctivitis and marginal keratitis.
- Tear substitutes for tear film instability.

Chronic posterior blepharitis

1. Pathogenesis – meibomian gland dysfunction with alterations in secretions.

2. Signs

- Capping of meibomian gland orifices with oil globules.
- Pouting or plugging of the meibomian gland orifices (*Fig. 4.72*).
- Oily and foamy tear film with accumulation of froth on the lid margins or inner canthi.
- Secondary papillary conjunctivitis and inferior corneal punctate epithelial erosions.

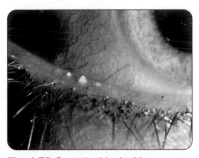

Fig. 4.72 Posterior blepharitis

3. Treatment

- Lid hygiene and topical treatment as for staphylococcal disease.
- Systemic tetracyclines for 6–12 weeks.

Phthiriasis palpebrarum

1. Pathogenesis – infestation of lashes by the crab louse *Phthirus pubis*.

2. Signs

- Lice anchored to the lashes.
- Oval, brownish, opalescent pearls adherent to the base of the cilia (*Fig. 4.73*).

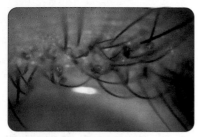

Fig. 4.73 Phthriasis palpebrarum

3. Treatment – mechanical removal of the lice and topical yellow mercuric oxide or petroleum jelly.

Angular blepharitis

1. **Pathogenesis** – usually infection with *Moraxella lacunata* or *S. aureus*.
2. **Signs** – often unilateral red, scaly, macerated skin at the lateral and medial canthus (*Fig. 4.74*).

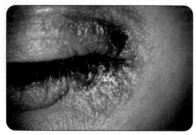

Fig. 4.74 Angular blepharitis

3. Treatment – topical chloramphenicol, bacitracin or erythromycin cream.

Childhood blepharokeratoconjunctivitis

1. **Signs**
   - Chronic blepharitis often associated with recurrent styes or meibomian cysts (*Fig. 4.75*).
   - Conjunctival hyperaemia, phlyctens, and follicular or papillary hyperplasia.
   - Superficial punctate keratopathy, marginal keratitis, peripheral vascularization, and axial subepithelial haze.

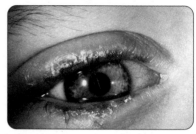

Fig. 4.75 Childhood blepharokerato-conjunctivitis

2. Treatment – lid hygiene and topical antibiotic ointment, weak topical steroids, and oral erythromycin syrup.

Ptosis

Classification

1. **Neurogenic** – innervational defect such as third nerve and oculosympathetic palsy (Horner syndrome).
2. **Myogenic**
   a. *Myopathic* – myopathy of the levator muscle itself.
   b. *Neuromyopathic* – impairment of transmission of impulses at the neuromuscular junction.
3. **Aponeurotic** – defect in the levator aponeurosis.
4. **Mechanical** – gravitational effect of a mass or scarring.

Simple congenital ptosis

1. **Pathogenesis** – failure of neuronal migration or development with muscular sequelae; minority of cases are hereditary.
2. **Signs**
   - Unilateral or bilateral ptosis of variable severity.
   - Absent upper lid crease and poor levator function (*Fig. 4.76*).
   - In down-gaze the ptotic lid is higher than the normal.

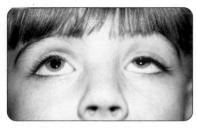

Fig. 4.76 Right congenital ptosis

3. **Associations** – superior rectus weakness, compensatory chin elevation in severe bilateral cases, and refractive errors.
4. **Treatment** – levator resection during preschool years.

Marcus Gunn jaw-winking syndrome

1. **Pathogenesis** – branch of the mandibular division of the 5th nerve is misdirected to the levator muscle.

2. **Signs** – unilateral retraction of the ptotic lid in conjunction with stimulation of the ipsilateral pterygoid muscles (chewing, sucking, opening the mouth (*Fig. 4.77*), or contralateral jaw movement).

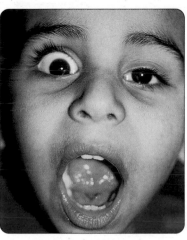

Fig. 4.77 Marcus Gunn jaw-winking syndrome

3. **Treatment** – surgery for a significant functional or cosmetic problem.

Third nerve misdirection syndromes

1. **Pathogenesis** – congenital or following acquired 3rd nerve palsy.
2. **Signs** – bizarre movements of the upper lid that accompany eye movements (*Fig. 4.78*).

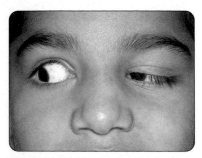

Fig. 4.78 Third nerve misdirection syndrome

3. Treatment – levator disinsertion and brow suspension.

Involutional ptosis

1. Pathogenesis – bilateral age-related dehiscence, disinsertion or stretching of the levator aponeurosis.
2. Signs
- High or absent upper lid crease and good levator function.
- Very thin lid above the tarsal plate and deep upper sulcus (*Fig. 4.79*).

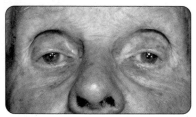

Fig. 4.79 Involutional ptosis

3. Treatment – levator resection, reinsertion or anterior levator repair.

Mechanical ptosis

Mechanical ptosis is the result of impaired mobility of the upper lid. It may be caused by dermatochalasis, large tumours such as neurofibromas (see *Fig. 4.29*), scarring, severe oedema, and anterior orbital lesions.

Measurements

1. Margin–reflex distance
- Distance between the upper lid margin and the corneal light reflex.
- Unilateral ptosis is quantified by comparison with the contralateral normal side which is 4–4.5 mm (*Fig. 4.80a*); mild ptosis = up to 2 mm (*Fig. 4.80b*); moderate ptosis = 3 mm (*Fig. 4.80c*); severe ptosis = 4 mm or more (*Fig. 4.80d*).

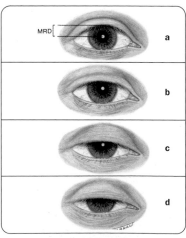

Fig. 4.80 Margin–reflex distance

2. Palpebral fissure height – distance between upper and lower lid margins (*Fig. 4.81*); normal in males is 7–10 mm and in females 8–12 mm.

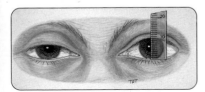

Fig. 4.81 Measurement of vertical fissure height

3. Levator function – normal = 15 mm or more; good = 12–14 mm; fair = 5–11 mm; poor = 4 mm or less (*Fig. 4.82*).

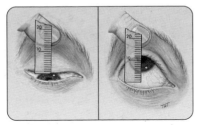

Fig. 4.82 Measurement of levator function

4. Upper lid crease – vertical distance between the lid margin and the lid crease in down-gaze.

5. Pretarsal show – distance between the lid margin and the skin fold with the eyes in the primary position.

Surgery

Conjunctival–Müller resection

1. Indications – mild ptosis with levator function of at least 10 mm, such as Horner syndrome and very mild congenital ptosis.

2. Technique – excision of Müller muscle and overlying conjunctiva, and reattachment of resected edges (*Fig. 4.83*); maximal lift is 2–3 mm.

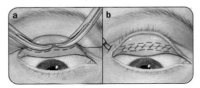

Fig. 4.83 Conjunctival–Müller resection

Levator resection

1. Indications – any ptosis provided levator function is at least 5 mm; amount of resection is determined by levator function and the severity of ptosis.

2. Technique – shortening of the levator complex through either an anterior (skin – *Fig. 4.84*) or posterior (conjunctival) approach.

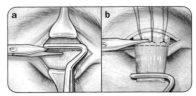

Fig. 4.84 Levator resection

Brow suspension

1. Indications – severe ptosis with very poor levator function.

2. Technique – suspension of the tarsus from the frontalis muscle with a sling (*Fig. 4.85*).

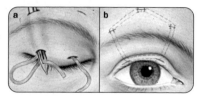

Fig. 4.85 Brow suspension

Ectropion

Involutional ectropion

1. **Pathogenesis** – age-related horizontal lid and canthal tendon laxity (*Fig. 4.86*), and disinsertion of lower lid retractors.

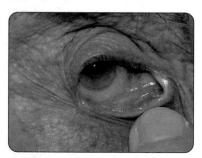

Fig. 4.86 Lid laxity in involutional ectropion

2. **Complications** – epiphora and conjunctival keratinization.
3. **Treatment**
   a. *Mild medial* – medial tarsoconjunctival diamond excision usually combined with a lateral canthal sling.

   b. *Severe generalized* – horizontal lid shortening (Kuhnt–Szymanowski procedure – *Fig. 4.87*) usually combined with a lateral canthal sling.

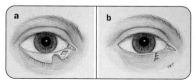

Fig. 4.87 Kuhnt–Szymanowski procedure

Cicatricial ectropion

1. **Pathogenesis** – scarring or contracture of the skin and underlying tissues (*Fig. 4.88*).

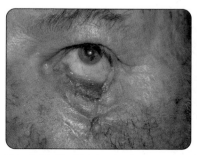

Fig. 4.88 Cicatricial ectropion

2. **Treatment**
   a. *Mild localized* – excision of the offending scar tissue combined with Z-plasty (*Fig. 4.89*).
   b. *Severe generalized* – transposition flaps or free skin grafts.

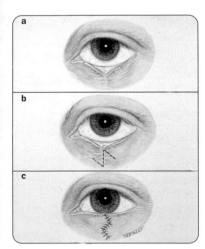

Fig. 4.89 Z-plasty for cicatricial ectropion

Paralytic ectropion

1. **Pathogenesis** – ipsilateral facial nerve palsy (*Fig. 4.90*).

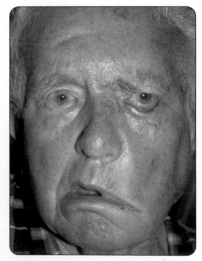

Fig. 4.90 Left paralytic ectropion

2. **Complications** – exposure keratopathy and epiphora.
3. **Treatment**
   a. *Temporary* – lubrication, botulinum toxin injection to induce ptosis, and temporary lateral tarsorrhaphy in patients with poor Bell phenomenon.
   b. *Permanent* – medial canthoplasty and lateral canthal sling.

Mechanical ectropion

1. **Pathogenesis** – tumours on or near the lid margin which mechanically evert the lid (*Fig. 4.91*).

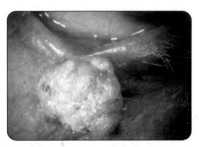

Fig. 4.91 Mechanical ectropion

2. **Treatment** – removal of the cause, if possible, and correction of significant horizontal lid laxity.

Entropion

Involutional entropion

1. **Pathogenesis** – age-related degeneration of elastic and fibrous tissues resulting in horizontal lid laxity, vertical lid instability and overriding of the pretarsal by the preseptal orbicularis during lid closure.

2. Complications – punctate corneal erosions, and ulceration if severe (*Fig. 4.92*).

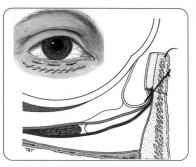

Fig. 4.94 Wies procedure

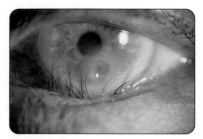

Fig. 4.92 Corneal ulceration due to involutional entropion

3. Treatment
   a. *Conservative* – lubricants, taping, soft bandage contact lenses or orbicularis chemodenervation with botulinum toxin injection.
   b. *Surgical* – lateral canthal sling, full-thickness wedge excision, transverse everting suture (*Fig. 4.93*), Wies procedure (*Fig. 4.94*), or Jones procedure (*Fig. 4.95*).

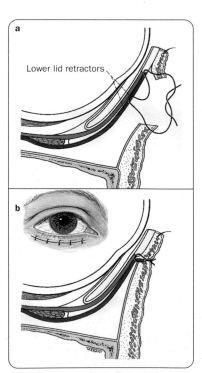

a

Lower lid retractors

b

Fig. 4.95 Jones procedure

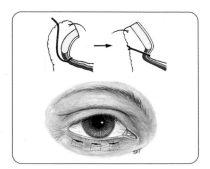

Fig. 4.93 Transverse everting suture

Cicatricial entropion

1. **Pathogenesis** – severe scarring of the palpebral conjunctiva (*Fig. 4.96*) caused by cicatrizing conjunctivitis, trachoma, and trauma.

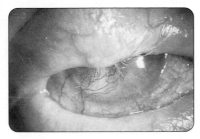

Fig. 4.96 Cicatricial upper lid entropion

2. **Treatment** – bandage contact lenses and transverse tarsotomy with lateral rotation of lid margin.

Miscellaneous disorders

Dermatochalasis

1. **Signs** – redundant loose upper lid skin with indistinct creases and pseudo-ptosis (*Fig. 4.97*).

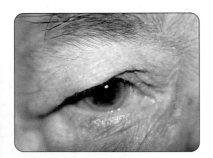

Fig. 4.97 Dermatochalasis

2. **Treatment** – blepharoplasty.

Blepharochalasis

1. **Presentation** – around puberty with recurrent episodes of bilateral, upper lid non-pitting oedema that resolves after a few days.
2. **Signs** – redundant, wrinkled and atrophic upper lid skin, and aponeurotic ptosis in severe cases (*Fig. 4.98*).

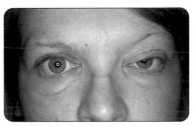

Fig. 4.98 Left aponeurotic ptosis and thin upper lid skin resulting from blepharochalasis

3. **Differential diagnosis** – drug-induced urticaria and angioedema.
4. **Treatment** – blepharoplasty and correction of ptosis.

Floppy eyelid syndrome

1. **Predispositions** – middle-aged, obese men who sleep face down with their lids everted by the pillow.
2. **Signs** – redundant upper lid skin, and loose and rubbery tarsal plates that evert easily (*Fig. 4.99*).

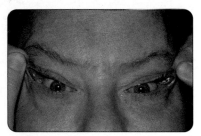

Fig. 4.99 Floppy eyelid syndrome

3. Complications
- Chronic papillary conjunctivitis, punctate keratopathy, and filamentary keratitis.
- Lash ptosis, lacrimal gland prolapse, ectropion, and aponeurotic ptosis.
4. Associations – keratoconus, skin hyperelasticity, joint hypermobility, obstructive sleep apnoea, diabetes, and mental retardation.
5. Treatment
  a. *Mild* – lubrication and nocturnal eye shields or taping of the lids.
  b. *Severe* – horizontal lid shortening.

Eyelid retraction

Lid retraction is suspected when the upper lid margin is either level with (*Fig. 4.100*) or above the superior limbus; causes are listed in *Table 4.4*.

Table 4.4 **Causes of lid retraction**
1. *Thyroid eye disease*
2. *Neurogenic*
· Contralateral unilateral ptosis
· Unopposed levator action due to facial palsy
· Third nerve misdirection
· Marcus Gunn jaw-winking syndrome
· Collier sign of the midbrain (Parinaud syndrome)
· Infantile hydrocephalus (setting sun sign)
· Parkinsonism
· Topical sympathomimetic drops
3. *Mechanical*
· Surgical over-correction of ptosis
· Scarring of upper lid skin
4. *Congenital*
· Isolated
· Duane retraction syndrome
· Down syndrome
· Transient 'eye popping' reflex in normal infants
5. *Miscellaneous*
· Prominent globe (pseudo-lid retraction)
· Uraemia (Summerskill sign)

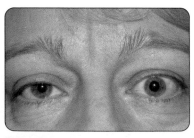

Fig. 4.100 Left lid retraction

Lacrimal Drainage System

Imaging

1. Dacryocystography (DCG)
- Radio-opaque dye is injected into both canaliculi and magnified images are taken.
- A normal dacryocystogram in the presence of epiphora indicates either functional obstruction or lacrimal pump failure.
- Failure of dye to reach the nose indicates an anatomical obstruction, the site of which is usually evident (Fig. 5.1).
- Digital subtraction provides a higher quality image (Fig. 5.2).

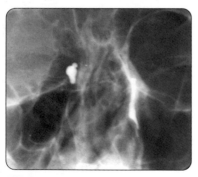

Fig. 5.1 Conventional DCG showing right nasolacrimal duct obstruction

2. Nuclear lacrimal scintigraphy
- Radioactive technetium-99 is delivered to the lateral conjunctival sac.
- Sequential images are taken (Fig. 5.3).
- More physiological than DCG.
- More sensitive than DCG in assessing incomplete blocks.

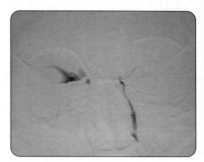

Fig. 5.2 Subtraction DCG showing a right sac obstruction

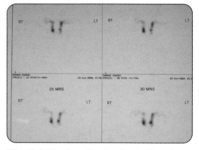

Fig. 5.3 Nuclear lacrimal scintigraphy showing tracer in both nasolacrimal ducts

Acquired obstruction

Primary punctal stenosis

Primary stenosis occurs in the absence of punctal eversion.
1. Causes – in order of frequency:
- Idiopathic primary stenosis.
- Chronic blepharitis.
- Herpes simplex and herpes zoster lid infection.

- Irradiation of malignant lid tumours.
- Cicatrizing conjunctivitis.
- Systemic cytotoxic drugs.
- Rare – porphyria cutanea tarda and acrodermatitis enteropathica.

2. Treatment – punctoplasty (*Fig. 5.4*).

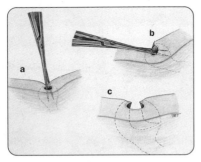

Fig. 5.4 Punctoplasty

Secondary punctal stenosis

1. Cause – punctal eversion (*Fig. 5.5*).

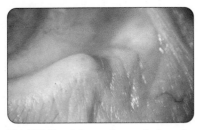

Fig. 5.5 Punctal eversion and stenosis

2. Treatment
   a. *Ziegler cautery* – for pure punctal eversion.
   b. *Medial conjunctivoplasty* (*Fig. 5.6*) – for medial ectropion not associated with lid laxity.
   c. *Lower lid tightening* – for lower lid laxity.

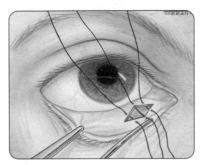

Fig. 5.6 Medial conjunctivoplasty

Canalicular obstruction

1. Causes – congenital, trauma, herpes simplex infection, drugs, irradiation, and chronic dacryocystitis.
2. Treatment – intubation, canaliculo-dacryocystorhinostomy, or Lester Jones tube.

Nasolacrimal duct obstruction

1. Causes – idiopathic, naso-orbital trauma, Wegener granulomatosis, and infiltration by nasopharyngeal tumours.
2. Treatment – usually dacryocysto-rhinostomy (DCR), occasionally balloon dilatation.

Dacryolithiasis

1. **Pathogenesis** – tear stagnation secondary to inflammatory obstruction and squamous metaplasia of the lacrimal sac epithelium.
2. **Presentation** – intermittent epiphora, recurrent attacks of acute dacryocystitis and lacrimal sac distension.
3. **Signs** – distended and relatively firm lacrimal sac.
4. **Treatment** – DCR.

Congenital obstruction

Nasolacrimal duct obstruction

1. **Pathogenesis** – delayed canalization of the lower end of the nasolacrimal duct at the valve of Hasner.
2. **Signs**
   - Epiphora and matting of lashes (*Fig. 5.7*).
   - Reflux of purulent material from the puncta on pressure over the sac.

3. **Differential diagnosis** – punctal atresia and fistula, and congenital glaucoma.
4. **Treatment**
   a. *Massage* (*Fig. 5.8*) – to rupture the membranous obstruction.
   b. *Probing* (*Fig. 5.9*) – at 12–18 months because spontaneous canalization occurs in about 95% of cases.

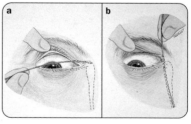

Fig. 5.8 Massage over lacrimal sac

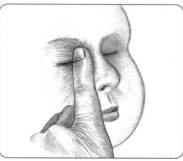

Fig. 5.9 Probing of nasolacrimal sac

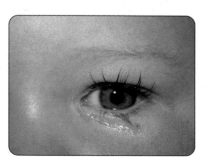

Fig. 5.7 Epiphora and matting of lashes

Congenital dacryocele (amniontocele)

1. **Definition** – collection of amniotic fluid or mucus in the lacrimal sac caused by an imperforate Hasner valve.
2. **Signs** – bluish cystic swelling at or below the medial canthal area, accompanied by epiphora (*Fig. 5.10*).

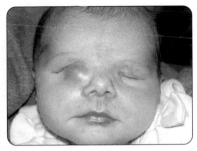

Fig. 5.10 Congenital dacryocele

3. **Treatment** – probing.
4. **Differential diagnosis** – encephalocele.

Lacrimal surgery

Conventional DCR

1. **Indications** – obstruction beyond the medial opening of the common canaliculus.
2. **Technique** – anastomosis between the lacrimal sac and the nasal mucosa of the middle nasal meatus (*Fig. 5.11*).

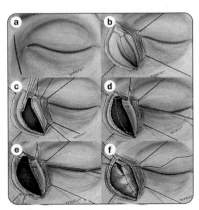

Fig. 5.11 Technique of DCR

3. **Results** – over 90% success.
4. **Causes of failure** – inadequate size and position of the ostium, scarring and the 'sump syndrome'.
5. **Complications** – injury to medial canthal structures, cellulitis, and CSF rhinorrhoea.

Lester Jones tube insertion

1. **Indications** – absence of canalicular function, lacrimal pump failure, and failed DCR.
2. **Technique** – DCR is performed as far as suturing the posterior flaps and then the tube is inserted between the inner canthus and the lacrimal sac (*Fig. 5.12*).

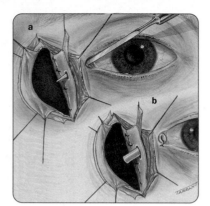

Fig. 5.12 Lester Jones intubation

Endoscopic DCR

1. **Indications** – obstruction beyond the medial opening of the common canaliculus, particularly following failed conventional DCR.
2. **Technique**
   - Light pipe is passed into the lacrimal sac and viewed from within the nasal cavity with an endoscope.
   - Remainder of the procedure is performed from within the nasal cavity.
3. **Results** – 80–85% success.

Endolaser DCR

1. **Indications** – mainly elderly patients because it is a quick procedure that can be performed under local anaesthesia.
2. **Results** – 70% success.

Infections

Chronic canaliculitis

1. **Pathogenesis** – infection with *Actinomyces israelii* usually without any identifiable predisposition.
2. **Presentation** – unilateral epiphora and chronic mucopurulent conjunctivitis, refractory to conventional treatment.
3. **Signs**
   - 'Pouting' punctum associated with pericanalicular oedema (*Fig. 5.13*).
   - Mucopurulent discharge on pressure over the canaliculus.
   - Concretions can be expressed (*Fig. 5.14*) or become evident following canaliculotomy.

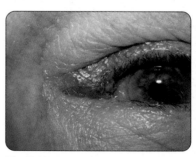

Fig. 5.13 Pericanalicular oedema in chronic canaliculitis

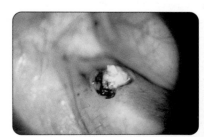

Fig. 5.14 Expressed concretions

4. **Treatment** – canaliculotomy.
5. **Differential diagnosis** – giant fornix syndrome, lacrimal diverticulum, and dacryolithiasis.

Acute dacryocystitis

1. **Pathogenesis** – obstruction of the nasolacrimal duct.
2. **Presentation** – epiphora and pain over the medial canthus.
3. **Signs** – tender, red, tense swelling at the medial canthus that may be associated with mild preseptal cellulitis (*Fig. 5.15*).

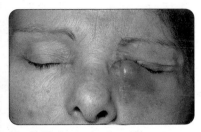

Fig. 5.15 Acute dacryocystitis

4. **Treatment** – oral antibiotics followed by DCR.

Chronic dacryocystitis

1. **Pathogenesis** – obstruction of the nasolacrimal sac.
2. **Presentation** – epiphora associated with a chronic or recurrent unilateral conjunctivitis.
3. **Signs** – subtle painless swelling at the inner canthus (*Fig. 5.16*) with reflux of mucopurulent material on pressure over the sac.
3. **Treatment** – DCR.

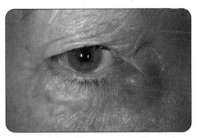

Fig. 5.16 Chronic dacryocystitis

Thyroid eye disease

Pathogenesis

Thyroid ophthalmopathy involves an organ-specific autoimmune reaction in which a humoral agent (IgG antibody) produces the following changes (*Fig. 6.1*):

1. **Inflammatory cellular infiltration** of interstitial tissues, orbital fat and lacrimal glands with accumulation of glycosaminoglycans and retention of fluid.
2. **Inflammation of extraocular muscles** – initially leading to hypertrophy (see *Fig. 6.9*) and later fibrosis and tethering effects.
3. **Secondary changes** – increase in the volume of orbital contents and elevation of intraorbital pressure, which may itself cause further fluid retention within the orbit.

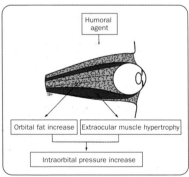

Fig. 6.1 Pathogenesis of thyroid ophthalmopathy

Soft tissue involvement

1. **Symptoms** – grittiness, photophobia, and retrobulbar discomfort.
2. **Signs** – epibulbar hyperaemia, periorbital swelling, chemosis (*Fig. 6.2*), superior limbic keratoconjunctivitis, and KCS.

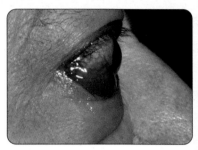

Fig. 6.2 Periorbital oedema and chemosis

3. **Treatment** – lubricants, head elevation during sleep, and eyelid taping.

Lid retraction

1. **Signs** – unilateral or bilateral, symmetrical or asymmetrical.
   a. *Dalrymple* – lid retraction in primary gaze (*Fig. 6.3*).
   b. *Kocher* – frightened appearance on attentive fixation (*Fig. 6.4*).
   c. *Von Graefe* – retarded descent of the upper lid on down-gaze (lid lag – *Fig. 6.5*).

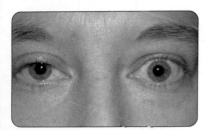

Fig. 6.3 Dalrymple sign

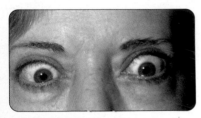

Fig. 6.4 Kocher sign

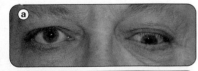
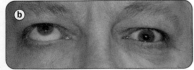

Fig. 6.5 (a) Left von Graefe sign;
(b) defective left elevation

2. Treatment

  a. *Mullerotomy* – for mild cases.
  b. *Recession of the levator aponeuro-sis* – for severe cases.
  c. *Recession of lower lid retractors* – when retraction of the lower lid is 2 mm or more.
  d. *Botulinum toxin injection* – temporary measure.

Proptosis

1. Signs – axial, unilateral or bilateral, symmetrical or asymmetrical (*Fig. 6.6*).

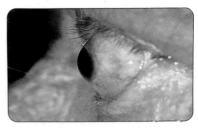

Fig. 6.6 Proptosis

2. Management

  a. *Oral steroids* – for rapidly progressive painful proptosis.
  b. *Radiotherapy* – combination with steroids or when steroids are contraindicated or ineffective.
  c. *Combined therapy* – irradiation, azathioprine and low-dose steroids may be more effective than steroids or radiotherapy alone.
  d. *Surgical decompression* (*Fig. 6.7*) – as primary treatment or when non-invasive methods fail.

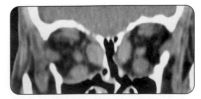

Fig. 6.7 Coronal CT following bilateral orbital decompression

Restrictive myopathy

1. **Signs** – in order of frequency the four ocular motility defects are: deficiency of elevation (see *Fig. 6.5b*), abduction (*Fig. 6.8*), depression and adduction.

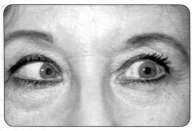

Fig. 6.8 Defective left abduction

2. **Treatment**
   a. *Surgery* – for diplopia in the primary or reading positions, provided the angle has been stable for at least 6 months.
   b. *Botulinum toxin injection* – into the involved muscle.

Optic neuropathy

1. **Pathogenesis** – compression of the optic nerve or its blood supply at the orbital apex by the congested and enlarged recti (*Fig. 6.9*).

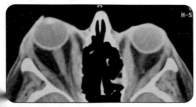

Fig. 6.9 Axial CT scan shows right proptosis and bilateral enlargement of extraocular muscles

2. **Signs** – optic nerve dysfunction with a normal, swollen or atrophic optic disc.
3. **Treatment**
   a. *Intravenous methylprednisolone.*
   b. *Orbital decompression* – if medical therapy fails or is inappropriate.

Infections

Preseptal cellulitis

1. **Definition** – infection of the subcutaneous tissues anterior to the orbital septum caused by *S. aureus* or *S. pyogenes*.
2. **Causes**
   - Skin laceration or insect bites.
   - Spread of local infection from an acute hordeolum or dacryocystitis.
   - Haematogenous spread from the upper respiratory tract or middle ear.
3. **Signs** – tender and red periorbital oedema (*Fig. 6.10*).

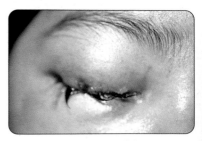

Fig. 6.10 Preseptal cellulitis

4. **CT** – opacification anterior to the orbital septum (*Fig. 6.11*).

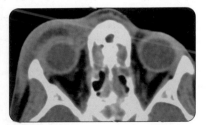

Fig. 6.11 Axial CT in right preseptal cellulitis

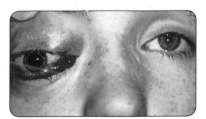

Fig. 6.12 Orbital cellulitis

5. Treatment – oral co-amoxiclav, or intramuscular benzylpenicillin and oral flucloxacillin if severe.

Bacterial orbital cellulitis

1. **Definition** – infection of soft tissues behind the orbital septum usually caused by *S. pneumoniae*, *S. aureus*, *S. pyogenes* and *H. influenzae*.
2. **Causes**
   - Sinus-related – usually ethmoidal.
   - Extension of preseptal cellulitis through the orbital septum.
   - Local spread from adjacent structures.
   - Haematogenous spread.
   - Post-traumatic.
   - Post-surgical.
3. **Presentation** – rapid onset of severe malaise, fever, pain, and visual impairment.
4. **Signs**
   - Tender, warm and red periorbital swelling.
   - Proptosis, usually lateral and downwards (*Fig. 6.12*).
   - Painful ophthalmoplegia.
   - Optic nerve dysfunction.
5. **CT** – opacification anterior to the orbital septum and orbit (*Fig. 6.13*).

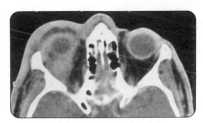

Fig. 6.13 Axial CT in right orbital cellulitis

6. **Ocular complications** – exposure keratopathy, raised intraocular pressure, retinal vascular occlusion, endophthalmitis, and optic neuropathy.
7. **Systemic complications** – meningitis, brain abscess, cavernous sinus thrombosis, subperiosteal orbital abscess.
8. **Treatment**
   a. *Medical* – intramuscular ceftazidime and oral metronidazole.
   b. *Surgery* – in unresponsive or vision-threatening cases.

Fungal orbital cellulitis

1. **Definition** – infection caused by *Mucor* or *Aspergillus*, which typically

affects patients with diabetic ketoacidosis or immunosuppression.

2. **Presentation** – gradual onset of facial and periorbital swelling, diplopia and visual loss.
3. **Signs** – black eschar on the palate, turbinates, nasal septum, skin and eyelids (*Fig. 6.14*).

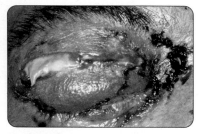

Fig. 6.14 Fungal orbital cellulitis

4. **Complications** – retinal vascular occlusion, cranial nerve palsies, and cerebrovascular occlusion.
5. **Treatment**
   a. *Medical* – intravenous amphotericin and excision of devitalized tissues.
   b. *Surgery* – exenteration in unresponsive cases.

Inflammatory disease

Idiopathic orbital inflammatory disease

1. **Definition** – non-neoplastic, non-infectious, space-occupying lesions that may involve any or all of the orbital soft tissues.
2. **Presentation** – 3rd–6th decade with usually unilateral acute periorbital redness, swelling, and pain.
3. **Signs** – congestive proptosis (*Fig. 6.15*).

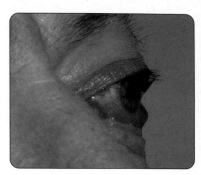

Fig. 6.15 Idiopathic orbital inflammatory disease

4. **CT** – ill-defined orbital opacification and loss of definition of contents (*Fig. 6.16*).

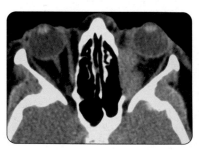

Fig. 6.16 Axial CT in left idiopathic orbital inflammatory disease

5. **Course**
   • Spontaneous remission after a few weeks.
   • Prolonged intermittent activity with eventual remission.
   • Severe prolonged activity resulting in fibrosis of orbital tissues (frozen orbit).
6. **Treatment**
   a. *NSAIDs* – initial therapy.
   b. *Oral steroids* – later tapered and discontinued.

c. *Radiotherapy* – if no improvement after 2 weeks of steroids.

d. *Antimetabolites* – if resistant to sterolds and radiotherapy.

e. *Systemic infliximab* – in cases that have failed to respond to conventional therapy.

Acute dacryoadenitis

1. **Presentation** – acute discomfort in the region of the lacrimal gland.
2. **Signs**
   - Tender swelling of the lateral aspect of the eyelid giving rise to a characteristic S-shaped ptosis and mild downward and inward globe displacement (*Fig. 6.17*).
   - Injection of the palpebral portion of the lacrimal gland and adjacent conjunctiva (*Fig. 6.18*).
   - Lacrimal secretion may be reduced.

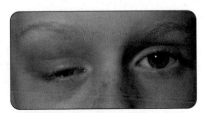

Fig. 6.17 Acute dacryoadenitis

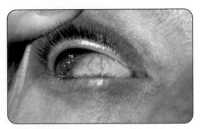

Fig. 6.18 Acute dacryoadenitis with injection of the lacrimal gland

3. **Treatment** – usually not required because spontaneous resolution is the rule.

Orbital myositis

1. **Definition** – idiopathic, non-specific inflammation of one or more extraocular muscles is considered a subtype of IOID.
2. **Presentation** – early adult life with diplopia and acute pain exacerbated by eye movement.
3. **Signs**
   - Lid oedema, ptosis and chemosis.
   - Diplopia and worsening of pain on attempted gaze into the field of action of the involved muscle(s).
   - Restrictive myopathy in chronic disease.
4. **CT** – enlargement of the affected muscles (*Fig. 6.19*), with or without involvement of the tendons of insertion.

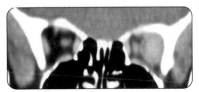

Fig. 6.19 Coronal CT shows enlargement of the left lateral rectus muscle

5. **Course** – acute non-recurrent involvement lasting a few weeks, recurrent attacks, or chronic disease.
6. **Treatment**
   a. *NSAIDs* – in mild disease.
   b. *Systemic steroids* – produce dramatic improvement.
   c. *Radiotherapy* – to limit recurrence.

Tolosa–Hunt syndrome

1. **Pathogenesis** – non-specific granulomatous inflammation of the cavernous sinus, superior orbital fissure and/or orbital apex.
2. **Presentation** – diplopia with ipsilateral periorbital or hemicranial pain.
3. **Signs**
   - Ocular motor nerve palsies often with involvement of the pupil.
   - Sensory loss along the distribution of the first and second divisions of the trigeminal nerve.
4. **Treatment** – systemic steroids.

Wegener granulomatosis

1. **Pathogenesis** – usually bilateral orbital involvement by contiguous spread from the paranasal sinuses or nasopharynx.
2. **Signs**
   - Congestive proptosis and ophthalmoplegia.
   - Dacryoadenitis and nasolacrimal duct obstruction.
3. **Treatment** – cyclophosphamide and steroids.

Vascular malformations

Varices

1. **Definition** – weakened segments of the orbital venous system which enlarge with increased venous pressure, such as the Valsalva manoeuvre (*Fig. 6.20*).

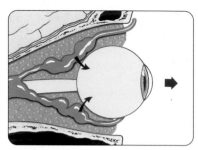

Fig. 6.20 Orbital varices causing intermittent proptosis

2. **Presentation** – from early childhood to late middle age.
3. **Signs**
   - Intermittent non-pulsatile proptosis not associated with a bruit.
   - Visible lesions in the eyelid (*Fig. 6.21*) or conjunctiva (*Fig. 6.22*), or both.

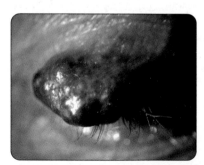

Fig. 6.21 Eyelid varices

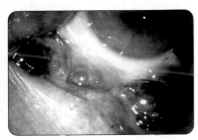

Fig. 6.22 Conjunctival varices

4. Complications
- Acute haemorrhage (*Fig. 6.23*) and thrombosis.
- Atrophy of surrounding fat (*Fig. 6.24*) and enophthalmos.

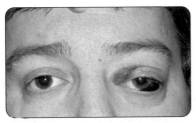

Fig. 6.23 Haemorrhage from varices

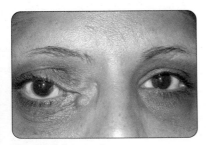

Fig. 6.24 Fat atrophy

Lymphangioma

1. **Definition** – abortive, non-functional, vascular malformations.
2. **Presentation** – early childhood.
3. **Signs**
   - Soft bluish masses in the upper nasal quadrant with a cystic conjunctival component.
   - Slowly progressive proptosis.
   - Sudden painful proptosis secondary to spontaneous haemorrhage (*Fig. 6.25*).
   - Encysted blood forms 'chocolate cysts' which may regress spontaneously.
   - Involvement of the oropharynx.

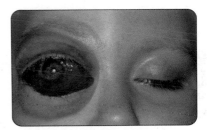

Fig. 6.25 Acute proptosis due to haemorrhage from lymphangioma

4. **Treatment** – sight-threatening 'chocolate cysts' should be drained or removed sub-totally by controlled vaporization using a carbon dioxide laser.

Direct carotid–cavernous fistula

1. **Definition** – high-flow shunt in which carotid artery blood passes directly into the cavernous sinus through a defect in the wall of the intracavernous portion of the internal carotid artery.

2. **Causes** – spontaneous or basal skull fracture.
3. **Presentation** – triad of pulsatile proptosis, conjunctival chemosis, and a whooshing noise in the head.
4. **Signs**
   - Ptosis, severe epibulbar injection and haemorrhagic chemosis (*Fig. 6.26*).
   - Pulsatile proptosis associated with a bruit, abolished by carotid compression (*Fig. 6.27*).
   - Ophthalmoplegia, most frequently 6th nerve palsy.
   - Optic disc swelling, venous dilatation, and intraretinal haemorrhages.

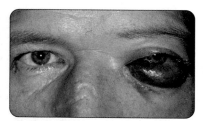

Fig. 6.26 Direct carotid–cavernous fistula

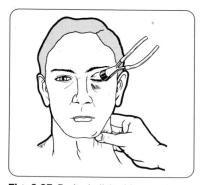

Fig. 6.27 Bruit abolished by carotid compression

5. **Complications** – exposure keratopathy, elevation of intraocular pressure, central retinal vein occlusion, and anterior segment ischaemia.
6. **Treatment** – interventional radiology in which a detachable balloon is used to occlude the fistula.

Indirect carotid–cavernous fistula (dural shunt)

1. **Definition** – slow-flow shunt in which arterial blood flows through the meningeal branches of the external or internal carotid arteries indirectly into the cavernous sinus.
2. **Causes** – congenital malformations, and spontaneous rupture which may be precipitated by minor trauma.
3. **Presentation** – gradual onset of redness of one or both eyes.
4. **Signs**
   - Dilated epibulbar vessels (*Fig. 6.28*).
   - Exaggerated ocular pulsation on applanation tonometry.
   - Elevation of intraocular pressure.
   - Mild proptosis occasionally associated with a soft bruit.
   - Ophthalmoplegia caused by 6th nerve palsy or swelling of extraocular muscles.
   - Fundus – normal or moderate venous dilatation.

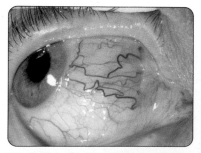

Fig. 6.28 Indirect carotid–cavernous fistula

5. Treatment – interventional radiology to occlude the feeding arteries, although some patients recover spontaneously.

Cystic lesions

Dacryops

1. **Definition** – ductal cyst of the lacrimal gland.
2. **Signs** – round, cystic lesion originating from the palpebral portion of the lacrimal gland which protrudes into the superior fornix (*Fig. 6.29*).

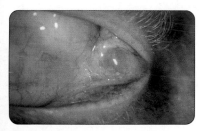

Fig. 6.29 Dacryops

3. **Treatment** – aspiration.

Superficial dermoid cyst

1. **Presentation** – in infancy.
2. **Signs** – firm, smooth, freely mobile subcutaneous mass most commonly located supero-temporally (*Fig. 6.30*) and occasionally supero-nasally.
3. **CT** – heterogeneous well-circumscribed lesion.
4. **Treatment** – excision.

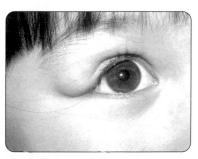

Fig. 6.30 Superficial dermoid cyst

Deep dermoid cyst

1. **Presentation** – in adolescence or adult life.
2. **Signs** – proptosis, globe displacement or a mass with indistinct posterior margins.
3. **CT** – well-circumscribed cystic lesion (*Fig. 6.31*).

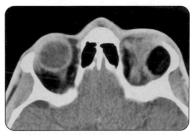

Fig. 6.31 Axial CT of a left deep dermoid

4. **Treatment** – excision.

Sinus mucocele

1. **Pathogenesis** – obstruction to drainage of normal frontal or ethmoidal sinus secretions caused by infection, allergy, trauma, tumour or congenital narrowing.
2. **Presentation** – adult life with proptosis, displacement (*Fig. 6.32*), diplopia or epiphora.

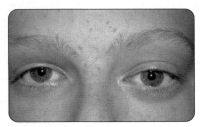

Fig. 6.32 Slight proptosis and inferior displacement due to left frontal mucocele

3. **CT** – soft tissue mass with thinning of the bony walls of the sinus (*Fig. 6.33*).

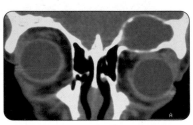

Fig. 6.33 Coronal CT of left frontal mucocele

4. **Treatment** – complete removal of the mucocele.

Encephalocele

1. **Pathogenesis** – herniation of intracranial contents into the orbit through a congenital basal skull defect (*Fig. 6.34*).

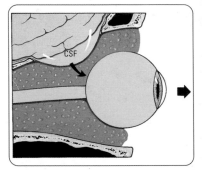

Fig. 6.34 Encephalocele giving rise to pulsatile proptosis

2. **Presentation** – infancy.
3. **Signs**
   - Anterior encephaloceles – forward and lateral displacement (*Fig. 6.35*).
   - Posterior encephaloceles – forward and downward displacement.
   - Cyst increases in size on straining or crying and may be reduced by manual pressure.
   - Pulsating proptosis without a thrill or bruit.

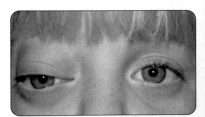

Fig. 6.35 Anterior encephalocele

4. CT – bony defect responsible for the herniation (*Fig. 6.36*).

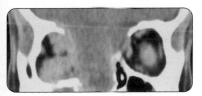

Fig. 6.36 Coronal CT shows a right bony defect and orbital opacification

5. Associations
   a. *Other bony abnormalities* – hypertelorism, broad nasal bridge, and cleft palate.
   b. *Ocular* – microphthalmos, colobomas, and morning glory anomaly.
   c. *NF 1* – with posterior encephalo-cele.

Tumours

Capillary haemangioma

1. Histology – varying-sized small vascular channels without true encapsulation.
2. Presentation – first few weeks of life.
3. Signs
   • Preseptal tumours appear dark blue through the overlying skin and are most frequently located superiorly (*Fig. 6.37*).
   • Deep orbital tumours give rise to unilateral proptosis without skin discoloration.
   • Involvement of the palpebral or forniceal conjunctiva (*Fig. 6.38*).
   • Coexisting lesions on the eyelids or elsewhere are common.

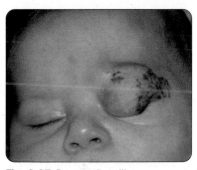

Fig. 6.37 Preseptal capillary haemangioma

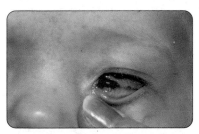

Fig. 6.38 Involvement of forniceal conjunctiva

4. Course – rapid growth followed by a slower phase of natural resolution in which 30% of lesions resolve by the age of 3 years and 70% by the age of 7 years.
5. Treatment
   a. *Indications* – amblyopia, optic nerve compression, exposure keratopathy, cosmesis, necrosis, and infection.
   b. *Steroid injection* – for early cutaneous or preseptal lesions.
   c. *Systemic steroids* – particularly if there is a large orbital component.
   d. *Subcutaneous injection of interferon alpha-2b* – for steroid-

resistance, organ interfering and/or life-threatening giant haemangiomas.

6. **Systemic associations** – of large lesions, particularly if associated with visceral involvement, are: high-output heart failure, Kasabach–Merritt syndrome, and Maffuci syndrome.

Cavernous haemangioma

1. **Histology** – endothelial-lined vascular channels of varying size separated by fibrous septae.
2. **Presentation** – 4th–5th decade with slowly progressive proptosis.
3. **Signs**
   - Axial proptosis (*Fig. 6.39*) which may be associated with optic disc oedema and choroidal folds.
   - Apical tumour may compress the optic nerve without causing significant proptosis.

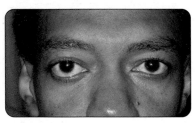

Fig. 6.39 Axial proptosis due to cavernous haemangioma

4. **CT** – well-circumscribed oval lesion just behind the globe (*Fig. 6.40*).
5. **Treatment** – excision is required in most cases.

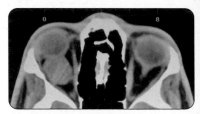

Fig. 6.40 Axial CT of a right cavernous haemangioma

Pleomorphic lacrimal gland adenoma (benign mixed cell tumour)

1. **Histology** – inner layer of cells forms glandular tissue that may be associated with squamous differentiation and keratin production; outer cells undergo metaplastic change leading to formation of myxoid tissue.
2. **Presentation** – 2nd–5th decade with a painless, slowly progressive proptosis or swelling in the supero-lateral part of the orbit.

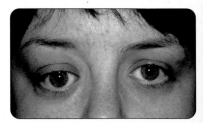

Fig. 6.41 Pleomorphic lacrimal gland adenoma

3. Signs
- Smooth, firm, non-tender mass in the lacrimal gland fossa with inferonasal displacement (*Fig. 6.41*).
- Tumour arising from the palpebral lobe may be visible on inspection.

4. CT – oval mass that may indent the lacrimal gland fossa and the globe (*Fig. 6.42*).

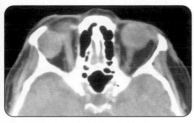

Fig. 6.42 Axial CT of a right pleomorphic lacrimal gland adenoma

5. Prognosis – excellent provided excision is complete and without disruption of the capsule.

Lacrimal gland carcinoma

1. Histology – adenoid cystic carcinoma (malignant mixed-cell tumour) is characterized by nests of basaloid cells with numerous mitoses.

2. Presentation – 4th–5th decade as follows:
- After incomplete excision of a pleomorphic adenoma, followed by recurrences and eventual malignant transformation.
- Long-standing proptosis which suddenly starts to increase.
- Without a previous history of pleomorphic adenoma as a rapidly growing lacrimal gland mass.

3. Signs
- Mass in the lacrimal area causing infero-nasal displacement.

- Epibulbar congestion, proptosis, periorbital oedema, and ophthalmoplegia due to posterior extension (*Fig. 6.43*).
- Hypoaesthesia in the region supplied by the lacrimal nerve.

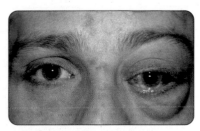

Fig. 6.43 Posterior extension of lacrimal gland carcinoma

4. CT – globular lesion with irregular edges that may show flecks of calcification and contiguous erosion or invasion of bone (*Fig. 6.44*).

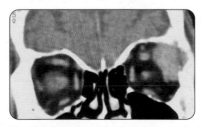

Fig. 6.44 Coronal CT of a left lacrimal gland carcinoma shows contiguous bony erosion

5. Treatment – biopsy followed by excision of the lesion and adjacent tissues, or orbital exenteration.

Optic nerve glioma

1. Histology – spindle-shaped pilocytic astrocytes and glial filaments.

2. Presentation – 1st decade with slowly progressive visual loss followed by proptosis.

3. Signs
- Proptosis often with inferior displacement.
- Optic nerve head is initially swollen and subsequently atrophic.
- Opticociliary collaterals and central retinal vein occlusion.

4. CT – fusiform enlargement of the optic nerve (*Fig. 6.45*).

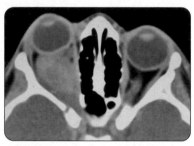

Fig. 6.45 Axial CT of a right optic nerve glioma

5. MR – may show intracranial extension (*Fig. 6.46*).

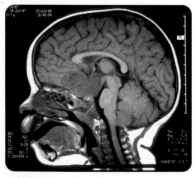

Fig. 6.46 Sagittal T1-weighted MR shows invasion of the hypothalamus

6. Treatment
- **a.** *Observation* – if no growth, good vision, and no cosmetic deformity.
- **b.** *Excision* – large or growing tumours confined to the orbit.
- **c.** *Radiotherapy* – may be combined with chemotherapy for tumours with intracranial extension.

7. Prognosis – indolent course with little growth in some cases; others may extend intracranially and threaten life.

8. Systemic association – NF 1 in 30%.

Optic nerve sheath meningioma

1. Histology
- **a.** *Meningothelial* – varying-sized irregular lobules of meningothelial cells separated by fibrovascular strands.
- **b.** *Psammomatous* – psammoma bodies among proliferating meningothelial cells.

2. Presentation – usually in middle-age, occasionally earlier, with gradual unilateral visual impairment.

3. Signs in chronological order:
- Optic nerve dysfunction and chronic disc swelling followed by atrophy.
- Opticociliary collaterals in 30% (*Fig. 6.47*).
- Restrictive motility defects, particularly in up-gaze.
- Proptosis usually develops after the onset of visual loss.

4. CT – thickening and calcification of the optic nerve (*Fig. 6.48*).

5. MR – T1-signal is hypointense, T2-signal is hyperintense (*Fig. 6.49*).

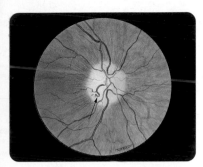

Fig. 6.47 Opticociliary collaterals

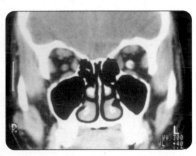

Fig. 6.48 Coronal CT shows thickening and calcification of the left optic nerve

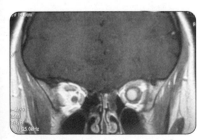

Fig. 6.49 T2-weighted coronal MR shows a left hyperintense signal

6. Treatment
   a. *Observation* – slow-growing tumours in middle-aged patients.
   b. *Excision* – in young patients with aggressive tumours.
7. Prognosis – good in adults and guarded in children.

Secondary meningioma

Secondary orbital meningiomas arise intracranially, usually from the sphenoidal ridge, tuberculum sellae or olfactory groove and subsequently invade the optic canal and orbit (see Chapter 21).

Plexiform neurofibroma

1. Presentation – early childhood with periorbital swelling.
2. Signs
   • Diffuse involvement with disfiguring hypertrophy of periocular tissues (*Fig. 6.50*).
   • On palpation the involved tissues feel like a bag of worms.

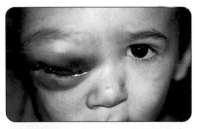

Fig. 6.50 Periorbital neurofibroma

3. Treatment – often unsatisfactory and complete surgical removal is extremely difficult.
4. Systemic association – NF 1 in 100%.

Isolated neurofibroma

1. **Presentation** – 3rd–4th decade with insidious mildly painful proptosis unassociated with visual impairment or ocular motility dysfunction.
2. **Treatment** – excision.
3. **Association** – NF 1 in 10%.

Lymphoma

1. **Classification** – based on the overall histological appearance (diffuse or nodular) and the cell type (B, T and NK cells); most orbital lesions are extranodal marginal B cell lymphomas and many are derived from lacrimal gland-associated MALT (Mucosa-Associated Lymphoid Tissue).
2. **Presentation** – insidious and usually in old age.
3. **Signs**
   - Any part of the orbit may be affected and occasionally involvement is bilateral (*Fig. 6.51*).
   - Anterior lesions have a rubbery consistency.
   - Occasionally disease may be confined to the conjunctiva or lacrimal glands.

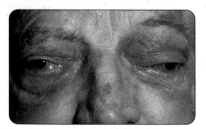

Fig. 6.51 Bilateral orbital lymphoma

4. **Treatment** – radiotherapy for localized lesions and chemotherapy for disseminated disease.

Embryonal sarcoma

1. **Histology**
   a. *Undifferentiated tumour* – mass of loosely arranged mesenchymal cells.
   b. *Differentiated tumour* – elongated and strap-like cells with a 'tadpole' or 'tennis-racket' configuration with (*Fig. 6.52*) or without cross-striations.

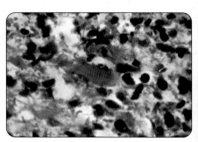

Fig. 6.52 Differentiated embryonal sarcoma with striations

2. **Presentation** – 1st decade with rapidly progressive proptosis.
3. **Signs**
   - Most frequent sites are supero-nasal (*Fig. 6.53*) and retrobulbar, followed by superior and inferior.
   - Swelling and hyperaemia of overlying skin without warmth.
4. **CT** – poorly defined mass of homogeneous density often with adjacent bony destruction (*Fig. 6.54*).

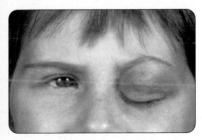

Fig. 6.53 Embryonal sarcoma

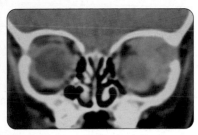

Fig. 6.54 Coronal CT of a left embryonal sarcoma

5. Treatment – radiotherapy and chemotherapy.
6. Prognosis – 95% cure for localized disease.

Adult metastatic tumours

1. Primary sites – in order of frequency are breast, bronchus, prostate, skin melanoma, gastrointestinal tract, and kidney.
2. Presentation
   - Proptosis and displacement.
   - Infiltration of orbital tissues causing ptosis, diplopia, brawny indurated periorbital skin and a firm orbit.

- Enophthalmos with scirrhous tumours (*Fig. 6.55*).
- Chronic orbital inflammation.
- Primarily with involvement of the cranial nerves at the orbital apex and only mild proptosis.

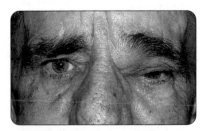

Fig. 6.55 Enophthalmos due to scirrhous metastatic carcinoma

3. CT – non-encapsulated mass (*Fig. 6.56*).

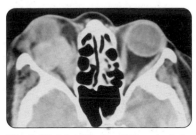

Fig. 6.56 Axial CT of a right metastatic carcinoma

4. Treatment – radiotherapy.

Childhood metastatic tumours

1. Neuroblastoma
   - Arises from primitive neuroblasts of the sympathetic chain, most

commonly in the abdomen, followed by the thorax and pelvis.
- Presentation is in infancy with an abrupt onset of proptosis and a superior orbital mass, sometimes bilateral, and often associated with lid ecchymosis (*Fig. 6.57*).

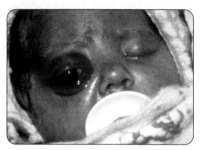

Fig. 6.57 Metastatic neuroblastoma

2. Myeloid sarcoma
- Localized tumour composed of malignant cells of myeloid origin that may occur as a manifestation of established myeloid leukaemia or it may precede the disease.
- Presentation is at about 7 years with rapid onset of proptosis, sometimes bilateral (*Fig. 6.58*).

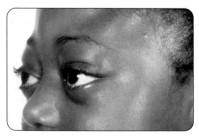

Fig. 6.58 Myeloid sarcoma

3. Langerhans cell granulomatosis
- Multisystem disease characterized by destructive inflammatory lesions that primarily involve bone.
- Orbital involvement consists of unilateral or bilateral osteolytic lesions and soft-tissue involvement, typically in the supero-temporal quadrant (*Fig. 6.59*).

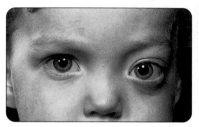

Fig. 6.59 Langerhans-cell histiocytosis

Orbital invasion by sinus tumours

1. Maxillary carcinoma – upward displacement (*Fig. 6.60*), diplopia and epiphora.

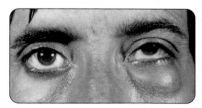

Fig. 6.60 Maxillary carcinoma

2. Ethmoidal carcinoma – lateral displacement.

3. Nasopharyngeal carcinoma – may spread to the orbit through the inferior orbital fissure; proptosis is a late finding.

Definitions

Dry eye occurs when there is inadequate tear volume or function resulting in an unstable tear film and ocular surface disease.

1. **Keratoconjunctivitis sicca** (KCS) – eye with some degree of dryness.
2. **Xerophthalmia** – dry eye due to vitamin A deficiency.
3. **Xerosis** – extreme dryness and ocular keratinization in severe cicatrizing conjunctivitis.
4. **Sjögren syndrome** – KCS and xerostomia.
   a. *Primary* – not associated with a distinct autoimmune disease.
   b. *Secondary* – associated with distinct autoimmune disease.

Classification

See *Table 7.1*.

Table 7.1 Classification of KCS

1. *Aqueous layer deficiency*
   · Sjögren syndrome
   · Non-Sjögren
2. *Evaporative*
   · Meibomian gland disease
   · Exposure
   · Defective blinking
   · Contact lens associated
   · Environmental factors

Causes

See *Tables 7.2 & 7.3*.

Table 7.2 Causes of non-Sjögren KCS

1. *Primary age-related*
2. *Lacrimal tissue destruction*
   · Tumour
   · Inflammation
3. *Absence or reduction of lacrimal gland tissue*
   · Surgical removal
   · Congenital
4. *Conjunctival scarring with obstruction of lacrimal gland ductules*
   · Chemical burns
   · Cicatricial pemphigoid
   · Stevens–Johnson syndrome
   · Old trachoma
5. *Neurological lesions with sensory or motor reflex loss*
   · Familial dysautonomia (Riley–Day syndrome)
   · Parkinson's disease
   · Reduced sensation after refractive surgery and contact lens wear
6. *Vitamin A deficiency*

Table 7.3 Causes of evaporative KCS

1. *Meibomian gland dysfunction*
   · Posterior blepharitis
   · Rosacea
   · Atopic keratoconjunctivitis
   · Congenital meibomian gland absence
2. *Lagophthalmos*
   · Severe proptosis
   · Facial nerve palsy
   · Eyelid scarring
   · Following blepharoplasty
3. *Miscellaneous*
   · Contact lens wear
   · Environmental factors such as air conditioning

- Mucous debris that moves with each blink (*Fig. 7.2*).
- Froth in the tear film or along the eyelid margin (*Fig. 7.3*).

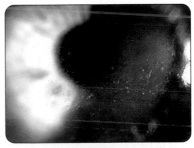

Fig. 7.2 Mucous debris in the tear film

Clinical features

1. **Symptoms** – dryness, grittiness and burning.
2. **Conjunctiva** – mild keratinization and redness.
3. **Tear film**
   - Marginal tear meniscus is less than 1 mm in height and may be absent (*Fig. 7.1*).

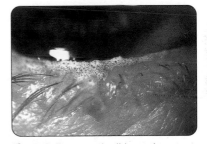

Fig. 7.3 Foam on the lid margin

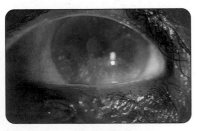

Fig. 7.1 Very thin marginal tear meniscus and inferior punctate erosions stained with fluorescein

4. Cornea

- Interpalpebral and inferior punctate epithelial erosions (see *Fig. 7.1*).
- Filaments (*Fig. 7.4*) and mucous plaques that stain with Rose Bengal (*Fig. 7.5*).

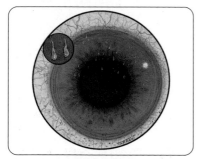

Fig. 7.4 Filaments

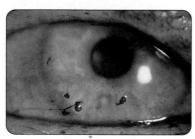

Fig. 7.5 Mucous plaques stained with Rose Bengal

5. Complications – peripheral superficial corneal neovascularization, epithelial breakdown, melting (*Fig. 7.6*), perforation (*Fig. 7.7*), and bacterial keratitis.

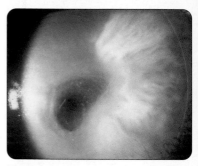

Fig. 7.6 Corneal melt with a bandage contact lens

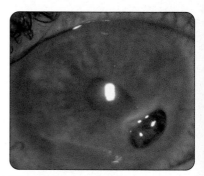

Fig. 7.7 Corneal perforation

Investigations

1. **Tear film break-up time** (BUT) – less than 10 sec in aqueous tear deficiency and meibomian gland disorders (*Fig. 7.8*).

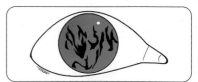

Fig. 7.8 Dry spots in the tear film

2. Schirmer test – less than 10 mm of wetting after 5 min without anaesthesia and less than 6 mm with anaesthesia is abnormal (*Fig. 7.9*).

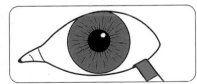

Fig. 7.9 Schirmer test

3. Fluorescein – stains damaged corneal and conjunctival epithelium.
4. Rose Bengal – interpalpebral staining of the cornea and conjunctiva in aqueous tear deficiency (*Fig. 7.10*).

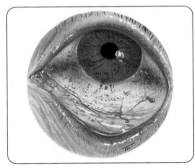

Fig. 7.10 Rose Bengal staining

Treatment

Topical

1. Tear substitute drops and gels
   - Cellulose derivatives for mild cases.
   - Carbomers are longer lasting.
   - Polyvinyl alcohol in mucin deficiency.
   - Sodium hyaluronate to promote epithelial healing.
   - Autologous serum in severe cases.
   - Povidone and sodium chloride.

2. Mucolytic agents – acetylcysteine drops for filaments and mucous plaques.
3. Weak topical steroids – supplementary treatment for acute exacerbations.
4. Topical ciclosporin – increases number of goblet cells and reverses squamous conjunctival metaplasia.

Punctal occlusion

1. Temporary – insertion of collagen plugs into the canaliculi that dissolve in 1–2 weeks to ensure that epiphora does not occur following permanent occlusion.
2. Reversible prolonged – silicone or long-acting collagen plugs that dissolve in 2–6 months (*Fig. 7.11*).

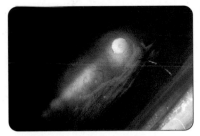

Fig. 7.11 Punctal plug in situ

3. Permanent – cauterization of the canaliculi in severe dry eye and positive response to temporary plugs without epiphora.

Other options

1. **Tarsorrhaphy** – diminishes surface evaporation by reducing the palpebral aperture.
2. **Botulinum toxin injection** – to control blepharospasm in severe dry eye.
3. **Oral cholinergic agonists** – pilocarpine may also benefit xerostomia.
4. **Zidovudine** – in primary Sjögren syndrome.
5. **Submandibular gland transplantation** – for extreme dry eye requires extensive surgery and tends to produce unacceptable levels of mucus in the tear film.

Bacterial conjunctivitis

Acute bacterial conjunctivitis

1. **Pathogenesis** – direct contact with infected secretions; most common isolates are *H. influenzae*, *S. pneumoniae*, *S. aureus*, and *Moraxella catarrhalis*.
2. **Symptoms** – acute onset of grittiness, and discharge.
3. **Signs** – crusty lids (*Fig. 8.1*), mucopurulent discharge and conjunctival injection most intense away from the limbus (*Fig. 8.2*).

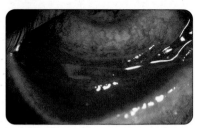

Fig. 8.1 Crusty eyelids

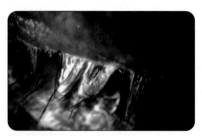

Fig. 8.2 Acute bacterial conjunctivitis

4. **Investigations** – not routinely performed.
5. **Treatment** – topical antibiotics drops every 2 hours for 5–7 days and ointment at bedtime.

Gonococcal keratoconjunctivitis

1. **Pathogenesis** – venereal infection with *N. gonorrhoeae* which is capable of invading the intact corneal epithelium.
2. **Signs**
   • Severe eyelid oedema and tenderness.
   • Intense conjunctival hyperaemia, chemosis, profuse purulent discharge and pseudomembrane formation (*Fig. 8.3*).
   • Preauricular lymphadenopathy.
   • Corneal ulceration and perforation (*Fig. 8.4*) if conjunctivitis is not treated appropriately.

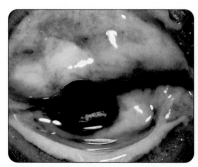

Fig. 8.3 Gonococcal conjunctivitis

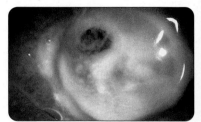

Fig. 8.4 Corneal perforation

3. Laboratory investigations
- Gram stain – Gram-negative kidney-shaped diplococci (*Fig. 8.5*).
- Culture – chocolate agar or Thayer–Martin medium.

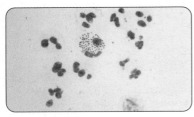

Fig. 8.5 Gram stain showing diplococci

4. Treatment
- **a.** *Topical* – hourly gentamicin or bacitracin.
- **b.** *Systemic* – ceftriaxone.

Meningococcal conjunctivitis

1. Signs
- Acute conjunctivitis, usually in a child, often associated with subconjunctival haemorrhages (*Fig. 8.6*).
- Preauricular lymphadenopathy.

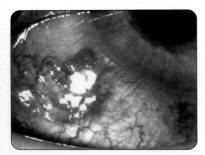

Fig. 8.6 Haemorrhagic meningococcal conjunctivitis

- Keratitis that may lead to ulceration and perforation.

2. Treatment
- **a.** *Topical* – penicillin or cefotaxime drops.
- **b.** *Systemic prophylaxis* – oral ciprofloxacin, or intramuscular ceftriaxone or cefotaxime to reduce the risk of meningitis.

Adult chlamydial conjunctivitis

1. Pathogenesis – oculogenital infection caused by serotypes D–K of *C. trachomatis* transmitted by autoinoculation from genital secretions and occasionally by eye-to-eye spread.

2. Presentation – subacute onset of unilateral or bilateral redness, watering, and discharge.

3. Signs
- Mucopurulent discharge.
- Large follicles often most prominent in the inferior fornix (*Fig. 8.7*).
- Peripheral corneal infiltrates may appear with 2–3 weeks.
- Preauricular lymphadenopathy.

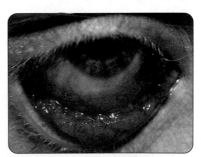

Fig. 8.7 Adult chlamydial conjunctivitis

4. Special investigations
- PCR for chlamydial DNA.
- Direct monoclonal fluorescent antibody microscopy of conjunctival smears.
- McCoy cell culture shows glycogen-positive inclusion bodies (*Fig. 8.8*).

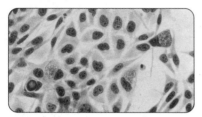

Fig. 8.8 McCoy cell culture showing inclusion bodies

5. Treatment
- **a.** *Topical* – erythromycin or tetracycline ointment.
- **b.** *Systemic* – doxycycline for 10 days, or a single dose of azithromycin 1 g.

Trachoma

1. **Pathogenesis** – chronic conjunctival infection with *C. trachomatis* in which the fly is the major vector.
2. **Signs** in chronological order:
   - Mixed follicular/papillary conjunctivitis (*Fig. 8.9*).
   - Herbert pits (*Fig. 8.10*).
   - Superior tarsal conjunctival linear or stellate scarring (*Fig. 8.11*) or broad confluent scars (Arlt lines) in severe disease (*Fig. 8.12*).
   - Superior pannus (*Fig. 8.13*).

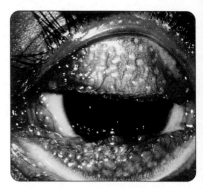

Fig. 8.9 Trachomatous conjunctivitis

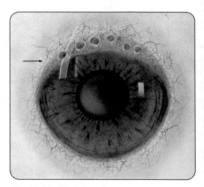

Fig. 8.10 Herbert pits

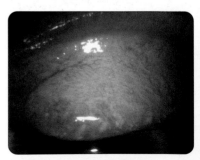

Fig. 8.11 Conjunctival scarring

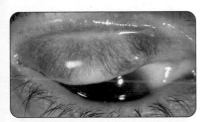

Fig. 8.12 Arlt line

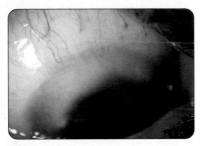

Fig. 8.13 Pannus

3. **Complications** – dry eye, trichiasis, distichiasis, cicatricial entropion, and corneal vascularization (*Fig. 8.14*).

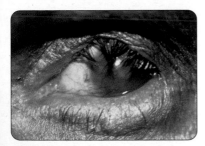

Fig. 8.14 Complications of trachoma

4. **Treatment** – single oral dose of azithromycin 1 g.

Table 8.1 Modified WHO grading of trachoma	
TF	Trachoma follicles with five or more (>0.5 mm) present on the superior tarsus.
TI	Trachomatous inflammation diffusely involving the tarsal conjunctiva, which obscures 50% or more of the normal deep tarsal vessels.
TS	Trachomatous conjunctival scarring
TT	Trachomatous trichiasis (at least one lash) touching the globe
CO	Corneal opacity over the pupil sufficient to blur iris details

Ophthalmia neonatorum

1. **Pathogenesis** – infection is transmitted from mother to infant during delivery that develops within 2 weeks of birth.
   a. *N. gonorrhoeae* – rare in developed countries.
   b. *C. trachomatis* — most common.
   c. *Other pathogens* – S. aureus, S. pneumoniae, H. influenzae, and Enterobacteriaceae.
2. **Prophylaxis** – single dose at birth of povidone-iodine 2.5%.
3. **Signs**
   • Usually bilateral eyelid oedema and mucopurulent discharge (*Fig. 8.15*).
   • Papillary conjunctival reaction.

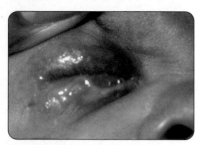

Fig. 8.15 Ophthalmia neonatorum

4. Treatment
  a. *Chlamydial* – oral erythromycin ethyl succinate for 2 weeks and erythromycin or tetracycline ointment.
  b. *Gonococcal* – parenteral ceftriaxone or cefotaxime.
  c. *Other bacterial* – chloramphenicol or neomycin ointment

Viral conjunctivitis

Adenoviral keratoconjunctivitis

1. **Pathogenesis** – spread by respiratory or ocular secretions, and disseminated by contaminated towels or equipment such as tonometer heads.
  a. *Pharyngoconjunctival fever (PCF)* – caused by serotypes 3, 7 and 11; keratitis develops in 30%.
  b. *Epidemic keratoconjunctivitis (EKC)* – caused by serotypes 8, 19 and 37; keratitis develops in 80%.
2. **Presentation** – unilateral watering, redness, discomfort and photophobia; the contralateral eye is typically affected 1–2 days later, but less severely.
3. **Signs**
   - Eyelid oedema and tender pre-auricular lymphadenopathy.

- Follicular conjunctivitis (*Fig. 8.16*).
- Conjunctival haemorrhages, chemosis, and pseudomembranes in severe cases (*Fig. 8.17*).

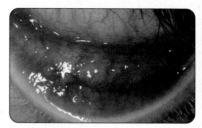

Fig. 8.16 Follicular adenoviral conjunctivitis

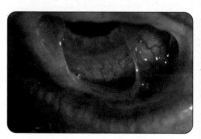

Fig. 8.17 Severe adenoviral conjunctivitis

4. Keratitis
- *Stage 1* – punctate epithelial lesions that resolves within 2 weeks (*Fig. 8.18a*).
- *Stage 2* – white, subepithelial opacities that develop beneath the fading epithelial lesions.
- *Stage 3* – anterior stromal infiltrates that gradually fade over many months (*Fig. 8.18b*).
5. **Treatment** – topical steroids only for severe conjunctivitis, and stage 3 keratitis causing visual disability.

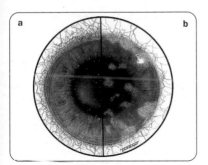

Fig. 8.18 Adenoviral keratitis; (a) stage 1; (b) stage 3

Molluscum contagiosum conjunctivitis

1. **Pathogenesis** – poxvirus transmitted by contact with infected people and then by autoinoculation.
2. **Presentation** – chronic, unilateral, ocular irritation and mild discharge.
3. **Signs**
   * Pale, waxy, umbilicated nodule on the lid margin associated with follicular conjunctivitis (*Fig. 8.19*).
   * Fine epithelial keratitis or pannus in longstanding cases.

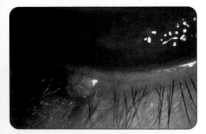

Fig. 8.19 Molluscum contagiosum

4. **Treatment** – physical expression.

Acute haemorrhagic conjunctivitis

1. **Pathogenesis** – enterovirus 70 or coxsackievirus A24 spread by direct inoculation.
2. **Presentation** – acute onset of usually bilateral burning, watering, discharge and lid swelling.
3. **Signs**
   * Subconjunctival haemorrhages and follicular conjunctivitis.
   * Preauricular lymphadenopathy.
4. **Treatment** – not possible.

Allergic conjunctivitis

Acute allergic rhinoconjunctivitis

1. **Classification**
   a. *Seasonal allergic conjunctivitis* (hay fever) – onset during the spring and summer caused by tree and grass pollens.
   b. *Perennial allergic conjunctivitis* – symptomatic throughout the year and caused by house dust mites, animal dander, and fungal allergens.
2. **Presentation** – transient, acute attacks of redness, watering and itching, associated with sneezing and nasal discharge.
3. **Signs** – lid oedema, chemosis, and mild papillary reaction (*Fig. 8.20*).

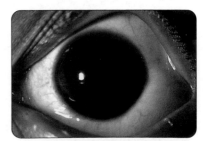

Fig. 8.20 Acute allergic conjunctivitis

4. Treatment – topical mast cell stabilizers for long-term use and antihistamines when the patient is symptomatic.

Vernal keratoconjunctivitis

1. Pathogenesis – recurrent disorder in which IgE and cell-mediated immune mechanisms play important roles; primarily affects boys and presents in the 1st decade; in temperate regions about 75% of patients have associated atopy and 60% a family history of atopy.

2. Classification

a. *Palpebral* – involves the upper tarsal conjunctiva and may be associated with significant corneal disease.

b. *Limbal* – affects black and Asian patients.

c. *Mixed.*

3. Symptoms – intense itching, lacrimation, photophobia, foreign body sensation, burning and thick mucoid discharge.

4. Conjunctivitis

- Superior tarsal papillary conjunctivitis (*Fig. 8.21*).
- Cobblestone macropillae (>1 mm) associated with mucus deposits (*Fig. 8.22*).
- Very large (giant papillae) – uncommon (*Fig. 8.23*).

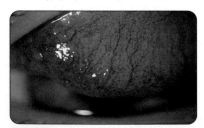

Fig. 8.21 Micropapillary conjunctivitis

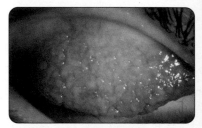

Fig. 8.22 Cobblestone papillae

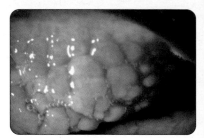

Fig. 8.23 Giant papillae

5. Limbitis

- Gelatinous limbal papillae often associated with discrete white spots at their apices (Trantas dots – *Figs 8.24 & 8.25*).
- Pseudogerontoxon in recurrent limbal disease (*Fig. 8.26*).
- Peripheral superficial neovascularization (*Fig. 8.27*).

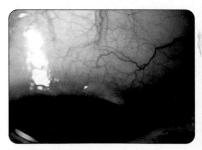

Fig. 8.24 Limbitis

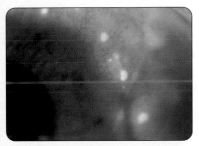

Fig. 8.25 Trantas dots

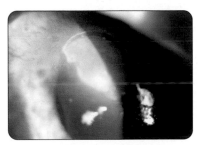

Fig. 8.28 Shield ulcer and plaque

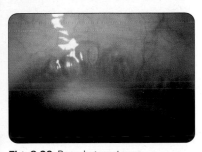

Fig. 8.26 Pseudogerontoxon

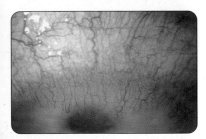

Fig. 8.27 Superficial neovascularization

6. Keratopathy
- Superior punctate epithelial erosions.
- Epithelial macroerosions.
- Shield ulcers and plaques (*Fig. 8.28*).

7. Topical treatment
  a. *Mast cell stabilizers and antihistamines* – rarely effective as sole treatment, but they reduce the need for steroids.
  b. *Steroids* – for keratopathy and short-term for severe discomfort.
  c. *Acetylcysteine* – for mucus deposition and early plaque formation.
  d. *Ciclosporin* – in steroid-resistant cases.

8. Supratarsal steroid injection – for non-compliant patients and those resistant to conventional therapy.

9. Systemic treatment
  a. *Immunosuppressive agents* – in severe unremitting disease unresponsive to maximum topical therapy.
  b. *Oral antihistamines* – help sleep and reduce nocturnal eye rubbing.

10. Surgery
  a. *Superficial keratectomy* – to remove plaques.
  b. *Excimer laser phototherapeutic keratectomy* – an alternative.
  c. *Amniotic membrane overlay graft* – for severe persistent epithelial defects with ulceration.

Atopic keratoconjunctivitis

1. **Pathogenesis** – affects young men following a long history of severe atopic dermatitis; sensitivity to a wide range of environmental airborne allergens.
2. **Symptoms** – similar to VKC but often more severe and unremitting.
3. **Eyelids**
   - Red, thickened, macerated and fissured lids with chronic staphylococcal blepharitis and madarosis (*Fig. 8.29*).
   - Tightening of skin may cause lower lid ectropion and epiphora.

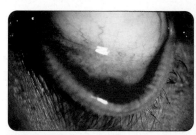

Fig. 8.30 Inferior papillary conjunctivitis

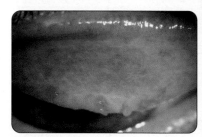

Fig. 8.31 Conjunctival scarring

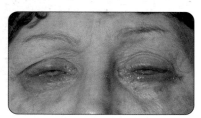

Fig. 8.29 Atopic dermatitis

4. **Conjunctivitis**
   - Papillary conjunctivitis involving the tarsal plates and inferior fornix (*Fig. 8.30*).
   - Macropapillae may develop with time.
   - Scarring results in flattening of papillae (*Fig. 8.31*).
   - Forniceal shortening and symblepharon in severe cases (*Fig. 8.32*).
5. **Keratopathy**
   - Inferior punctate epithelial erosions.
   - Persistent epithelial defects, plaque formation, and peripheral superficial vascularization (*Fig. 8.33*).

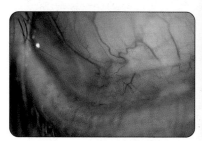

Fig. 8.32 Forniceal shortening

   - Predisposition to keratoconus, secondary bacterial and fungal infection, and aggressive herpes simplex.

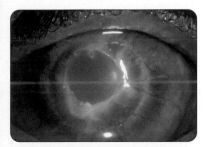

Fig. 8.33 Epithelial defect and peripheral vascularization

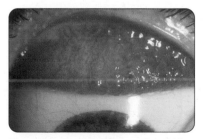

Fig. 8.34 Giant papillary conjunctivitis associated with ocular prosthesis

6. Topical treatment
   a. *Mast cell stabilizers* – prophylaxis against exacerbation and as steroid-sparing agents.
   b. *Ketolorac* – combined with a mast cell stabilizer.
   c. *Antihistamines* – more effective than in VKC.
   d. *Steroids* – short-term for severe exacerbations and keratopathy.
   e. *Acetylcysteine* – for corneal mucus deposits.
   f. *Ciclosporin* – steroid-sparing agent in severe disease.

7. Systemic treatment
   a. *Antihistamines* – for severe itching.
   b. *Antibiotics* – to reduce inflammation aggravated by blepharitis.
   c. *Ciclosporin* – in severe cases.

Giant papillary conjunctivitis

1. Aetiology – contact lens wear, ocular prosthesis (*Fig. 8.34*), exposed sutures, and filtering blebs; risk is increased by deposition of mucus and cellular debris on the contact lens surface (lens spoliation – *Fig. 8.35*).

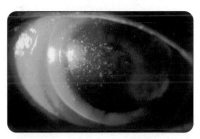

Fig. 8.35 Contact lens deposits

2. Symptoms – foreign body sensation, redness, itching and loss of contact lens tolerance, often worse when the lens has been removed.

3. Signs
   • Excessive mobility of the contact lens with upper lid lens capture.
   • Increased mucus production and coating of the contact lens.
   • Small papillae on the superior tarsal conjunctiva.
   • Macropapillae with focal scarring on the apices in advanced cases.

4. Treatment – removal of the stimulus, cleaning of contact lenses or prostheses, topical mast cell stabilizers, and occasionally topical steroids.

Cicatrizing conjunctivitis

Mucous membrane pemphigoid

1. **Pathogenesis** – autoimmune mucocutaneous blistering disease affecting elderly patients; conjunctival disease (ocular cicatricial pemphigoid – OCP) is seen in 75% of cases with oral involvement but only 25% of those with skin lesions; occasionally OCT occurs in isolation.
2. **Presentation** – insidious onset of non-specific conjunctivitis.
3. **Conjunctivitis**
   - Diffuse hyperaemia and oedema which may be associated with necrosis (*Fig. 8.36*).
   - Lines of subconjunctival fibrosis and shortening of the inferior fornices (*Fig. 8.37*).

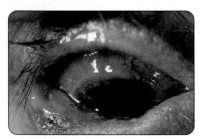

Fig. 8.36 Acute stage of cicatricial pemphigoid

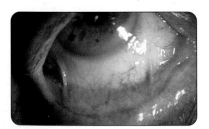

Fig. 8.37 Subconjunctival fibrosis and forniceal shortening

- Flattening of the plica, keratinization of the caruncle, and symblepharon formation (*Fig. 8.38*).

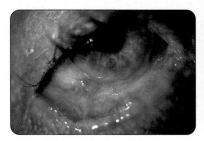

Fig. 8.38 Symblepharon formation

4. **Keratopathy**
   - Epithelial defects and peripheral vascularization.
   - Corneal keratinization (*Fig. 8.39*).
   - End-stage – total symblepharon and corneal opacification (*Fig. 8.40*).

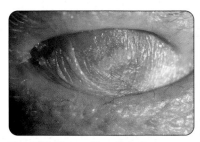

Fig. 8.39 Corneal keratinization

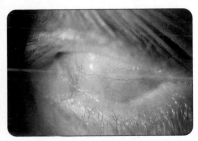

Fig. 8.40 End-stage disease

5. Eyelids
- Aberrant lashes (acquired distichiasis).
- Blepharitis and keratinization of the lid margin.
- Ankyloblepharon.

6. Treatment
- **a.** *Systemic steroids* – but not as sole long-term therapy.
- **b.** *Cyclophosphamide* – as steroid-sparing agent.
- **c.** *Azathioprine or mycophenolate mofetil* – for long-term therapy.
- **d.** *Other* – of aberrant lashes, punctal occlusion for dry eye, mucous membrane and limbal stem cell transplantation, and keratoprostheses in end-stage disease (*Fig. 8.41*).

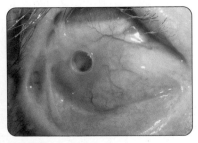

Fig. 8.41 Keratoprosthesis

Stevens–Johnson syndrome

1. **Pathogenesis** – delayed hypersensitivity response to drugs or a response to epithelial cell antigens modified by drug exposure.
2. **Acute disease**
   - Crusty eyelids associated with a transient, self-limiting papillary conjunctivitis.
   - Severe membranous or pseudomembranous conjunctivitis (*Fig. 8.42*).

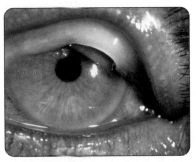

Fig. 8.42 Pseudomembranous conjunctivitis

3. **Late disease**
   - Reticular scarring of the superior tarsal conjunctiva (*Fig. 8.43*).
   - Conjunctival scarring and keratinization (*Fig. 8.44*).
   - Posterior lid margin disease with exposure of the meibomian orifices (*Fig. 8.45*).
   - Symblepharon formation and corneal keratinization.
   - Keratopathy secondary to dry eye, cicatricial entropion, aberrant lashes, and infection.

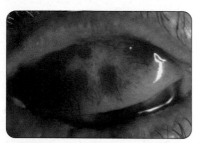

Fig. 8.43 Reticular conjunctival scarring

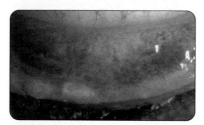

Fig. 8.44 Conjunctival scarring and keratinization

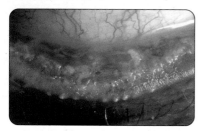

Fig. 8.45 Opening of meibomian gland orifices

4. Treatment

   a. *Systemic disease* – maintenance of hydration, and debridement and replacement of sloughing skin; efficacy of systemic steroids is debatable.

   b. *Eye disease* – topical steroids and retinoic acid, scleral ring to prevent symblepharon, mucous membrane grafting and limbal cell transplantation, and keratoprosthesis in end-stage disease.

Miscellaneous conjunctivitis

Superior limbic keratoconjunctivitis

1. **Pathogenesis** – blink-related mechanical trauma between the upper lid and superior bulbar conjunctiva, probably precipitated by tear film insufficiency.
2. **Signs**
   - Superior tarsal and limbal papillary hypertrophy, hyperaemia of the superior bulbar conjunctiva, superior corneal filaments (*Fig. 8.46*).
   - Downward pressure on the upper lid results in the appearance of a fold of redundant conjunctiva crossing the upper limbus (*Fig. 8.47*).
   - Superior punctate corneal epithelial erosions and dry eye.

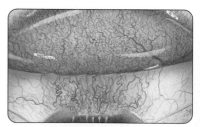

Fig. 8.46 Superior limbic keratoconjunctivitis

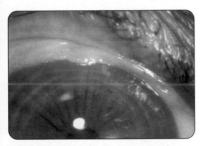

Fig. 8.47 Redundant conjunctiva

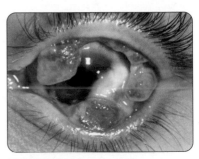

Fig. 8.48 Ligneous lesions

3. Treatment
   a. *Topical* – lubricants, mast cell stabilizers, steroids, ciclosporin, acetylcysteine, and retinoic acid.
   b. *Other measures* – temporary superior punctal occlusion, soft contact lenses, resection of the superior limbal conjunctiva and Tenon capsule, and transconjunctival thermocautery.

Ligneous conjunctivitis

1. Pathogenesis – plasminogen deficiency.
2. Presentation – usually in childhood with chronic conjunctivitis.
3. Signs
   • Gradual formation of wood-like masses on the palpebral conjunctiva associated with membranes or pseudomembranes (*Fig. 8.48*).
   • Profuse mucoid discharge (*Fig. 8.49*).
   • Lesions may also develop in the mouth, respiratory tract, middle ear, and cervix.
4. Treatment – surgical removal followed by hourly heparin and steroids; recurrences require

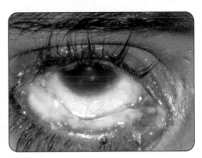

Fig. 8.49 Mucoid discharge

long-term systemic ciclosporin and steroids.

Parinaud oculoglandular syndrome

1. Causes – cat-scratch disease, tularaemia, sporotrichosis, tuberculosis, chancroid, and lymphogranuloma venereum.
2. Signs – chronic fever, unilateral granulomatous conjunctivitis with surrounding follicles (*Fig. 8.50*) and ipsilateral regional lymphadenopathy.

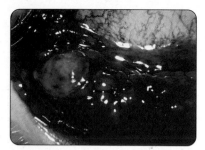

Fig. 8.50 Granulomatous conjunctivitis

Factitious conjunctivitis

1. **Pathogenesis** – self-injury that may be intentional or inadvertent.
2. **Signs**
   - Inferior conjunctival injection and staining with Rose Bengal (*Fig. 8.51*) with normal superior bulbar conjunctiva.
   - Linear corneal abrasions and persistent epithelial defects.
3. **Treatment** – exclusion of all other diagnoses and elimination of the underlying cause.

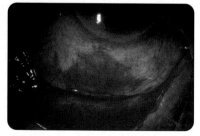

Fig. 8.51 Factitious conjunctivitis

Degenerations

Pinguecula

1. **Signs** – bilateral yellow-white deposits on the bulbar conjunctiva adjacent to the nasal or temporal limbus (*Fig. 8.52*).

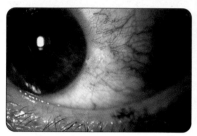

Fig. 8.52 Pinguecula

2. **Treatment** – usually unnecessary although occasionally the lesion may become acutely inflamed (pingueculitis) and require topical steroids.

Pterygium

1. **Pathogenesis** – response to chronic dryness and ultraviolet exposure.
2. **Classification**
   a. *Type 1* – extends less than 2 mm onto the cornea and may be associated with a deposit of iron (Stocker line) anterior to the advancing head of the pterygium.
   b. *Type 2* – involves up to 4 mm of the cornea (*Fig. 8.53*).
   c. *Type 3* – involves the visual axis.

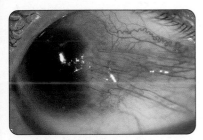

Fig. 8.53 Pterygium

3. Surgery – for types 2 and 3 involves excision of the ptcrygium and covering of the defect with either a conjunctival autograft or amniotic membrane.

Concretions

1. Signs – tiny, often multiple, chalky, deposits most commonly in the inferior tarsal and forniceal conjunctiva (*Fig. 8.54*).

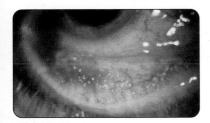

Fig. 8.54 Concretions

2. Treatment – usually unnecessary.

Conjunctivochalasis

1. Pathogenesis – normal ageing change that may be exacerbated by posterior lid margin disease.

2. Signs – fold of redundant conjunctiva interposed between the globe and lower eyelid that protrudes over the lid margin (*Fig. 8.55*).

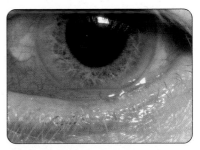

Fig. 8.55 Conjunctivochalasis

3. Treatment – conjunctival resection but only in severe cases.

Retention cyst

1. Signs – thin-walled lesion containing clear fluid (*Fig. 8.56*).

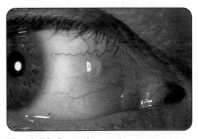

Fig. 8.56 Retention cyst

2. Treatment – simple puncture, if appropriate.

Benign pigmented lesions

Primary epithelial melanosis

1. **Presentation** – early childhood.
2. **Signs** – patchy, brownish pigmentation most intense at the limbus and around the perforating branches of the anterior ciliary vessels or an intrascleral nerve (Axenfeld loop – *Fig. 8.57*).

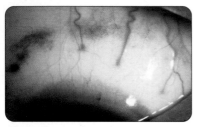

Fig. 8.57 Primary epithelial melanosis

Congenital ocular melanocytosis

1. **Histology** – increase in number, size and pigmentation of melanocytes.
2. **Classification**
   a. *Ocular* – involves only the eye (least common).
   b. *Dermal* – involves only facial skin in the distribution of the 1st and 2nd division of the trigeminal nerve (30% of cases).
   c. *Oculodermal (naevus of Ota)* – involves both facial skin and the eye (most common).

3. **Signs** – multifocal, slate-grey pigmentation in the episclera and cannot be moved over the globe (*Fig. 8.58*).

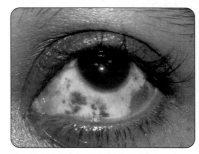

Fig. 8.58 Conjunctival melanocytosis

4. **Ipsilateral associations** – iris heterochromia (*Fig. 8.59*) and mammillations, trabecular hyperpigmentation, fundus hyperpigmentation, and increased risk of choroidal melanoma in Caucasians.

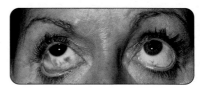

Fig. 8.59 Heterochromia iridis in naevus of Ota

Bacterial keratitis

1. **Risk factors** – contact lens wear, trauma, ocular surface disease, immunosuppression, diabetes, and vitamin A deficiency.
2. **Pathogens** – *P. aeruginosa*, *S. aureus*, *S. pyogenes*, and *S. pneumoniae*.
3. **Signs** in chronological order:
   - Epithelial defect associated with an infiltrate.
   - Enlargement of the infiltrate with stromal oedema (*Fig. 9.1*).
   - Severe infiltration with enlarging hypopyon (*Fig. 9.2*).
   - Progressive ulceration may lead to perforation and endophthalmitis.

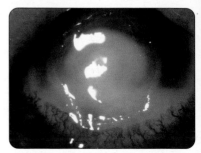

Fig. 9.2 Advanced bacterial keratitis

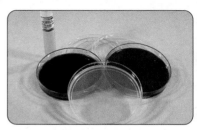

Fig. 9.3 Chocolate agar (left); blood agar (right); Sabouraud agar (centre)

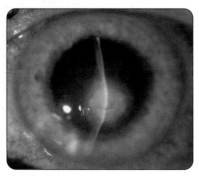

Fig. 9.1 Bacterial keratitis

4. **Culture media** (*Fig. 9.3*)
   - Blood agar – for fungi and bacteria except *Neisseria*, *Haemophilus* and *Moraxella* spp.
   - Chocolate agar – for *Neisseria*, *Haemophilus* and *Moraxella* spp.
   - Sabouraud agar – for fungi.
   - Brain–heart infusion broth or cooked meat broth – for fastidious organisms.

5. **Treatment**
   a. *Topical antibiotics* – hourly during day and night for 24–48 hours then reduced to 2-hourly during waking hours for 48 hours, and then q.i.d. for 1 week.
   b. *Oral antibiotics* (ciprofloxacin 750 mg twice daily for 7–10 days) – if perforation is threatened or has occurred.
   c. *Subconjunctival antibiotics* – if poor compliance with topical treatment.
   d. *Mydriatics*.
   e. *Topical steroids* – unproven value.

Fungal keratitis

1. **Risk factors** – trauma particularly with vegetable matter; others similar to bacterial keratitis.
2. **Pathogens**
   - In tropical climates – filamentous fungi (*Aspergillus* spp., *Fusarium solani*, and *Scedosporium* spp.).
   - In temperate climates – yeasts (*Candida* spp.).
3. **Signs**
   a. *Filamentous keratitis* – slowly progressive grey-yellow stromal infiltrate with indistinct margins often associated with satellite lesions and hypopyon (*Fig. 9.4*).

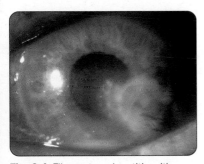

Fig. 9.4 Filamentous keratitis with satellite lesions

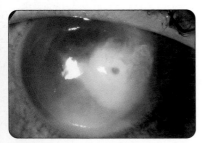

Fig. 9.5 Candida keratitis

   b. *Candida keratitis* – yellow-white infiltrate with dense suppuration (*Fig. 9.5*).
4. **Culture media** – Sabouraud agar, although most fungi will also grow on blood agar or in enrichment media at 27°C.
5. **Treatment**
   a. *Removal of overlying epithelium* – enhances penetration of antifungal agents.
   b. *Of filamentous*
   - Natamycin 5% or econazole 1%.
   - Alternatives – amphotericin B 0.15% and miconazole 1%.
   c. *Of candida*
   - Econazole 1%.
   - Alternatives – natamycin 5%, fluconazole 2%, amphotericin B 0.15% and clotrimazole 1%.

Herpes simplex keratitis

Epithelial keratitis

1. **Pathogenesis** – reactivation of latent HSV-1 which migrates down an axon of a branch of the trigeminal nerve to the cornea (*Fig. 9.6*).

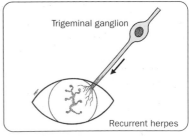

Trigeminal ganglion

Recurrent herpes

Fig. 9.6 Pathogenesis of epithelial keratitis

2. Signs in chronological order:
- Linear-branching (dendritic) ulcer (*Fig. 9.7*).
- The terminal buds and the bed of the ulcer stain with fluorescein (*Fig. 9.8*).
- The margin of the ulcer stains with Rose Bengal (*Fig. 9.9*).
- Progressive ulceration may give rise to a geographic (amoeboid) ulcer (*Fig. 9.10*).
- Reduced corneal sensation.

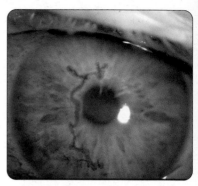

Fig. 9.9 Large dendritic ulcer stained with Rose Bengal

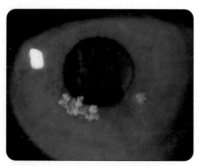

Fig. 9.7 Multiple small dendritic ulcers

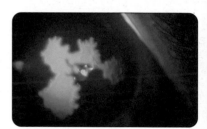

Fig. 9.10 Geographic ulcer

3. Treatment
   a. *Topical*
- Aciclovir 3% ointment 5 times daily.
- Alternatives – trifluorothymidine, vidarabine and ganciclovir.
   b. *Debridement* – for dendritic but not geographic ulcers.

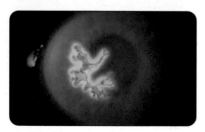

Fig. 9.8 Large dendritic ulcer stained with fluorescein

Disciform keratitis

1. **Pathogenesis** – immune reaction involving the endothelium.
2. **Signs**
   - Central stromal and epithelial oedema with underlying keratic precipitates (*Fig. 9.11*).
   - Surrounding (Wessely) ring of stromal haze (*Fig. 9.12*).
   - Folds in Descemet membrane in severe cases.
   - Reduced corneal sensation.
3. **Treatment** – topical steroids with antiviral cover, both q.i.d.

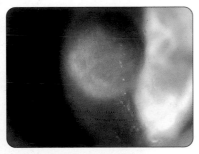

Fig. 9.11 Disciform keratitis

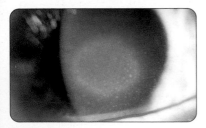

Fig. 9.12 Wessely ring

Stromal necrotic keratitis

1. **Pathogenesis** – direct viral stromal invasion with severe immune reaction.
2. **Signs**
   - Epithelial defect with stromal necrosis and opacification (*Fig. 9.13*).
   - Anterior uveitis with keratic precipitates underlying the area of active stromal infiltration.

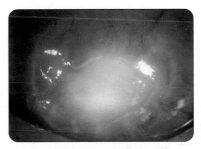

Fig. 9.13 Stromal necrotic keratitis

3. **Treatment** – topical lubricants and steroids.

Herpes zoster ophthalmicus

Pathogenesis

- Reactivation of VZV and migration down the first division of the trigeminal nerve to the skin and eye.
- Ocular damage may be caused by direct viral invasion, secondary inflammation, and occlusive vasculitis.
- Risks of ocular involvement – Hutchinson sign (*Fig. 9.14*), old age, and AIDS.

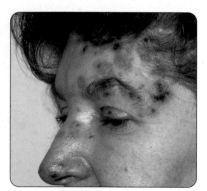

Fig. 9.14 Involvement of the side and tip of the nose (Hutchinson sign)

Acute disease

1. **Epithelial keratitis** – small, fine, pseudo-dendritic lesions with tapered ends (*Fig. 9.15*); resolves spontaneously within a few days.

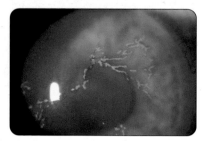

Fig. 9.15 Pseudo-dendrites

2. **Nummular keratitis** – granular subepithelial deposits surrounded by a halo of stromal haze (*Fig. 9.16*); treat with topical steroids if appropriate.

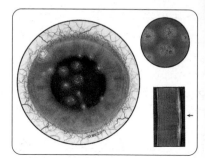

Fig. 9.16 Nummular keratitis

3. **Anterior stromal keratitis** (*Fig. 9.17*) – responds to topical steroids but often becomes chronic.

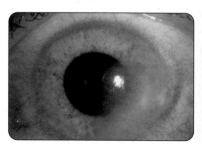

Fig. 9.17 Stromal keratitis

4. **Disciform keratitis** – topical steroids.
5. **Anterior uveitis** – often causes sectoral iris atrophy (see *Fig. 14.47*).
6. **Neurological complications** – cranial nerve palsies (*Fig. 9.18*), optic neuritis, encephalitis, Guillain–Barré syndrome, and contralateral hemiplegia.

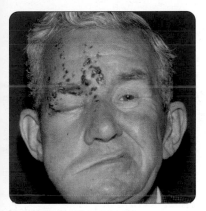

Fig. 9.18 Facial nerve palsy

Chronic disease

1. **Eyelids** – ptosis, cicatricial entropion, trichiasis, madarosis, and notching.
2. **Scleritis** – patchy scleral atrophy (*Fig. 9.19*).

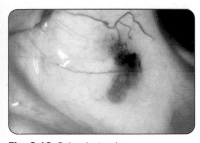

Fig. 9.19 Scleral atrophy

3. **Mucous plaque keratitis** – stains with Rose Bengal (*Fig. 9.20*).
4. **Neutrophic keratitis** – 50% of cases.
5. **Lipid keratopathy** – with persistent nummular or disciform keratitis.

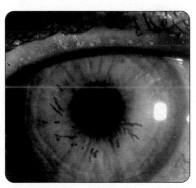

Fig. 9.20 Mucous plaques

Relapsing disease

Lesions may reappear years after acute disease. In some cases the acute episode may have been forgotten and lid scarring may be the only diagnostic clue.

Interstitis keratitis

Introduction

1. **Definition** – inflammation of the corneal stroma without primary involvement of the epithelium or endothelium.
2. **Causes** – congenital syphilis, tuberculosis, Lyme disease, leprosy, viral infection, and Cogan syndrome.

Syphilitic IK

1. **Pathogenesis** – transmission from the mother to child during primary, secondary, or early latent phases.

2. Presentation – acute bilateral pain and severe blurring of vision.

3. Signs in chronological order:
- Limbitis, and deep stromal vascularization and clouding (salmon-patch – *Fig. 9.21*).
- Anterior uveitis.
- Non-perfused (ghost vessels) and deep stromal scarring and thinning (*Fig. 9.22*).

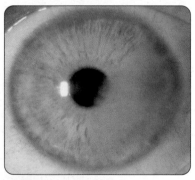

Fig. 9.21 'Salmon patch'

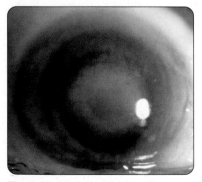

Fig. 9.22 Old interstitial keratitis

4. Treatment – systemic penicillin and topical steroids.

Cogan syndrome

1. Definition – systemic, autoimmune vasculitis characterized by intraocular inflammation and vestibulo-auditory dysfunction.

2. Systemic association – polyarteritis nodosa.

3. Signs of IK in chronological order:
- Faint bilateral peripheral anterior stromal opacities.
- Deeper opacities and neovascularization (*Fig. 9.23*).
- Uveitis, scleritis and retinal vasculitis.

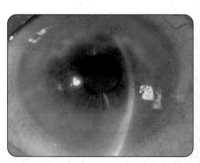

Fig. 9.23 Interstitial keratitis in Cogan syndrome

4. Treatment – topical steroids for keratitis; systemic steroids for other manifestations.

Protozoan keratitis

Acanthamoeba keratitis

1. Pathogenesis – *Acanthamoeba* spp. is found in soil, fresh or brackish water, and the upper respiratory tract; keratitis is most frequently associated with contact lens wear, especially if tap water is used for cleaning.

2. **Presentation** – blurred vision and pain, which may be severe and disproportionate to clinical signs.

3. **Signs** in chronological order:
   - Irregular greyish epithelium followed by pseudo-dendrite formation (*Fig. 9.24*).
   - Perineural infiltrates (radial keratoneuritis – *Fig. 9.25*) are pathognomonic.
   - Ring infiltrate (*Fig. 9.26*).
   - Slowly progressive stromal infiltration and vascularization (*Fig. 9.27*).
   - Corneal melting (*Fig. 9.28*) may occur at any stage.
   - Reduced corneal sensation.

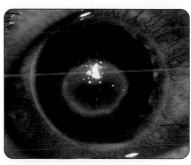

Fig. 9.26 Ring stromal infiltrate

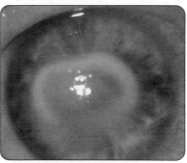

Fig. 9.27 Stromal infiltration

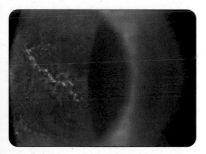

Fig. 9.24 Pseudo-dendrite

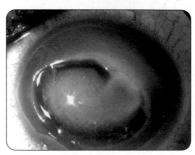

Fig. 9.28 Corneal melting

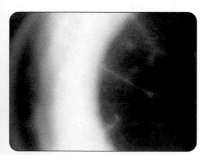

Fig. 9.25 Radial perineuritis

4. Investigations
   a. *Cultures* – non-nutrient agar later seeded with killed *E. coli*.
   b. *Staining* – periodic acid–Schiff or calcofluor white.
   c. *Other* – immunohistochemistry and PCR.

5. Treatment
   a. *Debridement* – of infected epithelium.
   b. *Topical amoebicides*
   • Propamidine isethionate 0.1% (Brolene) and polyhexamethylene biguanide 0.02% drops.
   • Alternative – hexamidine and chlorhexidine 0.02%.
   c. *Topical steroids* – for persistent inflammation which may be due to *Acanthamoeba* antigen rather than viable organisms.

Microsporidial keratitis

1. **Pathogenesis** – obligate intracellular, spore-forming opportunistic protozoa of the phylum *Microspora* that typically affect patients with AIDS.
2. **Signs** – bilateral chronic diffuse punctate epithelial keratitis (*Fig. 9.29*).

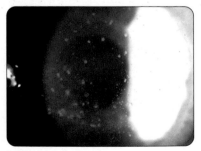

Fig. 9.29 Microsporidial keratitis

3. **Treatment** – topical fumagillin and oral albendazole.

Onchocercal keratitis

1. **Pathogenesis** – infestation with the parasitic helminth *Onchocerca volvulus*.
2. **Punctate keratitis** – at 3 and 9 o'clock in the anterior third of the stroma.
3. **Sclerosing keratitis** – full thickness scarring with superficial and deep vessels and pigment migration over the surface (*Fig. 9.30*).

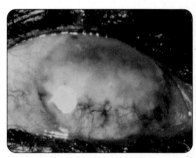

Fig. 9.30 Sclerosing onchocercal keratitis

4. **Treatment** – topical steroids for acute lesions.

Bacterial hypersensitivity-mediated corneal disease

Marginal keratitis

1. **Pathogenesis** – reaction against staphylococcal exotoxins and cell wall proteins with deposition of antigen–antibody complexes in the peripheral cornea.

2. Signs

- Subepithelial marginal infiltrates separated from the limbus by a clear zone (*Fig. 9.31*).
- Coalescence and circumferential spread (*Fig. 9.32*).
- Without treatment resolution occurs in 3–4 weeks.

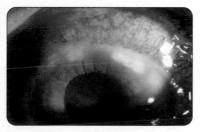

Fig. 9.31 Marginal keratitis

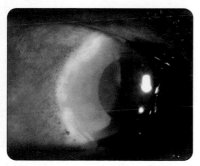

Fig. 9.32 Spreading marginal keratitis

3. Treatment – weak topical steroids to enhance resolution.

Phlyctenulosis

1. Pathogenesis – presumed delayed hypersensitivity reaction to staphylococcal cell wall antigen.

2. Presentation – in children or young adults with photophobia, lacrimation, and blepharospasm.

3. Signs

- Small white nodule with local hyperaemia on the conjunctiva or limbus (*Fig. 9.33*).
- A limbal lesion may extend onto the cornea (*Fig. 9.34*) and leave a triangular scar with superficial vascularization.

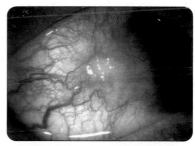

Fig. 9.33 Conjunctival phlycten

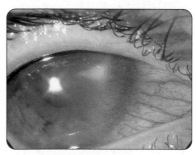

Fig. 9.34 Extending phlycten

4. Treatment – topical steroids; recurrent troublesome disease may require oral tetracycline.

Severe peripheral corneal ulceration

Mooren ulcer

1. **Pathogenesis** – autoimmune process directed against a specific target antigen in the corneal stroma, possibly triggered in genetically susceptible individuals by trauma.
2. **Symptoms** – severe pain, photophobia, and blurred vision.
3. **Signs** in chronological order:
   - Progressive circumferential stromal ulceration with an undermined and infiltrated leading edge (*Fig. 9.35*).
   - Central stromal thinning, opacification, and vascularization (*Fig. 9.36*).
   - Healing stage – thinning, vascularization, and scarring (*Fig. 9.37*).

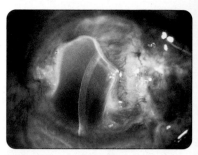

Fig. 9.36 Advanced Mooren ulcer

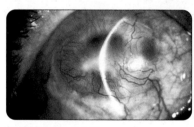

Fig. 9.37 Healed Mooren ulcer

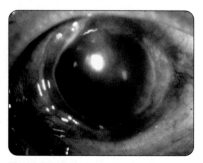

Fig. 9.35 Mooren ulcer

4. **Complications** – severe astigmatism, bacterial infection, cataract, and glaucoma.

5. **Treatment**
   a. *Topical* – steroids or ciclosporin, and collagenase inhibitors (acetylcysteine or L-cysteine).
   b. *Conjunctival resection* or *cryotherapy* – may be combined with excision of necrotic tissue.
   c. *Systemic ciclosporin*.
   d. *Surgery* – lamellar dissection of the residual central island in advanced disease.

Peripheral ulcerative keratitis

1. **Pathogenesis** – in patients with an underlying autoimmune disease there is immune complex deposition in peripheral cornea.

2. Signs

- Crescent-shaped ulceration and stromal infiltration at the limbus (Fig. 9.38).
- Circumferentially and occasionally central spread.
- Scleral spread may occur (unlike Mooren ulcer).
- End stage – 'contact lens' cornea (Fig. 9.39).

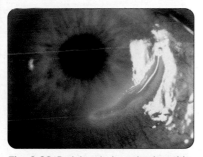

Fig. 9.38 Peripheral ulcerative keratitis

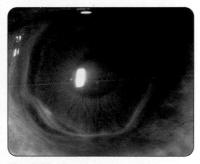

Fig. 9.39 'Contact lens' cornea

3. Associated systemic diseases

- Common – rheumatoid arthritis and Wegener granulomatosis.
- Rare – relapsing polychondritis and systemic lupus erythematosus.

4. Treatment – oral steroids and cytotoxic agents; cyclophosphamide for Wegener granulomatosis.

Neurotrophic keratitis

1. Pathogenesis – loss of the trigeminal innervation resulting in anaesthesia culminating in epithelial breakdown and persistent ulceration.

2. Causes

- **a.** *Acquired damage* – to the 5th nerve or trigeminal ganglion.
- **b.** *Systemic diseases* – diabetes and leprosy.
- **c.** *Ocular disease* – herpes simplex and zoster keratitis, abuse of topical anaesthetic, chemical burns, and refractive corneal surgery.
- **d.** *Congenital* – familial dysautonomia (Riley–Day syndrome), Möbius syndrome, Goldenhar syndrome, anhidrotic ectodermal dysplasia, and hereditary sensory neuropathy.

3. Signs

- Decreased corneal sensation.
- Interpalpebral punctate keratopathy with epithelial irregularity and oedema (Fig. 9.40).
- Persistent epithelial defect in which the edge appears rolled and thickened, and is poorly attached (Fig. 9.41).
- Enlargement of epithelial defect and stromal infiltration (Fig. 9.42).
- Stromal corneal melting (Fig. 9.43) but rarely perforation.

4. Treatment – topical lubricants and protection of the ocular surface with simple taping, bandage contact lenses, tarsorrhaphy, and botulinum toxin injection to induce ptosis.

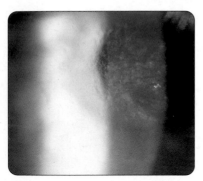

Fig. 9.40 Early neurotrophic keratitis

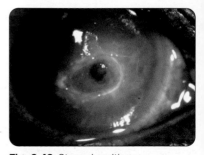

Fig. 9.43 Stromal melting

Exposure keratitis

1. **Pathogenesis** – incomplete lid closure (lagophthalmos) during blinking resulting in epithelial drying despite normal tear production.
2. **Causes**
   a. *Facial nerve palsy.*
   b. *Reduced muscle tone* – coma or Parkinsonism.
   c. *Mechanical* – eyelid scarring and tight facial skin (*Fig. 9.44*).
   d. *Severe proptosis.*

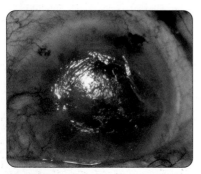

Fig. 9.41 Persistent epithelial defect

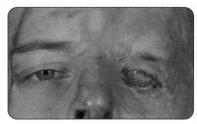

Fig. 9.44 Lagophthalmos due to scarring

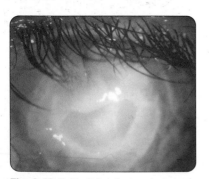

Fig. 9.42 Epithelial defect and stromal infiltration

3. Signs

- Inferior punctate epitheliopathy.
- Inferior epithelial breakdown (*Fig. 9.45*)
- Stromal thinning (*Fig. 9.46*) which may result in perforation.
- Secondary infection may supervene at any stage.

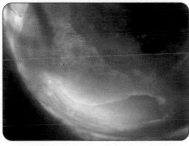

Fig. 9.45 Epithelial defect

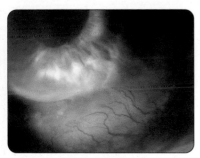

Fig. 9.46 Stromal thinning

4. Treatment

a. *Reversible exposure* – lubricants, taping of the eyelids at night, protective contact lenses, and temporary tarsorrhaphy or Frost suture.

b. *Permanent exposure* – permanent tarsorrhaphy.

Miscellaneous keratitis

Rosacea keratitis

1. **Symptoms** – non-specific irritation, burning and lacrimation.
2. **Lids** – margin telangiectasia, and intractable posterior blepharitis often associated with recurrent meibomian cyst formation.
3. **Conjunctiva** – hyperaemia, and rarely granulomas and phlyctenulosis.
4. **Cornea**
   - Inferior punctate epitheliopathy.
   - Peripheral vascularization and inferonasal and inferotemporal marginal keratitis (*Fig. 9.47*).
   - Circumferential spread and thinning (*Fig. 9.48*).
   - Perforation is rare.
   - Corneal scarring and vascularization (*Fig. 9.49*).

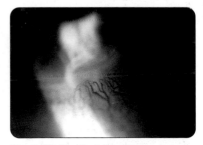

Fig. 9.47 Marginal keratitis

5. Treatment

a. *Topical* – lid hygiene, fusidic acid ointment at bedtime for 4 weeks, and fluorometholone 0.1% as a short-term measure.

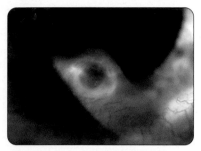

Fig. 9.48 Stromal thinning

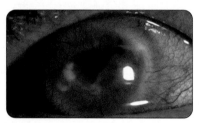

Fig. 9.49 Scarring and vascularization

b. *Systemic* – oxytetracycline 500 mg b.d. or doxycycline 100 mg daily.

Infectious crystalline keratitis

1. **Pathogenesis** – indolent infection, usually with *S. viridans,* associated with long-term topical steroid therapy most frequently following penetrating keratoplasty.
2. **Signs** – slowly progressive, grey-white, branching stromal opacities with intact overlying epithelium (*Fig. 9.50*).
3. **Treatment** – topical antibiotics for several weeks.

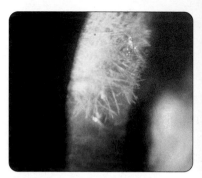

Fig. 9.50 Infectious crystalline keratitis

Thygeson superficial punctate keratitis

1. **Symptoms** – recurrent attacks of irritation, photophobia and tearing.
2. **Signs** – coarse, distinct, granular, greyish, elevated epithelial lesions (*Fig. 9.51*).

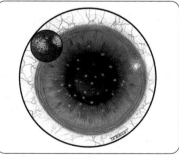

Fig. 9.51 Thygeson superficial punctate keratitis

3. Treatment
  a. *Topical* – lubricants, weak steroids, and ciclosporin.
  b. *Contact lenses* – if steroids are contraindicated.
  c. *Phototherapeutic keratectomy* – for short-term relief.

Filamentary keratitis

1. Causes
  - KCS.
  - Superior limbic keratoconjunctivitis.
  - Essential blepharospasm.
  - Corneal epithelial instability.
  - Prolonged patching of the eye.

2. Symptoms
  – discomfort and foreign body sensation.

3. Signs
  – strands of degenerating epithelial cells and mucus attached at one end to the cornea (*Fig. 9.52*).

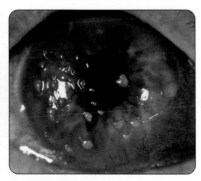

Fig. 9.52 Filaments

4. Treatment
  a. *General*
  - Treatment of underlying cause such as KCS.
  - Short-term topical steroids.
  - Topical diclofenac.

  b. *Specific for filaments*
  - Mechanical removal of filaments.
  - Hypertonic 5% saline to encourage adhesion of loose epithelium.
  - Mucolytic agents (acetylcysteine).
  - Bandage contact lenses.

Recurrent corneal epithelial erosions

1. Pathogenesis
  – weak attachment between the basal cells of the corneal epithelium and the basement membrane that may be associated with previous trauma, epithelial membrane dystrophy, or anterior stromal dystrophy.

2. Presentation
  – severe pain, spasm, and watering occurring during the night or on wakening.

3. Signs
  - Epithelial microcysts or a frank epithelial defect particularly in the interpalpebral zone and lower half of the cornea.
  - Extent of loose epithelium may be highlighted by epithelial pooling with fluorescein (*Fig. 9.53*).

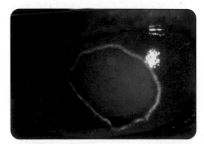

Fig. 9.53 Corneal erosion stained with fluorescein

4. Treatment

a. *Acute symptoms*
- Simple abrasions close faster without patching.
- A bandage contact lens to control pain.
- Topical antibiotics and cycloplegics.
- Topical diclofenac to reduce discomfort.

b. *Recurrent symptoms*
- Topical lubricant gel or ointment at night.
- Bandage contact lens.
- Excimer laser ablation after epithelial debridement.
- Anterior stromal puncture for localized areas off the visual axis.

Xerophthalmia

1. **Pathogenesis** – lack of vitamin A in the diet caused by malnutrition, malabsorption, chronic alcoholism, or highly selective dieting.
2. **Symptoms** – night blindness and ocular irritation.
3. **Conjunctiva**
   - Interpalpebral dryness and keratinization.
   - Patches of foamy keratinized epithelium in the interpalpebral zone (Bitot spot – *Fig. 9.54*).

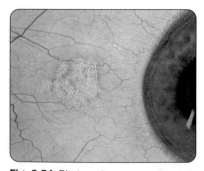

Fig. 9.54 Bitot spot

4. **Cornea**
   - Lustreless appearance due to secondary xerosis.
   - Epithelial defect and stromal liquefaction (keratomalacia).
5. **Retinopathy** – yellowish peripheral dots and decreased ERG amplitude in advanced cases.
6. **Treatment of keratomalacia** – oral or intramuscular vitamin A.

Corneal ectasias

Keratoconus

1. **Definition** – conical shaped cornea secondary to stromal thinning and protrusion.
2. **Presentation** – during puberty with unilateral impairment of vision due to progressive myopia and astigmatism.
3. **Signs** – usually bilateral but often asymmetrical.
   - 'Oil droplet' reflex on direct ophthalmoscopy.
   - Irregular 'scissor' reflex on retinoscopy.
   - Fine, vertical, deep stromal striae (Vogt lines – *Fig. 9.55*).
   - Epithelial iron deposits may surround the base of the cone (Fleischer ring).
   - Progressive corneal thinning and severe irregular myopic astigmatism (*Fig. 9.56*).
   - Bulging of the lower lid in downgaze (Munson sign – *Fig. 9.57*).
   - Acute hydrops caused by a rupture in Descemet membrane (*Fig. 9.58*).
   - Stromal scarring following resolution of hydrops (*Fig. 9.59*).

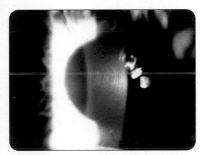

Fig. 9.55 Vogt lines

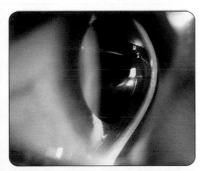

Fig. 9.56 Keratoconus

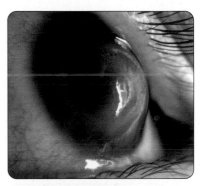

Fig. 9.58 Acute hydrops

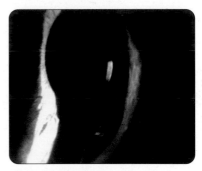

Fig. 9.59 Stromal scarring

4. **Corneal topography** – irregular astigmatism (*Fig. 9.60*).

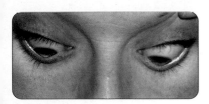

Fig. 9.57 Munson sign

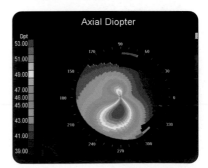

Fig. 9.60 Corneal topography showing 5.75 D of astigmatism

5. Associations

  a. *Systemic* – Down, Turner, Ehlers–Danlos and Marfan syndromes, atopy, and osteogenesis imperfecta.

  b. *Ocular* – vernal keratoconjunctivitis, blue sclera, aniridia, ectopia lentis, Leber congenital amaurosis, RP, and persistent eye rubbing.

6. Treatment

  a. *Rigid contact lenses* – for high astigmatism.

  b. *Keratoplasty* – in advanced progressive disease, especially with significant corneal scarring.

Pellucid marginal degeneration

1. Definition – progressive, peripheral corneal thinning involving the inferior cornea.

2. Presentation – 4th–5th decade with reduced visual acuity due to astigmatism.

3. Signs

  • Bilateral, slowly progressive, crescent-shaped band of inferior corneal thinning extending from 4 to 8 o'clock, 1 mm from the limbus (*Fig. 9.61*).

  • Ectatic cornea above the thin area.

  • Acute hydrops and spontaneous perforation are rare.

4. Corneal topography – 'butterfly' pattern (*Fig. 9.62*).

5. Treatment

  a. *Rigid gas-permeable contact lenses*.

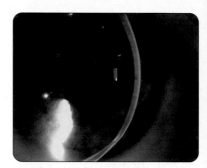

Fig. 9.61 Pellucid marginal degeneration

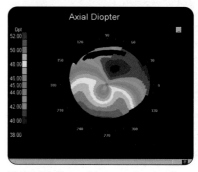

Fig. 9.62 Corneal topography showing severe astigmatism and inferior steepening

  b. *Surgery* – large eccentric penetrating keratoplasty, thermocauterization, crescentic lamellar keratoplasty, wedge resection of diseased tissue, epikeratoplasty, and intracorneal ring implantation.

Keratoglobus

1. **Definitions** – rare congenital condition in which the entire cornea is abnormally thin.
2. **Signs**
   - Generalized corneal thinning and global protrusion (*Fig. 9.63*).
   - Acute hydrops is uncommon.
   - Corneal rupture on relatively mild trauma.

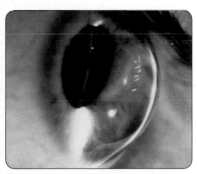

Fig. 9.63 Keratoglobus

3. **Corneal topography** – generalized steepening (*Fig. 9.64*).

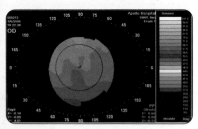

Fig. 9.64 Corneal topography showing generalized steepening

4. **Treatment** – scleral contact lenses.
5. **Systemic associations** – Leber congenital amaurosis and blue sclera.

Epithelial dystrophies

Epithelial basement membrane dystrophy

1. **Inheritance** – usually sporadic, rarely AD.
2. **Onset** – 10% of patients develop recurrent corneal erosions in the 3rd decade; the remainder are asymptomatic throughout life.
3. **Signs** (*Fig. 9.65*)
   - Dot-like opacities.
   - Epithelial microcysts.
   - Subepithelial map-like patterns surrounded by a faint haze.
   - Whorled fingerprint-like lines.

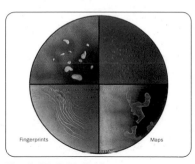

Fig. 9.65 Epithelial basement membrane dystrophy

4. **Histology** – thickening of the basement membrane with deposition of fibrillary protein between it and Bowman layer, and absence of hemidesmosomes of the basal epithelial cells.
5. **Treatment** – that of recurrent corneal erosions.

Meesmann dystrophy

1. **Inheritance** – AD (gene locus on 12q13 or 17q12).

2. **Onset** – early childhood with mild ocular irritation.
3. **Signs** – myriads of tiny intraepithelial cysts maximal centrally (*Fig. 9.66*).

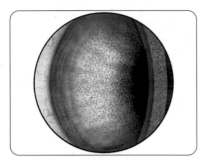

Fig. 9.66 Meesman dystrophy

4. **Histology** – irregular thickening of the epithelial basement membrane and intraepithelial cysts.
5. **Treatment** – lubrication.

Bowman layer dystrophies

Reis–Bückler dystrophy (Bowman layer 1 or corneal dystrophy of Bowman – CDB1)

1. **Inheritance** – AD (gene locus on 5q31).
2. **Onset** – 1st–2nd decade with painful recurrent corneal erosions.
3. **Signs** – fine, grey-white, round and polygonal opacities in Bowman layer (*Fig. 9.67*).
4. **Histology** – replacement of Bowman layer and the epithelial basement membrane with fibrous tissue.

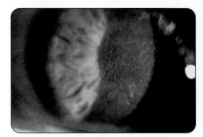

Fig. 9.67 Reis–Bückler dystrophy

5. **Treatment** – excimer laser keratectomy.

Thiel–Behnke dystrophy (Bowman layer 2 or corneal dystrophy of Bowman – CDB2)

1. **Inheritance** – AD (gene locus on 10q24).
2. **Onset** – end of the 1st decade with recurrent erosions.
3. **Signs** – that of Reis–Bückler except that the opacities have a more honeycomb pattern (*Fig. 9.68*).

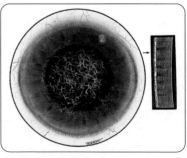

Fig. 9.68 Thiel–Behnke dystrophy

4. Histology – 'curly fibres' in Bowman layer.
5. Treatment – may not be necessary because visual impairment is less than in Reis–Bückler dystrophy.

Schnyder crystalline dystrophy

1. Pathogenesis – disorder of corneal lipid metabolism associated with raised serum cholesterol in approximately 50% of cases.
2. Inheritance – AD (gene locus on 1p36).
3. Onset – 2nd decade with visual impairment and glare.
4. Signs
- Central, oval, subepithelial 'crystalline' opacity.
- Diffuse corneal haze and prominent corneal arcus (*Fig. 9.69*).

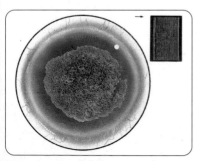

Fig. 9.69 Schnyder crystalline dystrophy

5. Histology – deposits of phospholipids and cholesterol.
6. Treatment – excimer laser keratectomy.

Stromal dystrophies

Lattice dystrophy type 1 (Biber–Haab–Dimmer)

1. Inheritance – AD (gene locus on 5q31).
2. Onset – end of the 1st decade with recurrent erosions which precede typical stromal changes.
3. Signs in chronological order:
- Glassy anterior stromal dots.
- Fine lattice lines best seen on retroillumination.
- Deep and outward spread sparing the periphery.
- Generalized stromal haze that may obscure the lattice lines (*Fig. 9.70*).

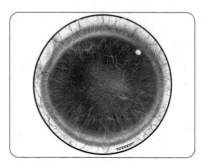

Fig. 9.70 Advanced lattice dystrophy type 1

4. Histology – amyloid that stains with Congo red and shows green birefringence when viewed with a polarized filter.
5. Treatment – keratoplasty before the 6th decade.

Lattice dystrophy type 2 (Meretoja syndrome)

1. **Inheritance** – AD (gene locus on 9q34).
2. **Onset** – 3rd decade with recurrent erosions.
3. **Signs** – sparse lattice lines which are more delicate and more radially orientated (*Fig. 9.71*) than in type 1 lattice.

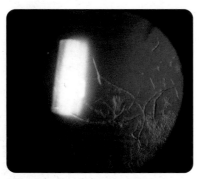

Fig. 9.71 Lattice dystrophy type 2

4. **Histology** – amyloid deposits in the corneal stroma.
5. **Treatment** – keratoplasty in the 7th decade.
6. **Systemic association** – amyloidosis.

Lattice dystrophy type 3 and 3A

1. **Inheritance** – type 3 is AR; type 3A is AD (gene locus on 5q31 in both).
2. **Onset**
   • Type 3 – 4th–6th decade with visual impairment.
   • Type 3A – presents later.
3. **Signs** – thick stromal lines with minimal intervening haze (*Fig. 9.72*).
4. **Treatment** – keratoplasty.

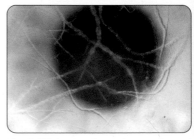

Fig. 9.72 Lattice dystrophy type 3

Granular dystrophy type 1

1. **Inheritance** – AD (gene locus on 5q31).
2. **Onset** – 1st decade but vision is not affected until later.
3. **Signs** in chronological order:
   • Small, white, deposits resembling crumbs, rings or snowflakes in the central anterior stroma (*Fig. 9.73*).
   • Gradual increase in number and size with deeper and outward spread but not reaching the limbus (*Fig. 9.74*).
   • Gradual confluence and diffuse haze of intervening stroma.

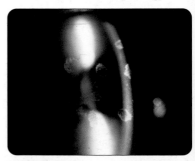

Fig. 9.73 Early granular dystrophy type 1

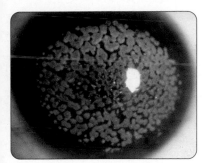

Fig. 9.74 Advanced granular dystrophy type 1

4. **Histology** – amorphous hyaline deposits which stain bright red with Masson trichrome.
5. **Treatment** – keratoplasty by the 5th decade.

Granular dystrophy type 2 (Avellino)

1. **Inheritance** – AD (gene locus on 5q31).
2. **Onset** – 2nd decade.
3. **Signs**
   * Superficial, fine, opacities similar to granular dystrophy type 1.
   * Deeper linear opacities reminiscent of lattice dystrophy (*Fig. 9.75*).

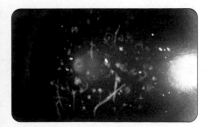

Fig. 9.75 Granular dystrophy type 2 (Avellino)

4. **Histology** – hyaline and amyloid in the stroma that stains with Masson trichrome and Congo red.
5. **Treatment** – not required.

Macular dystrophy

1. **Inheritance** – AR (gene locus on 16q22).
2. **Onset** – end of 1st decade with visual deterioration.
3. **Signs** in chronological order:
   * Central anterior stromal haze.
   * Greyish-white, dense, poorly delineated spots in the anterior stroma centrally and posterior stroma in the periphery (*Fig. 9.76*).
   * Full-thickness involvement associated with thinning (*Fig. 9.77*).

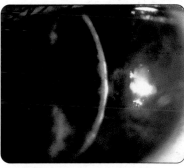

Fig. 9.76 Early macular dystrophy

4. **Histology** – abnormally close packing of collagen in the corneal lamellae and abnormal aggregations of glycosaminoglycans which stain with Prussian blue and colloidal iron.

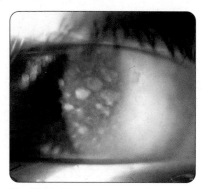

Fig. 9.77 Advanced macular dystrophy

5. Treatment – penetrating kerato-plasty.

Gelatinous drop-like dystrophy

1. **Inheritance** – AR.
2. **Onset** – 1st–2nd decade with severe photophobia, watering, and visual impairment.
3. **Signs** in chronological order:
   - Grey subepithelial nodules.
   - Gradual confluence and stromal involvement giving rise to a mulberry-like appearance (*Fig. 9.78*).
3. **Histology** – subepithelial and anterior stromal accumulation of amyloid.
4. **Treatment** – superficial keratectomy.

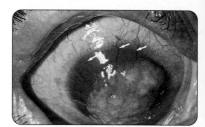

Fig. 9.78 Gelatinous dystrophy

Central cloudy dystrophy of François

1. **Inheritance** – AD.
2. **Signs** – non-progressive polygonal, cloudy grey opacities separated by relatively clear spaces, in the posterior stroma most prominent centrally, creating a leather-like appearance (*Fig. 9.79*).

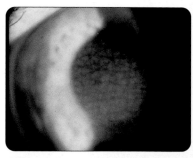

Fig. 9.79 Central cloudy dystrophy of François

3. **Treatment** – not required.

Endothelial dystrophies

Fuchs endothelial dystrophy

1. **Pathogenesis** – accelerated corneal endothelial cell loss.
2. **Inheritance** – usually sporadic, occasionally AD.
3. **Onset** – old age.
4. **Staging**
   a. *Stage 1* (cornea guttata).
   • Irregular excrescences of Descemet membrane (*Fig. 9.80a*).
   • 'Beaten metal' appearance which may be associated with melanin deposition in more advanced cases.
   b. *Stage 2* – central stromal oedema.
   c. *Stage 3* – bullous keratopathy (*Fig. 9.80b*).

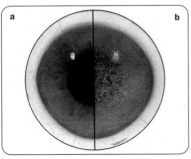

Fig. 9.80 Fuchs dystrophy. (a) Corneal guttata; (b) bullous keratopathy

5. **Treatment**
   a. *Topical* – sodium chloride 5% drops or ointment.
   b. *Bandage contact lenses* – for comfort.
   c. *Penetrating keratoplasty* – in advanced cases.
   d. *Other options* – conjunctival flaps and amniotic membrane transplants.

Posterior polymorphous dystrophy

1. **Pathogenesis** – endothelial cells display characteristics similar to epithelium.
2. **Inheritance** – AD (gene locus on 20q11 and 1p34–p32.2).
3. **Onset** – perinatal although identified much later.
4. **Signs** – vesicular, band-like or diffuse endothelial lesions which may be asymmetrical (*Fig. 9.81*).

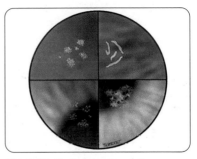

Fig. 9.81 Posterior polymorphous dystrophy

5. **Associations** – iris membranes, peripheral anterior synechiae, ectropion uveae, corectopia, polycoria, glaucoma, and Alport syndrome.
6. **Treatment** – not required.

Congenital hereditary endothelial dystrophy

1. **Pathogenesis** – focal or generalized absence of corneal endothelium; two types, CHED1 and CHED2, the latter being more severe.

2. Inheritance
- CHED1 is AD (gene locus on 20p11.2–q11.2).
- CHED2 is AR (gene locus on 20p13).

3. Onset – perinatal.

4. Signs
- Bilateral, symmetrical, diffuse corneal oedema.
- Corneal appearance varies from a blue-grey ground-glass (*Fig. 9.82*) to total opacification.

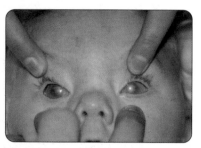

Fig. 9.82 Congenital hereditary endothelial dystrophy

5. Treatment – keratoplasty.

Age-related degenerations

Arcus senilis

1. Systemic associations
- Occasional – familial and non-familial dyslipoproteinaemias.
- Frequent – type 2 hyperlipoproteinaemia.

2. Signs
- Circumferential perilimbal 1mm wide band consisting of stromal lipid deposits separated from the limbus by a clear zone (*Fig. 9.83*).
- The clear zone may occasionally undergo mild thinning (senile furrow – *Fig. 9.84*).

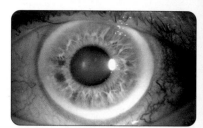

Fig. 9.83 Arcus senilis

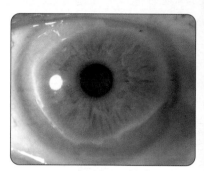

Fig. 9.84 Senile furrow

Vogt limbal girdle

This is a common, innocuous condition characterized by bilateral, narrow, crescentic lines composed of chalk-like flecks running in the interpalpebral fissure along the nasal and temporal limbus (*Fig. 9.85*). Type 1 is separated from the limbus by a clear interval but type 2 is not.

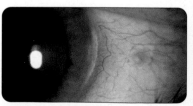

Fig. 9.85 Vogt limbal girdle

Cornea farinata

This is an innocuous condition characterized by minute, usually bilateral, flour-like deposits in the deep corneal stroma, most prominent centrally (*Fig. 9.86*).

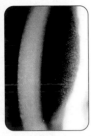

Fig. 9.86 Cornea farinata

Crocodile shagreen

This is a usually asymptomatic condition characterized by greyish-white, polygonal stromal opacities separated by relatively clear spaces (*Fig. 9.87*). The opacities most frequently involve the anterior two-thirds of the stroma (anterior crocodile shagreen), although on occasion they may be found more posteriorly (posterior crocodile shagreen).

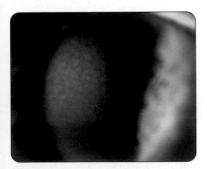

Fig. 9.87 Crocodile shagreen

Other degenerations

Lipid keratopathy

1. **Primary** – white or yellowish stromal deposits consisting of cholesterol, fats and phospholipids not associated with vascularization.
2. **Secondary** – associated with previous ocular injury or disease which has resulted in corneal vascularization (*Fig. 9.88*).

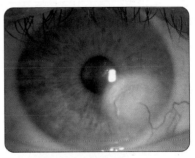

Fig. 9.88 Lipid keratopathy

3. **Treatment** – medical control of the underlying inflammatory disease; other options include:
   a. *Argon laser photocoagulation* – to arterial 'feeder' vessels.
   b. *Needle point cautery.*
   c. *Penetrating keratoplasty* – for advanced but quiescent disease.

Band keratopathy

1. **Causes**
   a. *Ocular* – chronic anterior uveitis (particularly in children), phthisis bulbi, silicone oil in the anterior chamber, chronic corneal oedema, and severe chronic keratitis.
   b. *Age-related.*
   c. *Metabolic* – raised serum calcium and phosphorus, hyperuricaemia, and chronic renal failure.
   d. *Hereditary* – familial cases and ichthyosis.
2. **Signs** in chronological order:
   • Peripheral interpalpebral calcification.
   • Gradual central spread to form a band-like chalky plaque containing small holes (*Fig. 9.89*).

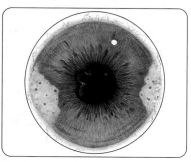

Fig. 9.89 Band keratopathy

3. **Histology** – deposition of calcium salts in Bowman layer, epithelial basement membrane and anterior stroma.
4. **Treatment options** – chelation, Nd:YAG laser removal, lamellar keratoplasty, and phototherapeutic keratectomy.

Spheroidal degeneration

1. **Predisposition** – exposure to ultraviolet light.
2. **Signs** in chronological order:
   • Amber-coloured granules in the superficial stroma of the peripheral interpalpebral cornea.
   • Increasing opacification, coalescence, and central spread.
   • Nodular lesions and surrounded by hazy stroma (*Fig. 9.90*).

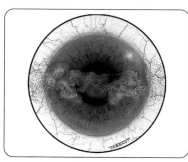

Fig. 9.90 Spheroidal degeneration

3. **Histology** – irregular protein deposits in the anterior stroma that replace Bowman layer.
4. **Treatment options** – superficial keratectomy or lamellar keratoplasty.

Salzmann nodular degeneration

1. **Predisposition** – chronic keratitis, especially trachoma.
2. **Signs** – discrete, nodular, superficial stromal opacities (*Fig. 9.91*).
3. **Treatment** – similar to that of spheroidal degeneration.

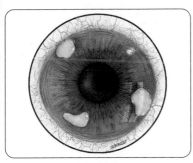

Fig. 9.91 Salzmann degeneration

Terrien marginal degeneration

1. **Definition** – uncommon, idiopathic, non-inflammatory thinning of the peripheral cornea.
2. **Presentation** – 4th decade initially without symptoms.
3. **Signs** in chronological order:
   - Fine, yellow-white, stromal opacities that spread circumferentially and are separated from the limbus by a clear zone.
   - Progressive guttering and vascularization (*Fig. 9.92*).
   - Formation of pseudopterygia.

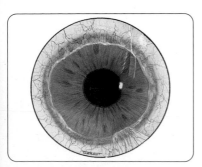

Fig. 9.92 Terrien marginal degeneration

4. **Treatment** – gas-permeable scleral contact lenses for early cases and excision of the gutter if advanced.

Metabolic keratopathies in systemic diseases

Cystinosis

1. **Pathogenesis** – AR metabolic disorder characterized by widespread deposition of cystine crystals as a result of a defect in lysosomal transport.
2. **Presentation** – in infancy with photophobia and blepharospasm.
3. **Keratopathy** – cystine crystals in the cornea and conjunctiva (*Fig. 9.93*).

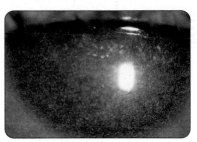

Fig. 9.93 Cystinosis

4. **Treatment** – topical cysteamine.

Mucopolysaccharidoses

1. **Pathogenesis** – inherited deficiencies of catabolic glycosidase necessary for hydrolysis of mucopolysaccharides of which there are six subtypes.
2. **Inheritance** – AR except with the two subtypes of Hunter syndrome which are X-LR.

3. Keratopathy
- Punctate corneal opacification and diffuse stromal haze in all except Hunter and Sanfilippo.
- In Hurler and Scheie syndromes opacification is most severe and present at birth (*Fig. 9.94*).

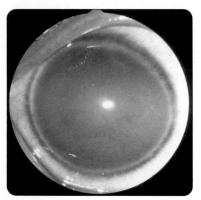

Fig. 9.94 Corneal opacification in Hurler syndrome

4. Other ocular features
  a. *Pigmentary retinopathy* – in all except Morquio and Maroteaux–Lamy.
  b. *Optic atrophy* – in all six MPS and most severe in Hurler.
  c. *Glaucoma* – uncommon.

Wilson disease

1. **Pathogenesis** – deficiency of caeruloplasmin resulting widespread deposition of copper.
2. **Presentation** – liver disease, basal ganglia dysfunction or psychiatric disturbances.

3. **Keratopathy** – zone of copper granules in the peripheral part of Descemet membrane (Kayser–Fleischer ring) which change colour under different types of illumination (*Fig. 9.95*).

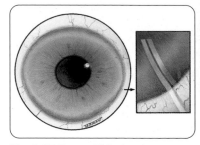

Fig. 9.95 Kayser–Fleischer ring

4. **Anterior capsular 'sunflower' cataract** – in some patients.

Lecithin-cholesterol-acyltransferase deficiency (Norum disease)

1. **Definition** – AR disease characterized by hyperlipidaemia, early atheroma, anaemia, and renal disease.
2. **Keratopathy** – minute, greyish dots throughout the stroma, often concentrated in the periphery in an arcus-like configuration (*Fig. 9.96*).

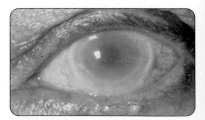

Fig. 9.96 Keratopathy in Norum disease

Fabry disease (angiokeratoma corporis diffusum)

1. **Pathogenesis** – X-L lysosomal storage disorder caused by deficiency of alpha-galactosidase A.
2. **Keratopathy** – faint but extensive vortex changes similar to chloroquine keratopathy (*Fig. 9.97*).

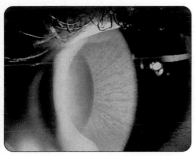

Fig. 9.97 Keratopathy in Fabry disease

3. **Other ocular manifestations** – wedge-shaped cataract, conjunctival vascular tortuosity, retinal vascular tortuosity (especially venous), 3rd nerve palsy, and nystagmus.

Tyrosinaemia type 2 (Richner–Hanhart syndrome)

1. **Pathogenesis** – AR disease in which deficiency of hepatic cytosolic tyrosine aminotransferase results in increase in plasma tyrosine levels.
2. **Keratopathy** – bilateral, pseudo-dendritic keratitis with crystalline edges but absence of terminal bulbs and poor staining with fluorescein.

Immunoprotein deposits

1. **Systemic associations** – multiple myeloma, Waldenström macroglobu-linaemia, idiopathic monoclonal gammopathy, lymphoproliferative disorders, and leukaemia.
2. **Signs** – bilateral bands of punctate, flake-like posterior stromal opacities (*Fig. 9.98*).

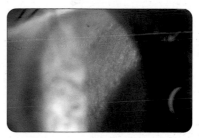

Fig. 9.98 Immunodeposit keratopathy

3. **Treatment** – chemotherapy or steroids for underlying systemic disease, and keratoplasty for severe keratopathy.

Contact lenses

Therapeutic indications
(*Fig. 9.99*)

1. **Optical** – to improve visual acuity when this cannot be achieved by spectacles in irregular astigmatism, anisometropia, aniseikonia, and prismatic effects.
2. **Promotion of epithelial healing** – persistent epithelial defects and recurrent corneal erosions.

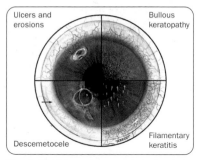

Fig. 9.99 Some therapeutic indications for contact lens wear

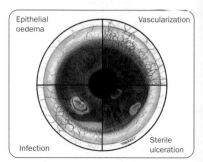

Fig. 9.100 Some complications of contact lens wear

3. **Pain relief** – bullous keratopathy, wet filamentary keratitis and Thygeson disease.
4. **Preservation of corneal integrity** – by capping a descemetocele to prevent perforation, or splinting of a small corneal wound.
5. **Miscellaneous** – ptosis props, maintenance of the fornices to prevent symblepharon formation, and to enhance drug delivery.

Complications (*Fig. 9.100*)

Mechanical and hypoxic keratitis

1. **Signs**
   a. *Superficial punctate keratitis.*
   b. *Tight lens syndrome* – indentation and staining of the conjunctival epithelium in a ring around the cornea.
   c. *Acute hypoxia* – epithelial microcysts and painful macro-erosions.
   d. *Chronic hypoxia* – vascularization and lipid deposition.

2. **Management**
   - Increasing oxygen permeability by changing the type of lens.
   - Modifying lens fit to increase movement.
   - Reduction of lens wearing time.

Immune response keratitis

1. **Signs** – red eye associated with marginal infiltrates with no or minimal epithelial defects.
2. **Management**
   - Contact lens wear should be stopped until resolution occurs.
   - Topical antibiotics and steroids may be used in severe cases and it is also important to review lens fit and hygiene.

Toxic keratitis

1. **Pathogenesis**
   - Acute chemical injury caused by placing a contact lens on the eye without neutralizing hydrogen peroxide or surfactant cleaners.
   - Chronic toxicity from disinfecting agents such as thiomersal or benzalkonium chloride.

2. Signs
- Acute pain, redness, and chemosis on lens insertion which may take 48 hours to resolve completely.
- Vascularization and scarring of the cornea and limbal conjunctiva in chronic cases.

3. Treatment
– fitting of daily disposable contact lenses and a non-preserved disinfectant used such as hydrogen peroxide or heat.

Suppurative keratitis

Contact lens wear is the greatest risk factor for the development of infectious keratitis particularly with *P. aeruginosa* and *Acanthamoeba* spp. Following an abrasion and hypoxia bacteria can attach and penetrate the epithelium with the potential to cause infection. Bacteria and amoebae may also be introduced onto the corneal surface by poor lens hygiene or the use of tap water.

Keratoplasty

Penetrating keratoplasty

1. **Definition** – operation in which abnormal host tissue is replaced by a full-thickness disc of healthy donor cornea.
2. **Indications** – optical, tectonic (to preserve corneal integrity), therapeutic (to remove infected tissue), and cosmetic.
3. **Technique**
   a. *Determination of graft size* – with trephines with different diameters or a caliper.
   b. *Preparation of donor cornea* – trephining of previously excised corneoscleral button.

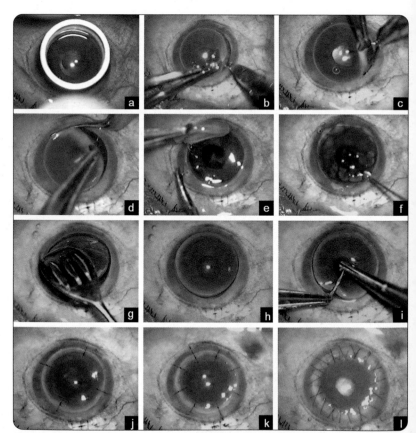

Fig. 10.1 Technique of penetrating keratoplasty

c. *Excision of diseased host tissue* (Fig. 10.1a–e).

d. *Insertion of viscoelastic substance* (Fig. 10.1f).

e. *Fixation of donor button* (Fig. 10.1g–l).

4. **Postoperative management**

   a. *Topical steroids* – initially 2-hourly then q.i.d. for a few weeks.

   b. *Mydriatics* – 2–3 weeks.

   c. *Removal of sutures* – after 12–18 months.

5. **Complications**

   a. *Early* – persistent epithelial defects, irritation by protruding sutures, wound leak, flat anterior chamber, iris prolapse, uveitis, elevation of intraocular pressure and infection.

   b. *Late* – astigmatism, recurrence of initial disease process on the graft, wound separation, retrocorneal membrane formation, glaucoma, and CMO.

   c. *Rejection* – endothelial rejection (Fig. 10.2) is the most common and most dangerous; epithelial (Fig. 10.3) and stromal rejection (Fig. 10.4) are less frequent and respond readily to topical steroids.

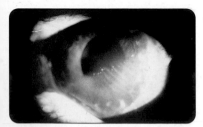

Fig. 10.2 Khodadoust line in endothelial rejection

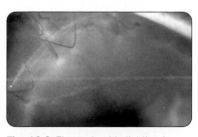

Fig. 10.3 Elevated epithelial line in epithelial rejection

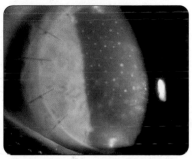

Fig. 10.4 Krachmer spots in stromal rejection

Superficial anterior lamellar keratoplasty

1. **Definition** – partial thickness excision of the corneal epithelium and stroma so that the endothelium and part of deep stroma are left behind.

2. **Indications**
   - Opacification of the superficial one-third of the corneal stroma.
   - Marginal corneal thinning or infiltration as in Terrien marginal degeneration.
   - Localized thinning or descemetocele formation.

3. Technique – similar to penetrating keratoplasty except that only a partial thickness of cornea is grafted.

Deep anterior lamellar keratoplasty

1. Definition – removal of opaque corneal tissue almost to the level of Descemet membrane.

2. Indications
- Disease involving the anterior 95% of corneal thickness with a normal endothelium and absence of breaks or scars in Descemet membrane.
- Chronic inflammatory disease such as atopic keratoconjunctivitis which carries an increased risk of graft rejection.

3. Advantages
- No risk of endothelial rejection although epithelial rejection may occur.
- Less astigmatism and a structurally stronger globe.
- Increased availability of graft material since endothelial quality is irrelevant.

4. Disadvantages – difficult and time-consuming.

Keratoprosthesis

1. Definition – artificial corneal implants consisting of the patient's own tooth root and alveolar bone which support the central optical cylinder.

2. Indications
- Severe bilateral visual impairment but normal optic nerve and retinal function.
- Severe, debilitating but inactive anterior segment disease with no realistic chance of success from conventional keratoplasty.

- Multiple previous failed corneal grafts or other types of ocular surface reconstruction such as amniotic membrane or stem cell grafting.

3. Complications – glaucoma, retroprosthesis membrane formation, tilting or extrusion of the cylinder (*Fig. 10.5*), RD, and endophthalmitis.

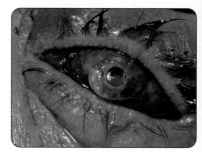

Fig. 10.5 Extrusion of keratoprosthesis

4. Results – improvement in 80% of cases.

Refractive surgery

Refractive surgery encompasses a range of procedures aimed at changing the refraction of the eye by altering the cornea and/or crystalline lens, which constitute the principal refracting components.

Non-laser refractive procedures

1. Clear lens extraction – carries a small risk of RD.

2. Iris clip (lobster claw) implant (*Fig. 10.6*) – may become subluxated and cause an oval pupil.

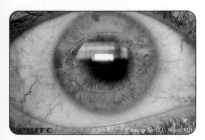

Fig. 10.6 Anterior chamber 'lobster claw' implant

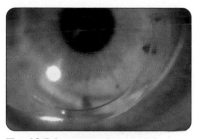

Fig. 10.8 Intrastromal corneal ring segment

3. **Phakic posterior chamber implant** – insertion behind the iris, in front of the crystalline lens and supported in the ciliary sulcus (*Fig. 10.7*).

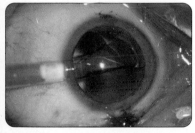

Fig. 10.7 Injection of posterior chamber implant

4. **Limbal relaxing incisions/arcuate keratotomy** – to correct astigmatism.
5. **Lens surgery** – toric IOL to correct astigmatism.
6. **Intrastromal corneal ring segments** (*Fig. 10.8*) – can be removed or replaced.

Laser refractive procedures

Photorefractive keratectomy (PRK)

1. **Principles** – excimer laser ablation to an exact depth with minimal disruption of surrounding tissue.
   - Myopia is treated by ablating the central anterior corneal surface so that it becomes flatter.
   - Hypermetropia is treated by ablation of the periphery so that the centre becomes steeper.
   - Can correct myopia up to 6 D, astigmatism up to 3 D, and low hypermetropia.
2. **Technique**
   - Corneal epithelium is scraped away to expose Bowman layer.
   - Excimer laser is applied to ablate Bowman layer and anterior stroma (*Fig. 10.9*).
3. **Complications**
   a. *Common* – slow-healing epithelial defects, corneal haze and haloes, poor night vision, and regression of refractive correction.

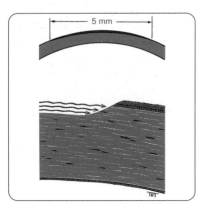

Fig. 10.9 Principles of PRK

b. *Uncommon* – decentred ablations, scarring, abnormal epithelial healing, irregular astigmatism, reduced corneal sensation, sterile infiltrates, infection, and acute corneal necrosis.

Laser in-situ keratomileusis (LASIK)

1. **Principles** – more versatile than PRK and can correct hypermetropia of up to 4 D, astigmatism of up to 5 D and myopia of up to 12 D depending on corneal thickness.
2. **Technique**
   - Very thin corneal flap is cut with an automated microtome (*Fig. 10.10*).
   - Bed is treated with excimer laser as for PRK.
   - Flap is repositioned.
3. **Complications**
   a. *Operative* – buttonholes, thin flaps, flap amputation, incomplete or irregular flaps, and rarely corneal perforation.

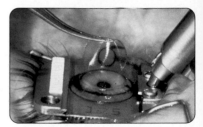

Fig. 10.10 LASIK

   b. *Postoperative* – dry eye, problems involving the flap, subepithelial haze, and granular deposits at the flap interface (sands of Sahara).

Laser epithelial keratomileusis

Laser epithelial keratomileusis (LASEK) can be used for low myopia and hypermetropia and in patients unsuitable for LASIK. The epithelial flap is formed using a solution of 18% alcohol, the bed is then treated with laser as for PRK, and the flap is repositioned. The procedure produces less haze than PRK and avoids potential flap complications of LASIK.

Femosecond assisted LASIK (IntraLASIK)

This 'all laser LESIK' is similar to conventional LASIK except that the corneal flap is created with femosecond laser rather than with a mechanical microtome. Advantages over conventional LASIK include more precise positioning of the flap, more accurate thickness of the flap, and lower probability of intraoperative complications such as buttonhole formation.

Episcleritis

Simple episcleritis

1. **Presentation** – sudden redness and discomfort.
2. **Signs** – interpalpebral sectoral or diffuse redness with maximal congestion within Tenon capsule (*Fig. 11.1*) that gradually fades over several days.

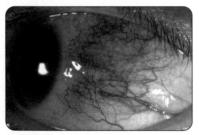

Fig. 11.1 Simple diffuse episcleritis

3. **Treatment** – topical steroids; systemic NSAID (flurbiprofen) for frequent attacks.

Nodular episcleritis

1. **Presentation** – red eye typically first noted on waking.
2. **Signs**
   - Tender nodule within the interpalpebral fissure that persists longer than simple episcleritis.
   - A slit beam shows a flat scleral surface (*Fig. 11.2*).
   - Instillation of 10% phenylephrine drops decongests the conjunctival and episcleral vessels allowing better visualization of underlying sclera.

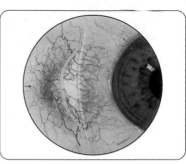

Fig. 11.2 Nodular episcleritis

3. **Treatment** – that of simple episcleritis.

Scleritis

Table 11.1 Classification of scleritis

1. **Anterior**
   a. *Non-necrotizing*
      - Diffuse
      - Nodular
   b. *Necrotizing with inflammation*
      - Vaso-occlusive
      - Granulomatous
      - Surgically-induced
   c. *Scleromalacia perforans*
2. **Posterior**

Diffuse anterior non-necrotizing scleritis

1. **Presentation** – 5th decade with redness and then aching.
2. **Signs**
   - Intense redness that may be diffuse (*Fig. 11.3*) or localized to one quadrant.
   - As the inflammation subsides scleral translucency ensues (*Fig. 11.4*).

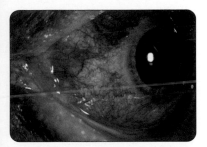

Fig. 11.3 Diffuse non-necrotizing scleritis

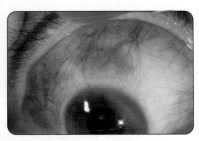

Fig. 11.4 Increased scleral translucency

Nodular anterior non-necrotizing scleritis

1. **Presentation** – insidious onset of pain followed by increasing redness.
2. **Signs**
   - One or more interpalpebral scleral nodules.
   - A slit beam is displaced by the nodule (*Fig. 11.5*).
   - Instillation of 10% phenylephrine drops will constrict the conjunctival and superficial episcleral vasculature but not the deep plexus over the nodule.
   - As the nodule subsides increased scleral translucency ensues.

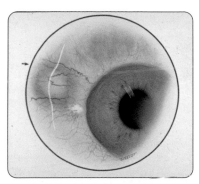

Fig. 11.5 Nodular non-necrotizing scleritis

Necrotizing anterior scleritis with inflammation

1. **Presentation** – gradual onset of pain which becomes severe and radiates to the temple, brow or jaw.
2. **Signs**
   - Nodular scleritis with deep vascular congestion.
   - Progressive scleral necrosis with exposure of underlying uvea (*Fig. 11.6*).
   - Inactive stage – uvea covered by atrophic conjunctiva (*Fig. 11.7*).

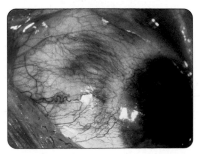

Fig. 11.6 Active necrotizing scleritis

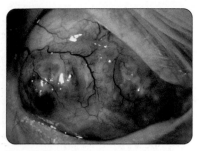

Fig. 11.7 Healed necrotizing scleritis

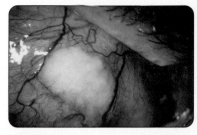

Fig. 11.9 Granulomatous necrotizing scleritis

3. Specific types of necrotizing disease

a. *Vaso-occlusive* – avascular areas of necrotic sclera, episclera, and conjunctiva (*Fig. 11.8*).

b. *Granulomatous* – raised and oedematous sclera, episclera, and conjunctiva (*Fig. 11.9*).

c. *Surgically-induced scleritis* – starts at the site of surgery and tends to remain localized to one segment (*Fig. 11.10*).

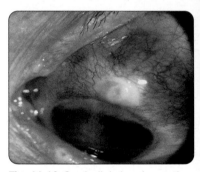

Fig. 11.10 Surgically-induced necrotizing scleritis following trabeculectomy

4. Complications

a. *Corneal* – infiltrative stromal keratitis, sclerosing keratitis (*Fig. 11.11*), and peripheral ulcerative keratitis.

b. *Other* – uveitis, uveal effusion, glaucoma, and hypotony.

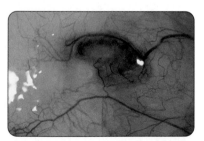

Fig. 11.8 Vaso-occlusive necrotizing scleritis

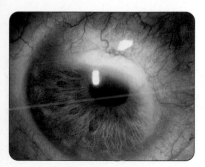

Fig. 11.11 Sclerosing keratitis

Scleromalacia perforans

1. **Definition** – specific type of necrotizing scleritis without inflammation that typically affects elderly women with longstanding rheumatoid arthritis.
2. **Signs** in chronological order:
   - Yellow scleral necrotic plaques near the limbus without vascular congestion that gradually coalesce (*Fig. 11.12*).
   - Very slow progression of scleral thinning and exposure of underlying uvea (*Fig. 11.13*).

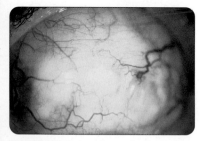

Fig. 11.12 Early scleromalacia perforans

3. **Treatment** – usually not appropriate.

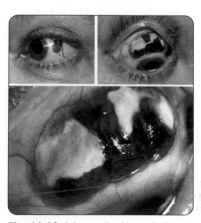

Fig. 11.13 Advanced scleromalacia perforans

Posterior scleritis

1. **Signs**
   a. *Exudative RD* – in about 25% of cases (*Fig. 11.14*).
   b. *Uveal effusion* – exudative RD and choroidal detachment.
   c. *Choroidal folds.*
   d. *Yellowish-brown subretinal mass* (*Fig. 11.15*).
   e. *Disc oedema.*
   f. *Myositis* – diplopia, pain on eye movement, tenderness to touch and redness around a muscle insertion.
   g. *Proptosis* – mild and frequently associated with ptosis.

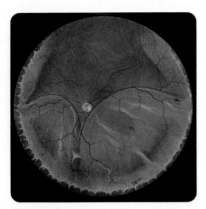

Fig. 11.14 Exudative retinal detachment

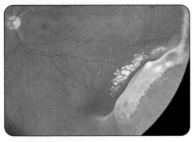

Fig. 11.15 Subretinal mass

2. US – scleral thickening and fluid in Tenon space gives rise to the characteristic 'T' sign (*Fig. 11.16*).

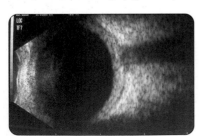

Fig. 11.16 Ultrasound of posterior scleritis

3. CT – scleral thickening and proptosis (*Fig. 11.17*).

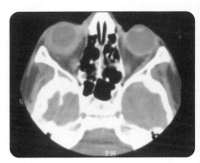

Fig. 11.17 Axial CT in right posterior scleritis

Systemic associations of scleritis

1. **Rheumatoid arthritis**
   - Non-necrotizing scleritis in mild joint disease.
   - Necrotizing scleritis in severe long-standing disease with extra-articular manifestations.
2. **Wegener granulomatosis** – rapidly progressive necrotizing granulomatous disease.
3. **Relapsing polychondritis** – intractable non-necrotizing or necrotizing disease.
4. **Polyarteritis nodosa** – aggressive necrotizing disease although other types may also occur.
5. **Systemic lupus erythematosus** – anterior diffuse or nodular disease.
6. **Other uncommon associations** – spondyloarthropathies, Behçet disease, sarcoidosis, and gout.

Treatment of scleritis

1. **Topical steroids** – for symptoms and oedema in non-necrotizing disease.
2. **Systemic NSAIDs** – in non-necrotizing disease.
3. **Periocular steroid injections** – in non-necrotizing and necrotizing disease.
4. **Systemic steroids** – when NSAIDs are inappropriate or ineffective.
5. **Cytotoxic agents** – whenever activity is not completely controlled with steroids alone, or as a steroid-sparing measure.
6. **Immune modulators** – short-term ciclosporin and tacrolimus in acute presentations before a cytotoxic agent exerts its action.

Scleral infection

1. **Herpes zoster** – necrotizing scleritis is resistant to treatment and may result in a punched-out area in the sclera (*Fig. 11.18*).

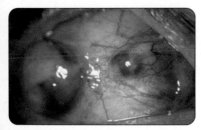

Fig. 11.18 Necrotizing herpes zoster scleritis

2. **Tuberculous** – nodular non-necrotizing (*Fig. 11.19*) or necrotizing disease.

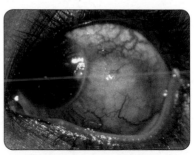

Fig. 11.19 Tuberculous scleritis

3. **Leprosy** – nodular scleritis in lepromatous leprosy; necrotizing disease a result of scleral infection or as part of an immune response.
4. **Secondary syphilis** – diffuse anterior scleritis.
5. **Lyme disease** – scleritis in late disease.

Scleral discoloration

1. **Scleral hyaline plaques** – innocuous, oval, dark-grey areas near the insertion of the horizontal rectus muscles (*Fig. 11.20*).

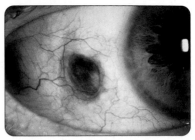

Fig. 11.20 Scleral hyaline plaque

2. Alcaptonuria – brown-black discoloration at the insertions of horizontal recti (ochronosis – *Fig. 11.21*).

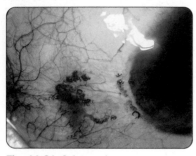

Fig. 11.21 Ochronosis

3. Haemochromatosis – rusty-brown discoloration.
4. Systemic minocycline – blue-grey paralimbal discoloration.

5. Metallic foreign body – rust staining.
6. Diffuse blue (*Fig. 11.22*) – osteogenesis imperfecta types 1 and 2, Ehlers–Danlos syndrome (usually type 6), pseudoxanthoma elasticum (dominant type 2), and Turner syndrome.

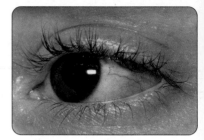

Fig. 11.22 Blue sclera

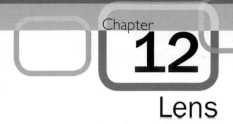

Acquired cataract

Age-related cataract

1. Subcapsular cataract – anterior or posterior (*Fig. 12.1*).

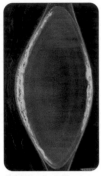

Fig. 12.1 Subcapsular cataract

2. Nuclear cataract – nucleus appears brown when advanced (*Fig. 12.2*).

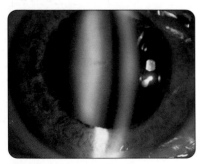

Fig. 12.2 Nuclear cataract

3. Cortical cataract – may involve the anterior, posterior or equatorial cortex (*Fig. 12.3*).

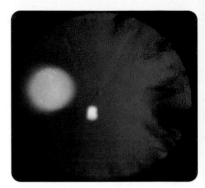

Fig. 12.3 Cortical cataract

4. Christmas tree cataract – polychromatic, needle-like deposits in the deep cortex and nucleus (*Fig. 12.4*).

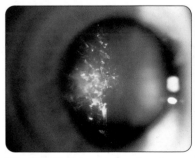

Fig. 12.4 Christmas tree cataract

Cataract maturity

1. Immature – lens is partially opaque.
2. Mature – lens is completely opaque (*Fig. 12.5*).
3. Hypermature – shrunken and wrinkled anterior capsule (*Fig. 12.6*).

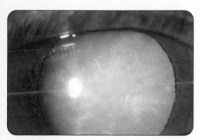

Fig. 12.5 Mature cataract

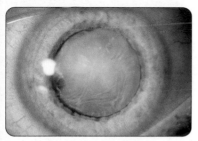

Fig. 12.6 Hypermature cataract

4. Morgagnian – hypermature cataract in which the nucleus has sunk inferiorly (*Fig. 12.7*).

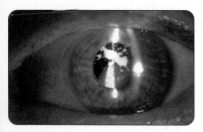

Fig. 12.7 Morgagnian cataract

Cataract in systemic diseases

1. Diabetes mellitus
   a. *Classical* – snowflake cortical opacities which may resolve spontaneously or mature within a few days.
   b. *Age-related* – occurs earlier and tend to progress rapidly.
2. Myotonic dystrophy – stellate posterior subcapsular opacities develop in the 5th decade (*Fig. 12.8*).

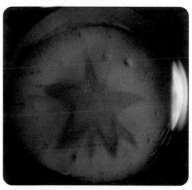

Fig. 12.8 Myotonic cataract

3. Atopic dermatitis – shield-like dense anterior subcapsular plaque which wrinkles the anterior capsule (*Fig. 12.9*); posterior subcapsular opacities may also occur.
4. NF 2 – posterior subcapsular or posterior cortical opacities.

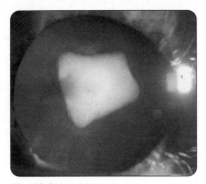

Fig. 12.9 Atopic cataract

Secondary (complicated) cataract

1. **Chronic anterior uveitis** – fine polychromatic granules at the posterior pole (*Fig. 12.10*) followed by posterior and anterior opacities.

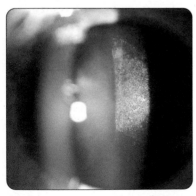

Fig. 12.10 Polychromatic opacities

2. **Acute congestive angle-closure** – grey-white, anterior, subcapsular or capsular opacities within the pupillary area (glaukomflecken – *Fig. 12.11*).

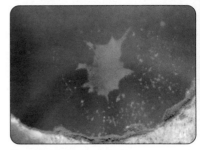

Fig. 12.11 Glaukomflecken

3. **High myopia** – posterior subcapsular lens opacities and early-onset nuclear sclerosis.
4. **Hereditary fundus dystrophies** – posterior subcapsular lens opacities.

Management of age-related cataract

Biometry

Biometry involves two parameters (a) *keratometry* – the curvature of the anterior corneal surface (steepest and flattest meridians), expressed in dioptres or millimetres of radius of curvature and (b) *axial length* – the anteroposterior dimension of the eye in millimetres. There are three main methods used to measure axial length.

1. **A-scan ultrasonic biometry** – display allows ocular structures to be identified and the distance from the front of the cornea to the retina determined.

2. Zeiss IOL Master – non-contact method that utilizes two coaxial laser beams which are partially coherent and produce an interference pattern. Measurements have high reproducibility and generally require less skill than ultrasonic biometry.

3. IOL power calculation formulae – numerous formulae, incorporating additional parameters such as anterior chamber depth and individualized surgeon factors have been developed to optimize the accuracy of preoperative prediction.

Anaesthesia

1. Peribulbar block – through the skin or conjunctiva (*Fig. 12.12*).

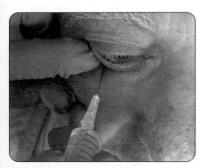

Fig. 12.12 Peribulbar block

2. Sub-Tenon block – blunt tipped cannula is passed through an incision in the conjunctiva and Tenon capsule and the anaesthetic is injected beyond the equator of the globe (*Fig. 12.13*).

3. Topical-intracameral anaesthesia – initial surface anaesthesia with

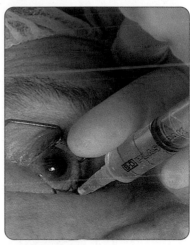

Fig. 12.13 Sub-Tenon block

drops or gel (proxymetacaine 0.5%, lignocaine 2%) which can be augmented with intracameral injection or infusion of diluted preservative-free lignocaine 1% usually during hydrodissection.

Phacoemulsification

1. Capsulorrhexis – with a cystitome or a bent needle (*Fig. 12.14a*).

2. Hydrodissection – to separate the nucleus and cortex from the capsule (*Fig. 12.14b*).

3. Removal of nucleus
- The nucleus is broken up using the 'divide and conquer' technique (*Fig. 12.14c,d*) or nuclear 'phaco chop'.
- Each fragment is emulsified and aspiration (*Fig. 12.14e*).

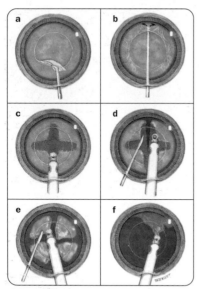

Fig. 12.14 Phacoemulsification

4. **Cortical clean up** – with Simcoe cannula (*Fig. 12.14f*).
5. **Insertion of IOL** (*Fig. 12.15*).
6. **Completion** – aspiration of viscoelastic, sealing of side port incisions with a jet of saline, and subconjunctival injection of steroid and antibiotic.

Operative complications

1. **Posterior capsular rupture**
   - May be accompanied by vitreous loss, posterior migration of lens material and rarely, expulsive haemorrhage.
   - Long-term complications of vitreous loss – updrawn pupil, uveitis, vitreous touch, endophthalmitis, elevation of IOP, posterior dislocation of the IOL, RD, and CMO.
2. **Loss of lens fragments** into vitreous (*Fig. 12.16*) – may result in elevation of IOP, chronic uveitis, RD and CMO; treatment involves pars plana vitrectomy.

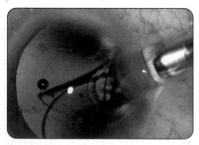

Fig. 12.15 Injection of intraocular lens

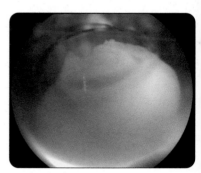

Fig. 12.16 IOL and lens material dislocated into the vitreous

3. **Dislocation of an IOL into vitreous** – treatment involves pars plana vitrectomy with removal, repositioning or exchange of the IOL depending on the extent of capsular support.

4. Suprachoroidal (expulsive) haemorrhage – may result in extrusion of intraocular contents or apposition of retinal surfaces; predispositions include old age, glaucoma, increased axial length, systemic cardiovascular disease, and vitreous loss.

Acute postoperative endophthalmitis

Pathogenesis

1. Risk factors – diabetes, secondary lens implantation, posterior capsule rupture, and cataract surgery combined with other procedures.

2. Pathogens – in order of frequency:
- Coagulase-negative staphylococci (*S. epidermidis*).
- Other Gram-positive organisms (*S. aureus* and *Streptococcus* spp.).
- Gram-negative organisms (*Pseudomonas* spp. and *Proteus* spp.).

3. Source of infection – flora of the eyelids and conjunctiva (most common), contaminated solutions and instruments, the air in theatre, and the surgeon or operating room personnel.

Clinical features

1. Presentation – pain and visual loss.

2. Signs vary according to severity.
- Chemosis, conjunctival injection and discharge.
- Relative afferent pupil defect.
- Corneal haze (*Fig. 12.17*).
- Fibrinous exudate and hypopyon (*Fig. 12.18*).
- Vitritis with impaired view of the fundus (*Fig. 12.19*).

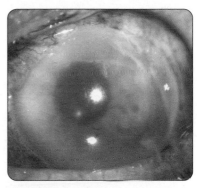

Fig. 12.17 Corneal haze

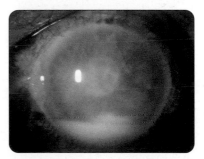

Fig. 12.18 Fibrinous exudate and hypopyon

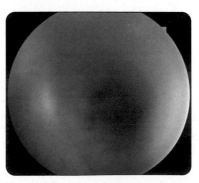

Fig. 12.19 Vitreous haze

Investigations

1. Aqueous samples – 0.1–0.2 ml of aqueous is aspirated via a limbal paracentesis using a 25G needle on a tuberculin syringe.

2. Vitreous samples
- A 2 ml syringe and a 23G needle may be used or a special disposable vitrector.
- About 0.2–0.4 ml are aspirated from the mid-vitreous cavity.

3. Culture media
- Blood agar.
- Cooked meat broth.
- Brain–heart infusion.
- Slide for Gram stain if sufficient sample is available.
- A blood culture bottle is an alternative if specific media are unavailable.

4. Polymerase chain reaction (PCR) – helpful in identifying unusual organisms.

Treatment

1. Intravitreal antibiotics
- Ceftazidime (2 mg in 0.1 ml) and vancomycin (2 mg in 0.1 ml).
- Amikacin (0.5 mg in 0.1 ml) as alternative to ceftazidime in patients allergic to penicillin.

2. Periocular antibiotic injections – doubtful additional benefit; vancomycin 50 mg and ceftazidime 125 mg (or amikacin 50 mg).

3. Oral antibiotics
- Moxifloxacin 400 mg daily for 10 days.
- Clarithromycin 500 mg b.d. for culture negative infections.

4. Steroids
- Oral prednisolone 60 mg daily in severe cases.

- Periocular injections (dexamethasone 12 mg or triamcinolone 1.0 mg) should be considered if systemic therapy is contraindicated.

5. Pars plana vitrectomy – for eyes with a visual acuity of perception of light (NOT hand movements or any better acuity level) at presentation.

Delayed-onset postoperative endophthalmitis

1. Pathogenesis – low virulence organisms trapped in the capsular bag such as *P. acnes* and occasionally *S. epidermidis*, *Corynebacterium* spp. or *Candida parapsilosis*.

2. Presentation – painless mild progressive visual deterioration ranging from 4 weeks to years (mean 9 months) postoperatively.

3. Signs
- Low-grade anterior uveitis, sometimes with mutton-fat keratic precipitates (*Fig. 12.20*).
- Vitritis is common but hypopyon infrequent.
- Enlarging capsular plaque (*Fig. 12.21*).

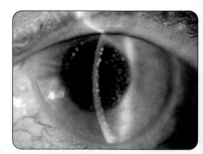

Fig. 12.20 Mutton fat keratic precipitates

2. Lamella
- Invol
  lens
  and
  exte
- May
  as
  and

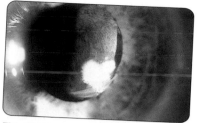
Fig. 12.21 Capsular plaque

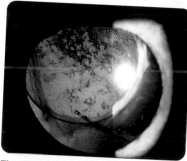
Fig. 12.22 Elschnig pearls

4. **Investigations** – as for acute endophthalmitis but anaerobic culture if *P. acnes* infection is suspected (isolates may take 10–14 days to grow).
5. **Clinical course** – inflammation initially responds well to topical steroids but recurs when treatment is stopped and eventually becomes steroid resistant.
6. **Treatment**
   - Removal of the capsular bag and IOL.
   - Vancomycin (1 mg in 0.1 ml) can be irrigated into capsular remnants.
   - *P. acnes* – is also sensitive to methicillin, cefazolin, and clindamycin.

Fig. 1:
riders

3. Co
- L

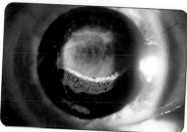
Fig. 12.23 Capsular fibrosis

Posterior capsule opacification

1. **Clinical features**
   a. *Elschnig pearls* – vacuolated appearance to the posterior capsule, best visualized on retroillumination (*Fig. 12.22*).
   b. *Capsular fibrosis* (*Fig. 12.23*) – less common and appears earlier than Elschnig pearls.
2. **Treatment** – Nd:YAG laser capsulotomy (*Fig. 12.24*).

Fig.

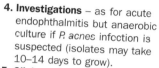

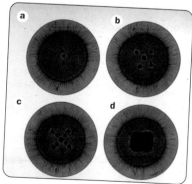
Fig. 12.24 Nd:YAG laser capsulotomy

3. Cor
   (pit
   and

Misc

1. Co
   int
   en
   ma
2. M
   us
   tic

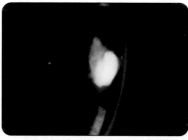

Fig. **12.32** Anterior polar pyramidal cataract

6. **Anterior polar** – flat or pyramidal (*Fig. 12.32*).
7. **Posterior polar** – may be associated with persistent hyaloid remnants (Mittendorf dot – *Fig. 12.33*), posterior lenticonus, and persistent anterior fetal vasculature.

Fi

3.

4.

5

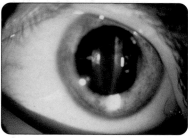

Fig. **12.33** Posterior polar cataract and Mittendorf dot

8. **Central 'oil droplet'** (*Fig. 12.34*) – in galactosaemia.

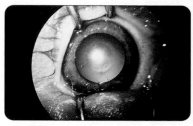

Fig. **12.34** 'Oil droplet' cataract

9. **Membranous** (*Fig. 12.35*) – in Hallermann–Streiff–François syndrome.

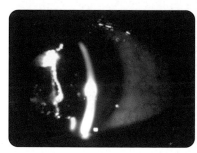

Fig. **12.35** Membranous cataract

Systemic associations

1. **Metabolic** – galactosaemia, Lowe oculorenal syndrome, Fabry disease, hypoparathyroidism, pseudo-hypoparathyroidism, mannosidosis, hypoglycaemia, and hyperglycaemia.
2. **Intrauterine infections** – toxoplasmosis, rubella, cytomegalovirus, and herpes simplex (TORCH).
3. **Chromosomal abnormalities** – Down syndrome (trisomy 21), Patau syndrome (trisomy 13), and Edward syndrome (trisomy 18).

4. Skeletal syndromes – Hallermann–Streiff–François and Nance–Horan syndrome.

Systemic investigations

Unless there is an established hereditary basis for the cataracts, the investigation of the infant with bilateral cataracts should include the following:

1. Serology – for TORCH.

2. Urinalysis – reducing substance after drinking milk (galactosaemia) and chromatography for amino acids (Lowe syndrome).

3. Other investigations – fasting blood glucose, serum calcium and phosphorus, red blood cell GPUT and galactokinase levels.

4. Referral to a paediatrician – for dysmorphic features or suspicion of other systemic diseases.

Surgery

1. Indications

  a. *Bilateral dense cataracts (Fig. 12.36)* – surgery within 4–6 weeks.

  b. *Unilateral dense cataract* – surgery within days.

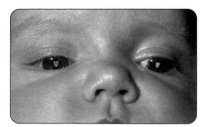

Fig. 12.36 Dense bilateral cataracts

2. Technique – anterior capsulorrhexis, aspiration of lens matter, posterior capsulorrhexis, limited anterior vitrectomy, and IOL implantation, if appropriate.

3. Complications – posterior capsular opacification, secondary pupillary membrane formation, glaucoma, and RD.

Visual rehabilitation

1. Spectacles – older children with bilateral aphakia.

2. Contact lenses – older children with unilateral and bilateral aphakia.

3. IOL implantation – increasingly being performed in young children and even infants.

4. Occlusion – to treat or prevent amblyopia is vital; atropine penalization may also be considered.

Ectopia lentis

Introduction

1. Definition – ectopia lentis refers to a displacement of the lens from its normal position. The lens may be completely dislocated, rendering the pupil aphakic (luxated), or partially displaced, still remaining in the pupillary area (subluxated).

2. Acquired causes – trauma, large eye (i.e. high myopia, buphthalmos), and anterior uveal tumours.

3. Hereditary causes – see below.

Without systemic associations

1. Familial ectopia lentis
  • AD – may manifest at birth or later.
  • Bilateral symmetrical superotemporal subluxation (*Fig. 12.37*).

Introduction

Definition

Glaucoma is a disease which exhibits a characteristic optic neuropathy which may result in progressive visual field loss. The most important risk factor is raised IOP secondary to reduced aqueous outflow through the filtration angle.

Classification

1. General
- Congenital (developmental) and acquired.
- Open-angle and angle-closure.
- Primary and secondary.

2. Secondary
- Open angle – pre-trabecular (Fig. 13.1a), trabecular (Fig. 13.1b), and post-trabecular.
- Angle closure – with pupil block (Fig. 13.1c) and without pupil block (Fig. 13.1d).

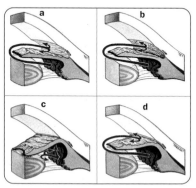

Fig. 13.1 Mechanisms of secondary glaucoma

Ocular hypertension

Definition

In the general population the mean IOP is 16 mmHg; two standard deviations on either side of this gives a 'normal' IOP range of 11–21 mmHg; individuals with IOP >21 mmHg without detectable glaucomatous damage are referred to as ocular hypertensives or glaucoma suspects.

Risk factors for developing glaucoma

1. Older age.
2. NFL defects – precede changes in visual field (pre-perimetric glaucoma).
3. High vertical cup–disc ratio – on the premise that it represents an early glaucomatous change.
4. High IOP – risk of damage increases as the IOP rises.
5. Parapapillary changes – present in over 50% of ocular hypertensive that convert to POAG.
6. Thin central corneal thickness.
7. Family history – POAG in a first-degree relative.
8. High myopia.

Management

Therapeutic decisions in individual patients are based on a combination of risk factors as follows:

1. High risk
- NFL defects.
- Parapapillary crescent.
- IOP 30 mmHg or more.
- IOP 26 mmHg or more and central corneal thickness <555 μm.
- Vertical cup–disc ratio 0.4 or more and central corneal thickness <555 μm.

Most patients with high risk factors should be treated to delay or prevent POAG.

2. Moderate risk

- IOP of 24–29 mmHg without NFL defects.
- IOP of 22–25 mmHg and central corneal thickness <555 μm.
- Vertical cup–disc ratio 0.4 or more and central corneal thickness 555–588 μm.
- Family history of POAG in a first-degree relative.
- High myopia.

Annual examination is appropriate and treatment is withheld until damage has been documented.

Primary open-angle glaucoma

Definition

A bilateral but not always symmetrical disease characterized by:

- Adult onset.
- IOP >21 mmHg.
- Open angle of normal appearance.
- Glaucomatous optic nerve head damage and visual field loss.

Despite this definition it should be emphasized that approximately 16% of all patients with otherwise characteristic POAG will have IOP consistently below 22 mmHg. Moreover, the majority of individuals with IOP >21 mmHg do not have POAG.

Glaucomatous optic neuropathy

Glaucomatous damage results in characteristic signs involving (a) *retinal nerve fibre layer*, (b) *parapapillary area* and (c) *optic nerve head*.

Retinal nerve fibre layer

Subtle NFL defects precede the characteristic optic disc and visual field changes. NFL dropout may be diffuse or localized. Localized damage is characterized by slit defects in the NFL which is best visualized with a green filter (*Fig. 13.2*).

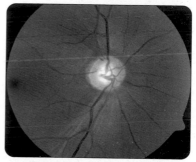

Fig. 13.2 Supero-temporal NFL defects

Parapapillary changes

- The inner 'beta' zone of chorioretinal atrophy bordering the disc margin is larger and occurs more frequently in glaucoma than in normals (*Fig. 13.3*).
- The outer 'alpha' zone of epithelial hypo- and hyperpigmentation is larger in glaucoma but not more frequent than in normals.
- In ocular hypertension, the presence and size of parapapillary changes correlates with the subsequent development of optic disc and visual field damage.

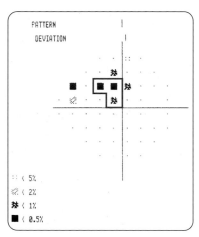

PATTERN
DEVIATION

∷ ‹ 5%
▨ ‹ 2%
✻ ‹ 1%
■ ‹ 0.5%

Fig. 13.9 Minimal criteria for glaucoma

3. CPSD – that occurs in less than 5% of normal individuals on two consecutive fields.

Progression of glaucomatous damage

1. Paracentral defects – small, relatively steep scotomas, most commonly supero-nasally (*Fig. 13.10a*).
2. Nasal (Roenne) step (*Fig. 13.10b*).
3. Arcuate-shaped defects
   - Develop between 10–20° of fixation (Bjerrum area).
   - Elongate circumferentially (Seidel scotoma).
   - Connect with the blind spot (arcuate scotoma) reaching to within 5° of fixation nasally (*Fig. 13.10c*).
4. Enlargement – due to damage to adjacent fibres (*Fig. 13.10d*).
5. Deepening (*Fig. 13.10e*).
6. Ring scotoma – due to joining of arcuate defects in upper and lower halves of the visual field (*Fig. 13.10f*).

7. End-stage – small island of central vision and an accompanying temporal island.

Medical therapy

1. Principles
   - Initial treatment is usually with one drug, usually a prostaglandin analogue or a beta-blocker.
   - If the response is satisfactory subsequent assessment is after 2 months and then 4-monthly intervals thereafter.
   - If the response is unsatisfactory the initial drug is withdrawn and another substituted.
   - If the response is still unsatisfactory yet another drug is added or a combined preparation substituted.
2. Perimetry – annually when control is good.
3. Causes of failure
   - Inappropriate target pressure.
   - Non-compliance with therapy.
   - Wide fluctuations in IOP.

Indications for laser trabeculoplasty

1. Avoidance of polypharmacy – usually with more than two preparations.
2. Avoidance of surgery
   - Elderly patients in whom laser therapy may defer the need for surgery to beyond life expectancy.
   - Black patients in whom filtration surgery carries a poorer prognosis.
3. Primary therapy – in poor compliance with medical therapy; since IOP reduction with laser is seldom greater than 30%, an IOP >28 mmHg is unlikely to be adequately controlled by laser alone.

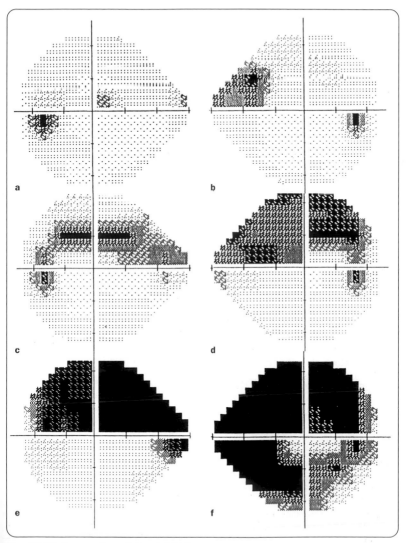

Fig. 13.10 Progression of visual field loss

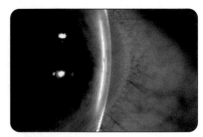

Fig. 13.13 Close proximity of iris to peripheral cornea

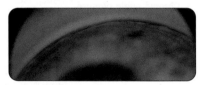

Fig. 13.14 Very narrow angle

3. Clinical course
- IOP may remain normal.
- Acute or subacute angle closure may ensue.
- Chronic angle closure may develop, without passing through subacute or acute stages.

4. Treatment
- If one eye has had acute or subacute angle closure, the fellow eye should undergo prophylactic peripheral laser iridotomy.
- If both eyes have occludable angles laser treatment may be considered.

Intermittent angle closure

1. Pathogenesis
- Rapid closure of the angle results in sudden increase in IOP.
- Pupillary block is then spontaneously relieved, the angle opens and the IOP returns to normal.

2. Symptoms
transient blurring of vision associated with haloes around lights.

3. Signs
during an attack the eye is usually white and the cornea oedematous; in between attacks it looks normal, although the angle is narrow.

4. Clinical course
some develop an acute attack and others chronic angle closure.

5. Treatment
prophylactic peripheral laser iridotomy.

Acute congestive angle closure

Diagnosis

1. Presentation – rapidly progressive unilateral visual loss associated with periocular pain.

2. Signs
- 'Ciliary' flush and corneal oedema.
- Shallow anterior chamber with flare and cells.
- Semi-dilated fixed pupil (*Fig. 13.15*).
- IOP 50–100 mmHg.
- Gonioscopy shows complete iridocorneal contact (Shaffer grade 0 – *Fig. 13.16*).

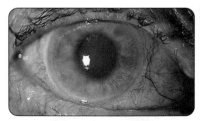

Fig. 13.15 Acute angle closure

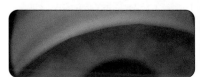

Fig. 13.16 Complete angle closure

Medical treatment

1. Immediate

- **a.** *Acetazolamide* – 500 mg intravenously and 500 mg orally (not slow-release).
- **b.** *Topical*
  - Predsol or dexamethasone q.i.d.
  - Timolol 0.5%.
- **c.** *Analgesia and anti-emetics.*

2. After one hour

- Pilocarpine 2% q.i.d.
- Pilocarpine 1% q.i.d to the fellow eye until prophylactic laser iridotomy is performed.

3. After a further 30 minutes

- Recheck IOP.
- If the IOP has not fallen to below 35 mmHg give oral 50% glycerol (with caution in diabetics).
- If the patient is unable to tolerate oral glycerol give 20% mannitol intravenously over 45 minutes.

Nd:YAG laser iridotomy

1. Purpose – to re-establish communication between the posterior and anterior chambers by making an opening in the peripheral iris.

2. Timing

- Usually after 48 hours when the cornea has cleared.
- It may be appropriate to perform a prophylactic laser iridotomy on the fellow eye in the interim period.

Post-congestive angle closure

Clinical settings

1. Post-surgical – the IOP is normalized by successful peripheral iridotomy.

2. Spontaneous angle re-opening – is uncommon.

3. Temporary ciliary body shutdown – subsequent recovery of ciliary function may lead to chronic elevation of IOP.

Diagnosis

1. Slit-lamp biomicroscopy

- Fine pigment granules on the corneal endothelium.
- Aqueous flare and cells.
- Glaukomflecken (see Fig. 12.11).
- Stromal iris atrophy with a spiral-like configuration (*Fig. 13.17*).
- Fixed semi-dilated pupil.
- IOP may be normal, subnormal or elevated.

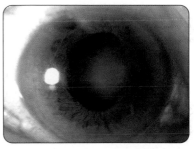

Fig. 13.17 Iris atrophy (note peripheral iridectomy

2. Gonioscopy – narrow angle which may be open or partly closed.

Chronic angle closure

Type 1 (creeping)

1. Pathogenesis – gradual progressive synechial angle closure.

2. Treatment – initially laser iridotomy followed by medical therapy or trabeculectomy as appropriate.

Type 2

1. Pathogenesis – synechial angle closure as a result of intermittent attacks.

2. Treatment – medical, preferably with a prostaglandin analogue.

6. Iris

- Fine surface pigment granules that may extend onto the lens.
- Mid-periphery radial slit-like retroillumination defects (*Fig. 13.24*).
- Partial loss of the pupillary ruff (frill).

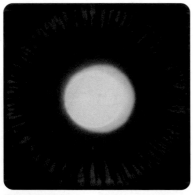

Fig. 13.24 Iris retroillumination defects

7. Gonioscopy – wide open angle with mid-peripheral iris concavity; trabecular hyperpigmentation is most marked over the posterior trabeculum (*Fig. 13.25*).

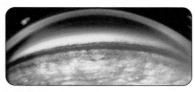

Fig. 13.25 Trabecular hyperpigmentation

Pigmentary glaucoma

1. **Pathogenesis** – trabecular blockage by pigment and damage to the trabeculum secondary to collapse and sclerosis.
2. **Risk factors** – about one-third of patients develop elevation of IOP after 15 years.
3. **Presentation** – chronic glaucoma in the 4th–5th decade.
4. **Treatment** – as for POAG.
5. **Prognosis** – good and over time the control of IOP becomes easier.

Neovascular glaucoma

Introduction

1. **Pathogenesis** – iris neovascularization (rubeosis iridis – *Fig. 13.26*) secondary to severe chronic retinal ischaemia.

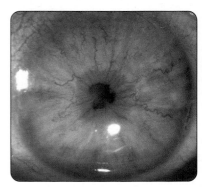

Fig. 13.26 Rubeosis iridis

2. Causes of rubeosis iridis –
ischaemic central retinal vein
occlusion, diabetes, chronic anterior
uveitis, intraocular tumours, longstanding RD, ocular ischaemic
syndrome, and occasionally central
retinal artery occlusion.

Rubeosis iridis

1. Signs
- Tiny dilated capillary tufts or red
  spots develop at the pupillary
  margin.
- The new vessels grow radially over
  the surface of the iris towards the
  angle (*Fig. 13.27*).

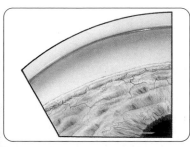

Fig. 13.27 Mild angle rubeosis

2. Treatment – panretinal photocoagulation.

Secondary open-angle glaucoma

1. Pathogenesis – trabecular block by a
fibrovascular membrane.
2. Treatment
- **a.** *Medical* – aqueous suppressants,
  atropine and steroids.
- **b.** *Panretinal photocoagulation* – even
  if the IOP is adequately controlled
  medically.

Secondary angle-closure glaucoma

1. Pathogenesis – synechial angle
closure by contraction of fibrovascular tissue (*Fig. 13.28*)

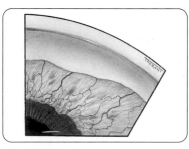

Fig. 13.28 Synechial rubeotic angle
closure

2. Signs
- Very high IOP, pain and severe
  visual impairment.
- Corneal oedema, mydriasis and
  severe rubeosis (*Fig. 13.29*).

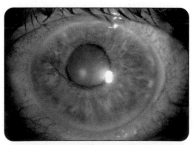

Fig. 13.29 Neovascular glaucoma

3. Treatment

  a. *Medical* – topical beta-blockers, atropine and steroids, and systemic acetazolamide.

  b. *Panretinal photocoagulation* – if fundus can be visualized.

  c. *Filtration surgery* – trabeculectomy with adjunctive mitomycin C or artificial filtering shunts.

  d. *Anti-VEGF agents* – as adjunct to filtration surgery.

  e. *Cyclodestruction* – may control IOP and render the eye more comfortable.

  f. *Retrobulbar alcohol injection* – to relieve pain.

  g. *Enucleation* – as last resort.

Inflammatory glaucoma

Classification

1. Angle-closure with pupil block.
2. Angle-closure without pupil block.
3. Open angle.
4. Posner–Schlossman syndrome.

Angle-closure glaucoma with pupil block

1. **Pathogenesis**
   - Seclusio pupillae obstructs aqueous flow from the posterior to the anterior chamber.
   - Increased pressure in the posterior chamber produces iris bombé and apposition of the peripheral iris to the trabeculum and peripheral cornea.
2. **Signs** – seclusio pupillae, iris bombé, shallow anterior chamber, and iridotrabecular contact (*Fig. 13.30*).

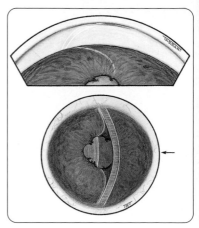

Fig. 13.30 Pupil block glaucoma

Angle-closure glaucoma without pupil block

1. **Pathogenesis** – organization and contraction of inflammatory cells and debris in the angle causes gradual and progressive synechial angle closure.
2. **Signs** – deep anterior chamber and extensive synechial angle closure (*Fig. 13.31*).

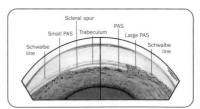

Fig. 13.31 Angle closure without pupil block

Open-angle glaucoma

1. In acute anterior uveitis
   a. *Trabecular obstruction* – by inflammatory cells and debris which may be associated with increased aqueous viscosity.
   b. *Acute trabeculitis* – with secondary diminution of intertrabecular porosity resulting in reduction in outflow facility.
2. In chronic anterior uveitis – reduced outflow facility caused by trabecular scarring and/or sclerosis secondary to chronic trabeculitis.

Treatment

1. Medical
   - Use of prostaglandin agonists as initial therapy is tempered by the small risk of precipitating uveitis or CMO.
   - A topical beta-blocker is therefore usually the first drug of choice.
   - If the IOP is very high, systemic acetazolamide may be required in the short-term.
   - If elevation of IOP is moderate (e.g. less than 35 mmHg on a beta-blocker) in the absence of significant damage, an alpha-adrenergic agonist, a topical CAI, or prostaglandin analogue may be appropriate.
2. Laser iridotomy – in eyes with pupil-block angle closure.
3. Surgery
   a. *Trabeculectomy* – with adjunctive antimetabolites in eyes unresponsive to medical therapy.
   b. *Artificial drainage shunts* – when trabeculectomy has failed.

c. *Cyclodestruction* – should be used with caution because it may exacerbate the uveitis and also induce hypotony.
d. *Angle procedures* – trabeculodialysis (*Fig. 13.32*) and goniotomy in children.

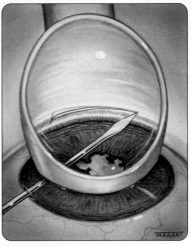

Fig. 13.32 Trabeculodialysis

Posner–Schlossman syndrome

1. Definition – recurrent attacks of unilateral, acute secondary open-angle glaucoma associated with mild anterior uveitis and trabeculitis.
2. Presentation – haloes around lights and slight blurring of vision.
3. Signs
   - Corneal epithelial oedema due to a high IOP.
   - Mild iritis and fine white central keratic precipitates (*Fig. 13.33*).
   - Gonioscopy shows an open angle.

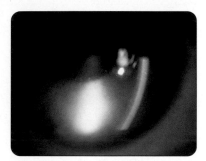

Fig. 13.33 Posner–Schlossman syndrome

4. Treatment – topical steroids, aqueous suppressants, and oral NSAIDs.

Lens-related glaucoma

Phacolytic glaucoma

1. Pathogenesis (*Fig. 13.34*)
- Trabecular obstruction by high molecular weight lens proteins which have leaked through the intact capsule of a hypermature cataract.
- Macrophages containing lens proteins may also contribute to trabecular blockage.

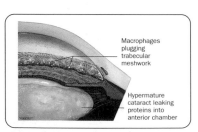

Macrophages plugging trabecular meshwork

Hypermature cataract leaking proteins into anterior chamber

Fig. 13.34 Pathogenesis of phacolytic glaucoma

2. Signs
- Corneal oedema, hypermature cataract, and deep anterior chamber.
- The aqueous may manifest floating white particles (*Fig. 13.35*).

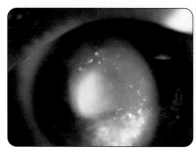

Fig. 13.35 Phacolytic glaucoma

3. Treatment – medical control of IOP followed by cataract removal.

Phacomorphic glaucoma

1. Pathogenesis – acute secondary angle closure precipitated by an intumescent cataract.
2. Presentation – similar to acute PACG.
3. Treatment – initially similar to acute PACG; cataract surgery is performed once the eye is quiet.

Dislocated lens into the anterior chamber

1. Pathogenesis – acute pupil block.
2. Causes
  a. *Blunt trauma*, particularly in eyes with weak zonules as in buphthalmos or homocystinuria (*Fig. 13.36*).
  b. *Small lenses* – microspherophakia.

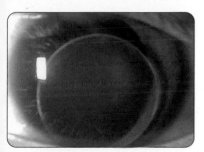

Fig. 13.36 Lens dislocation into anterior chamber

3. Signs – sudden severe elevation of IOP and visual impairment.
4. Treatment – reduction of IOP with osmotic agents followed by lens removal.

Incarcerated lens in the pupil

1. Pathogenesis – pupil block by a microspherical lens in which only part of the zonule has been disrupted so that the intact zonule acts as a hinge (*Fig. 13.37*).

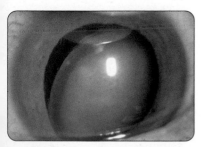

Fig. 13.37 Lens incarceration in the pupil

2. Treatment – Nd:YAG laser iridotomy.

Traumatic glaucoma

Red cell glaucoma

1. Pathogenesis – trabecular blockage by red blood cells.
2. Medical treatment
   - Beta-blockers and/or carbonic anhydrase inhibitors depending on the IOP.
   - Topical steroids and mydriatics.
3. Surgical evacuation of blood with or without trabeculectomy is indicated in the following circumstances:
   - IOP of >50 mmHg for 2 days or >35 mmHg for 7 days.
   - Early corneal blood staining.
   - Total hyphaema for more than 5 days (*Fig. 13.38*).

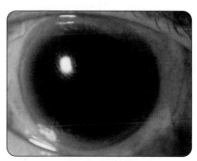

Fig. 13.38 Total hyphaema

Angle recession glaucoma

1. Pathogenesis
   - Disruption of the trabeculum and rupture of the face of the ciliary body due to blunt trauma (*Fig. 13.39*).
   - Chronic elevation of IOP is caused by subsequent trabecular damage.

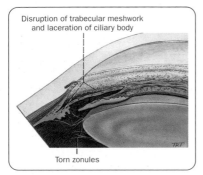

Disruption of trabecular meshwork and laceration of ciliary body

Torn zonules

Fig. 13.39 Pathogenesis of angle recession glaucoma

2. Signs – irregular widening of the ciliary body associated with scarring and pigment within the recess (*Fig. 13.40*).

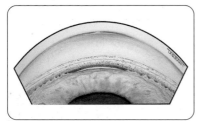

Fig. 13.40 Angle recession

3. Treatment
  a. *Medical* – frequently unsatisfactory (laser trabeculoplasty is ineffective).
  b. *Trabeculectomy with adjunctive antimetabolites.*
  c. *Artificial filtering shunt* – if trabeculectomy fails.

Iridocorneal endothelial syndrome

Classification

The iridocorneal endothelial (ICE) syndrome typically affects one eye of a middle-aged woman. It consists of the following three very rare and frequently overlapping disorders: (a) *progressive iris atrophy*, (b) *iris naevus (Cogan–Reese) syndrome* and (c) *Chandler syndrome*.

Pathogenesis

Abnormal corneal endothelial cells proliferate and migrate across the angle and onto the surface of the iris ('proliferative endotheliopathy') and may cause synechial angle closure glaucoma and corneal decompensation.

General features

1. Signs
  • Corectopia (malposition of the pupil – *Fig. 13.41*).

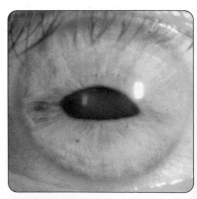

Fig. 13.41 Corectopia

- Pseudopolycoria (supernumerary false pupils – *Fig. 13.42*).
- Iris atrophy of varying severity (*Fig. 13.43*).
- Broad-based peripheral anterior synechiae that often extend anterior to Schwalbe line (*Fig. 13.44*).

2. Glaucoma – in about 50% of cases.

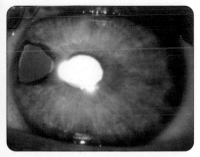

Fig. 13.42 Pseudopolycoria

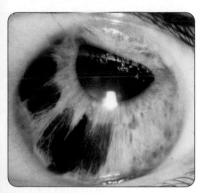

Fig. 13.43 Iris atrophy

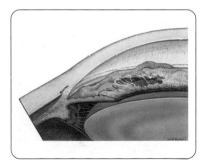

Fig. 13.44 Peripheral anterior synechiae

Specific features

1. Progressive iris atrophy – severe iris changes.

2. Iris naevus (Cogan–Reese) syndrome
- Diffuse iris naevus or iris nodules (*Fig. 13.45*).
- Iris atrophy is absent in 50% of cases and in the remainder it is mild to moderate.
- Corectopia may be severe.

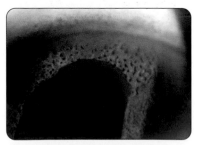

Fig. 13.45 Iris nodules in Cogan–Reese syndrome

3. Chandler syndrome
- 'Hammered-silver' endothelial abnormalities (*Fig. 13.46*).
- Blurred vision and haloes due to corneal oedema.
- Stromal atrophy is absent in about 60% of cases and in the remainder is variable.
- Corectopia is mild to moderate.

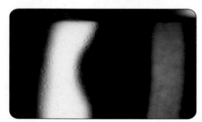

Fig. 13.46 Endothelial changes in Chandler syndrome

Treatment of glaucoma

1. **Medical** – often ineffective.
2. **Trabeculectomy** – even with adjunctive antimetabolites is frequently unsuccessful.
3. **Artificial filtering shunts** – frequently required.

Glaucoma in intraocular tumours

Depending on the location of the tumour one or more of the following mechanisms may be responsible:
1. **Angle invasion** – by solid iris melanoma (*Fig. 13.47*).

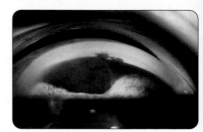

Fig. 13.47 Angle invasion by solid tumour

2. **Trabecular infiltration** – by neoplastic cells originating from an iris melanoma (*Fig. 13.48*).

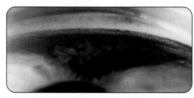

Fig. 13.48 Cellular trabecular invasion

3. **Melanomalytic glaucoma** – trabecular blockage by macrophages which have ingested pigment and tumour cells similar to phacolytic glaucoma (*Fig. 13.49*).

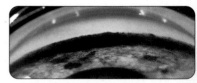

Fig. 13.49 Melanomalytic glaucoma

4. **Neovascular glaucoma** – most common mechanism in choroidal melanoma or retinoblastoma.
5. **Angle closure** – by ciliary body melanoma (*Fig. 13.50*).

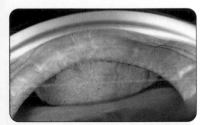

Fig. 13.50 Angle closure by ciliary body melanoma

Glaucoma in iridoschisis

1. **Pathogenesis** – acute or intermittent angle closure results in iris atrophy.
2. **Signs**
   - Shallow anterior chamber.
   - Iridoschisis usually involves the inferior iris (*Fig. 13.51*).
   - Narrow occludable angle with peripheral anterior synechiae.

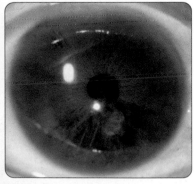

Fig. 13.51 Iridoschisis – note laser iridotomy

3. **Treatment** – initially peripheral laser iridotomy followed by medical therapy.

Primary congenital glaucoma

Introduction

1. **Inheritance** – mostly sporadic; 10% are AR (gene GLC3 on 1p36).
2. **Pathogenesis** – maldevelopment of the angle structures (isolated trabeculodysgenesis) characterized by absence of the ciliary body band due to translucent amorphous material that obscures the trabeculum (*Fig. 13.52*).

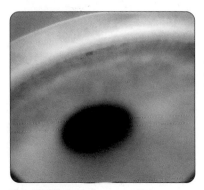

Fig. 13.52 Angle in congenital glaucoma

3. **Classification**
   a. *True congenital* (40%) – IOP becomes elevated during intrauterine life.
   b. *Infantile* (55%) – manifests prior to the 3rd birthday.
   c. *Juvenile* – manifests between the ages of 3 and 16 years.

Diagnosis

1. **Corneal haze** – associated with photophobia, lacrimation, and blepharospasm (*Fig. 13.53*).

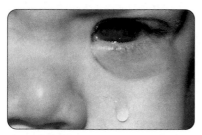

Fig. 13.53 Corneal haze, lacrimation, and blepharospasm

2. **Buphthalmos** – when IOP becomes elevated prior to the age of 3 years (*Fig. 13.54*).

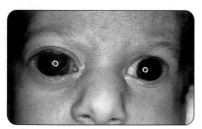

Fig. 13.54 Bilateral buphthalmos and corneal haze

3. **Breaks in Descemet membrane** – with sudden influx of aqueous into the corneal stroma.
4. **Haab striae** – healed breaks in Descemet membrane and appear as horizontal or transverse curvilinear lines (*Fig. 13.55*).

5. **Optic disc cupping** – in infants may regress in infants once the IOP is normalized.

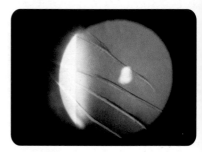

Fig. 13.55 Haab striae

Treatment

1. **Goniotomy** (*Fig. 13.56*) – provided the angle can be visualized.

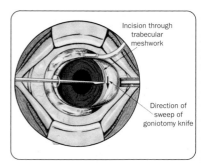

Incision through trabecular meshwork

Direction of sweep of goniotomy knife

Fig. 13.56 Goniotomy

2. **Trabeculotomy** (*Fig. 13.57*) – if corneal clouding prevents visualization of the angle or when repeated goniotomy has failed.
3. **Trabeculectomy** – often successful, particularly when combined with adjunctive antimetabolites.

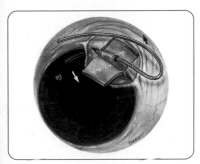

Fig. 13.57 Trabeculotomy

Glaucoma in phacomatoses

Sturge–Weber syndrome

1. **Pathogenesis** – trabeculodysgenesis or raised episcleral venous pressure.
2. **Presentation** – within the first 2 years in 60%; at any time in the remainder.
3. **Treatment**
   a. *Medical* – prostaglandin analogues.
   b. *Goniotomy* – in trabeculodysgenesis.
   c. *Combined trabeculotomy-trabeculectomy* – in early-onset cases.

NF 1

1. **Incidence of glaucoma** – uncommon, usually unilateral and congenital; about 50% have ipsilateral plexiform neurofibroma of the upper eyelid or facial hemiatrophy.

2. Pathogenesis
- Obstruction of the angle by neurofibromatous tissue,
- Developmental angle anomaly which may be associated with congenital ectropion uveae (*Fig. 13.58*).
- Secondary angle closure caused by forward displacement of the peripheral iris associated with neurofibromatous thickening of the ciliary body.
- Secondary synechial angle closure caused by contraction of a fibrovascular membrane.

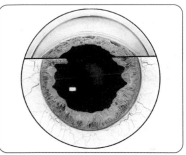

Fig. 13.58 Angle anomaly in congenital ectropion uveae

Glaucoma medications

Beta-blockers

Properties

- They antagonize the effects of catecholamines at beta receptors.
- Non-selective are equipotent at beta-1 and beta-2 receptors.
- Cardioselective (e.g. betaxalol) are more potent at beta-1 receptors.
- Reduce IOP by decreasing aqueous secretion.

- Effective in all types of glaucoma, irrespective of the state of the angle.

Preparations

1. Timolol
- Timoptol 0.25%, 0.5% b.d.
- Timoptol-LA 0.25%, 0.5% once daily.
- Nyogel 0.1% once daily.

2. Betaxolol (Betoptic) 0.5% b.d. – less potent than timolol.

3. Levobunolol (Betagan) 0.5% daily or b.d. – similar to timolol.

4. Carteolol (Teoptic) 1%, 2% b.d. – similar to timolol and also exhibits intrinsic sympathomimetic activity.

5. Metipranolol 0.1%, 0.3% b.d. – similar to timolol but may occasionally cause a granulomatous anterior uveitis.

Side-effects

1. Ocular – allergy, corneal punctate epithelial erosions and reduced aqueous tear secretion.

2. Systemic
- Bradycardia and hypotension from beta-1 blockade.
- Bronchospasm induced by beta-2 blockade.
- Miscellaneous – sleep disorders, hallucinations, confusion, depression, fatigue, headache, nausea, dizziness, and decreased libido.

3. Contraindications – congestive cardiac failure, 2nd or 3rd degree heart block, bradycardia, asthma and obstructive airways disease.

Alpha-2 agonists

1. Action – reduce IOP by decrease in aqueous secretion and enhancement of uveoscleral outflow.

2. Brimonidine (Alphagan) 0.2% b.d.
- Less potent than timolol but additive with beta-blockers.
- Side-effects – allergic conjunctivitis, xerostomia, drowsiness and fatigue.

Prostaglandin and prostamide analogues

Preparations

1. Latanoprost (Xalatan) 0.005% nocte – enhances outflow through the uveoscleral route; superior to timolol although some patients are unresponsive.

2. Travoprost (Travatan) 0.004% nocte – similar to latanoprost except in black patients where it appears to be more effective.

3. Bimatoprost (Lumigan) 0.03% nocte – similar to latanoprost but also enhances outflow through the trabecular route.

4. Unoprostone isopropyl (Rescula) 0.15% b.d. – enhances trabecular outflow but is less effective than latanoprost.

Side-effects

1. Ocular
- Conjunctival hyperaemia and a foreign body sensation are common.
- Eyelash lengthening, thickening, hyperpigmentation, and occasionally increase in number (*Fig. 13.59*).
- Iris hyperpigmentation in 11–23% of patients after 6 months.
- Hyperpigmentation of periorbital skin is uncommon.

2. Systemic – headache, precipitation of migraine, rash, and mild upper respiratory tract symptoms.

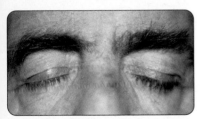

Fig. 13.59 Left lash changes due to prostaglandin analogue

Topical carbonic anhydrase inhibitors

1. **Dorzolamide** (Trusopt) 2% t.i.d. as monotherapy or b.d. as adjunctive treatment – side-effects are allergic blepharoconjunctivitis and a transient bitter taste.
2. **Brinzolamide** (Azopt) 1% b.d. or t.i.d. is similar to dorzolamide but with a lesser allergy.

Miotics

Mode of action

1. **In POAG** – contraction of the ciliary muscle increases the facility of aqueous outflow through the trabecular meshwork.
2. **In PACG** – miosis pulls the peripheral iris away from the trabeculum, thus opening the angle.

Preparations

1. **Pilocarpine**
   - Pilocarpine drops 1%, 2%, 3%, 4% is used q.i.d. as monotherapy and b.d. when combined with a beta-blocker.
   - Pilocarpine gel (Pilogel) nocte.
2. **Carbachol** 3% t.i.d.

Combined preparations

Combined preparations with similar ocular hypotensive effects to the sum of the individual components improve convenience and patient compliance.

1. **Cosopt** (timolol + dorzolamide) b.d.
2. **Xalacom** (timolol + latanoprost) daily.
3. **TimPilo** (timolol + pilocarpine) b.d.
4. **Combigan** (timolol + brimonidine) b.d.
5. **Extravan** (timolol + travoprost) daily.
6. **Duotrav** (timolol + travoprost) daily.
7. **Ganfort** (timolol + bimatoprost) daily.

Systemic carbonic acid inhibitors

Preparations

1. **Acetazolamide** is available in the following forms:
   - Tablets 250–1000 mg in divided doses; onset is within 1 hour, with a peak at 4 hours and duration up to 12 hours.
   - Sustained-release capsules 250–500 mg daily with duration of up to 24 hours.
   - Powder 500 mg vials for injection; onset is almost immediate, with a peak at 30 min and duration up to 4 hours.
2. **Dichlorphenamide** tablets 50–100 mg (2–3 times daily); onset is within 1 hour, with a peak at 3 hours and duration up to 12 hours.
3. **Methazolamide** tablets 50–100 mg (2–3 times daily); onset is within 3 hours, with a peak at 6 hours and duration up to 10–18 hours (not available in the UK).

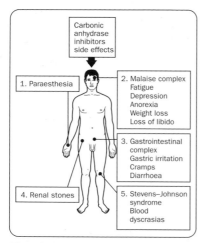

Fig. 13.60 Side-effects of systemic carbonic anhydrase inhibitors

Systemic side-effects (*Fig. 13.60*)

1. **Paraesthesia** – universal.
2. **Malaise complex** – malaise, fatigue, depression, weight loss and decreased libido.
3. **Gastrointestinal complex** – gastric irritation, abdominal cramps, diarrhoea and nausea.
4. **Renal stone formation** – uncommon.
5. **Stevens–Johnson syndrome** – rare.
6. **Blood dyscrasias** – extremely rare.

Osmotic agents

Clinical uses

When a temporary drop in IOP is required that cannot be obtained by other means.

- In acute angle-closure glaucoma.
- Prior to intraocular surgery when the IOP is very high, as may occur from dislocation of the lens into the anterior chamber.

Preparations

1. **Oral glycerol** – 1–2 g/kg body weight or 2 ml/kg body weight (50% solution). Peak action is within 1 hour, with duration up to 3 hours; must be diluted with pure lemon juice.
2. **Oral isosorbide** – same dose as glycerol.
3. **Intravenous mannitol** – 1 g/kg body weight or 5 ml/kg body weight (20% solution in water); peak of action is within 30 min with duration up to 6 hours.

Side-effects

1. **Cardiovascular overload** – due to increased extracellular volume.
2. **Urinary retention** – in elderly men following intravenous administration.
3. **Miscellaneous** – headache, backache, nausea and mental confusion.

Laser therapy

Argon laser trabeculoplasty

1. **Definition** – application of discrete laser burns to the trabecular meshwork to enhance aqueous outflow and lowers IOP.
2. **Indications** – open angle glaucomas, usually as an adjunct to medical therapy.
3. **Technique**
   - Laser settings – 50 μm spot size, 0.1 sec duration and 700 mW (can be increased later if necessary.
   - A goniolens is inserted with the mirror at 12 o'clock position to visualize the inferior angle.
   - Laser is fired at the junction of the pigmented and non-pigmented trabecular meshwork (*Fig. 13.61*).
   - Total of 50 burns are applied over 180° of the angle.

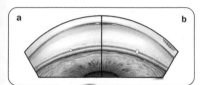

Fig. 13.61 Laser trabeculoplasty. (a) Correct focus of aiming beam; (b) incorrect focus

4. Complications – peripheral anterior synechiae (*Fig. 13.62*), acute elevation of IOP, and iritis.

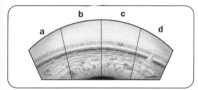

Fig. 13.62 Laser trabeculoplasty. (a) Blanching of trabecular meshwork – appropriate; (b) small bubble – also appropriate; (c) large bubble – excessive; (d) peripheral anterior synechiae

5. Results – good in POAG, pigmentary glaucoma and pseudoexfoliation glaucoma.

Selective laser trabeculoplasty

1. Definition – 532 nm frequency-doubled, Q-switched Nd:YAG laser is used which selectively targets melanin pigment in the trabecular meshwork cells, leaving non-pigmented cells and structures unscathed.

2. Efficacy – probably as effective as ALT although its exact place in the treatment of open-angle glaucoma is yet to be defined.

Nd:YAG laser iridotomy

1. Definition – procedure that produces a hole in the iris in order to re-establish communication between the posterior and anterior chambers.

2. Indications
- Pupil-block angle-closure glaucoma, both primary and secondary.
- Prophylaxis in fellow eyes of patients with primary angle-closure glaucoma.

3. Technique
- Laser settings – 4–8 mJ with 2–3 shots per burst.
- Special iridotomy lens is inserted.
- The opening is made in a peripheral site that is covered by the upper lid (*Fig. 13.63*).
- Successful penetration is characterized by a gush of pigment.

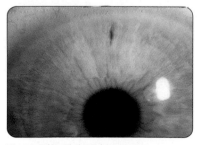

Fig. 13.63 Nd:YAG iridotomy

4. Complications – bleeding, elevation of IOP, iritis, lens opacities, glare and diplopia.

Diode laser cycloablation

1. **Definition** – procedure that lowers IOP by destroying part of the secretory ciliary epithelium.
2. **Indications** – mainly to control pain in uncontrolled secondary glaucoma with poor visual potential.
3. **Technique**
   - Sub-Tenon or peribulbar anaesthetic is given.
   - Laser settings – 1–2 sec and 1500–2000 mW.
   - Burns are applied 1.2 mm posterior to the limbus over 180° (*Fig. 13.64*).

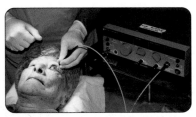

Fig. 13.64 Diode laser cycloablation

4. **Complications** – iritis, scleral thinning, hypotony, corneal decompensation, and retinal and choroidal detachment.

Surgery

Trabeculectomy

1. **Definition** – procedure in which a fistula is created which allows aqueous outflow from the anterior chamber to the sub-Tenon space.
2. **Indications** – when medical therapy (with or without laser trabeculoplasty) has failed to achieve adequate control of IOP.
3. **Technique**
   - Flap of conjunctiva and Tenon capsule is fashioned superiorly (*Fig. 13.65a–c*).
   - Superficial scleral flap is dissected (3 mm × 4 mm – *Fig. 13.65d–f*).

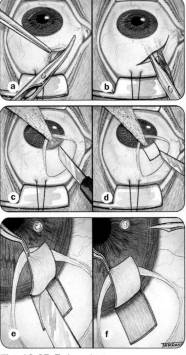

Fig. 13.65 Trabeculectomy

- Block of deep sclera (1.5 mm × 2 mm) is excised (*Fig. 13.66a–c*).
- Iridectomy (*Fig. 13.66d*).
- Superficial flap is sutured (*Fig. 13.66e*).
- Conjunctiva and Tenon capsule are sutured (*Fig. 13.66f*).

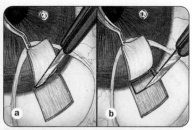
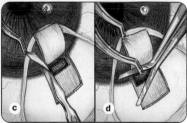
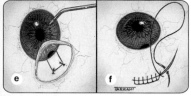

Fig. 13.66 Trabeculectomy

4. Complications – shallow anterior chamber (pupil block, overfiltration, malignant glaucoma), failure of filtration, bleb leakage, and bleb-associated bacterial infection.

Non-penetrating surgery

1. Definition – procedure in which the anterior chamber is not entered and the internal trabecular meshwork preserved, thus reducing the incidence of postoperative overfiltration and hypotony and its potential sequelae.

2. Indications – POAG not requiring very low IOP.

3. Technique
- Two lamellar scleral flaps are fashioned (*Fig. 13.67*).
- The deep flap is excised leaving behind a thin membrane consisting of trabeculum/ Descemet membrane through which aqueous diffuses from the anterior chamber to the subconjunctival space.

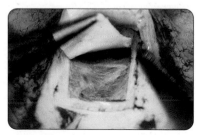

Fig. 13.67 Non-penetrating surgery – the deep flap is being held

4. Complications – similar to trabeculectomy except for shallow anterior chamber.

Adjunctive antimetabolites

1. **Definition** – agents that inhibit the natural healing response that may preclude successful filtration surgery.
2. **Indications** – risk factors for failure of trabeculectomy such as neovascular glaucoma, previous failed trabeculectomy or artificial filtering devices, and certain secondary glaucomas.
3. **Agents**
   a. *5-Fluorouracil* (5-FU) – can be used during surgery by applying a cellulose sponge soaked to the filtration site or postoperatively by subconjunctival injection.
   b. *Mitomycin C* (MMC) – more potent than 5-FU; can be used during surgery in the same way as 5-FU and can also be applied externally to the bleb postoperatively.
4. **Complications** – corneal epithelial defects, and cystic thin-walled blebs that predispose to chronic hypotony, late-onset bleb leak, blebitis (*Fig. 13.68*) and endophthalmitis.

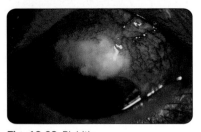

Fig. 13.68 Blebitis

Artificial drainage implants

1. **Definition** – plastic devices, which create a communication between the anterior chamber and sub-Tenon space (*Fig. 13.69*).

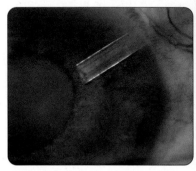

Fig. 13.69 Drainage implant

2. **Indications** – conditions where conventional surgery, even with adjunctive antimetabolites, is very unlikely to be successful.
3. **Implant types**
   a. *Molteno* – silicone tube connected to polypropylene plates.
   b. *Baerveldt* – silicone tube connected to a large area silicone plate impregnated with barium.
   c. *Ahmed* – silicone tube connected to a silicone sheet valve held in a polypropylene body.
4. **Complications** – excessive drainage, malposition, tube erosion, drainage failure, and bleb encapsulation.
5. **Results** – IOP <21 mmHg is achieved in 50–70% of cases but topical medication is often required to maintain the IOP at this level.

Introduction

Classification (*Fig. 14.1*)

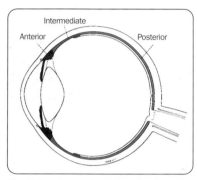

Fig. 14.1 Anatomical classification of uveitis

1. **Anterior uveitis**
   - Iritis – primarily involves the iris.
   - Iridocyclitis – involves the iris and ciliary body.
2. **Intermediate** – predominantly involving the vitreous.
3. **Posterior uveitis**.
   - Retinitis.
   - Choroiditis.
   - Vasculitis – may involve veins, arteries or both.
4. **Panuveitis (diffuse)** – involves the entire uveal tract without a predominant site of inflammation.
5. **Endophthalmitis** – involves all intraocular tissues except the sclera.
6. **Panophthalmitis** – involves the entire globe.

Definitions

1. **Onset** – sudden or insidious.
2. **Duration**
   a. *Limited* – 3 months or less.
   b. *Persistent* – longer.
3. **Course**
   a. *Acute* – sudden onset and limited duration.
   b. *Recurrent* – repeated episodes separated by periods of inactivity lasting at least 3 months.
   c. *Chronic* – persistent with prompt relapse (in less than 3 months) after discontinuation of treatment.
   d. *Remission* – inactive disease for at least 3 months after discontinuation of treatment.

Clinical features

Acute anterior uveitis

1. **Presentation** – sudden onset of unilateral, pain, and photophobia.
2. **Ciliary (circumcorneal) injection** (*Fig. 14.2*).

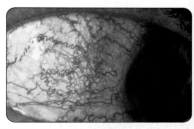

Fig. 14.2 Ciliary injection

3. **Endothelial cellular dusting** – gives rise to a 'dirty' appearance (*Fig. 14.3*).

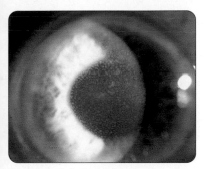

Fig. 14.3 Endothelial dusting

4. **Aqueous cells and flare** – vary according to activity (*Fig. 14.4*).

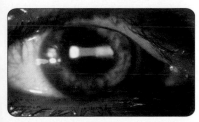

Fig. 14.4 Flare and cells

5. **Anterior vitreous cells** – in iridocyclitis.
6. **Aqueous fibrinous exudate** – in HLA-B27-associated uveitis (*Fig. 14.5*).

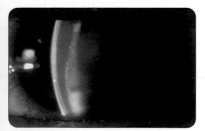

Fig. 14.5 Fibrinous exudate

7. **Hypopyon** – in severe uveitis (*Fig. 14.6*).

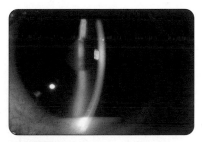

Fig. 14.6 Hypopyon

8. **Posterior synechiae** – may develop quickly (*Fig. 14.7*).

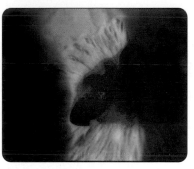

Fig. 14.7 Posterior synechiae

9. **Course** – 5–6 weeks.
10. **Prognosis** – good.

Chronic anterior uveitis

1. **Presentation** – insidious and may be occasionally asymptomatic until the development of complications.
2. **External** – usually white eye or occasionally pink during periods of exacerbation.
3. **Aqueous cells** – vary according to disease activity.

4. Aqueous flare – may be more marked than cells in eyes with prolonged activity.

5. Keratic precipitates (KP) – in granulomatous disease have a greasy ('mutton-fat') appearance (*Fig. 14.8*).

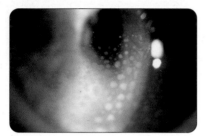

Fig. 14.8 'Mutton fat' keratic precipitates

6. Iris nodules – occur in granulomatous disease (*Fig. 14.9*).
- Koeppe nodules are small and situated at the pupillary border.
- Busacca nodules are stromal.
- Large pink nodules are characteristic of sarcoid uveitis.

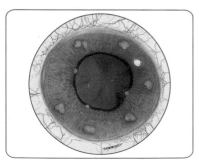

Fig. 14.9 Iris nodules

7. Course – longer than 6 weeks and many last many months.

8. Prognosis – guarded; complications such as band keratopathy, cataract, and glaucoma are common.

Posterior uveitis

1. Presentation – depends on the location of the inflammatory focus and the presence of vitritis.

2. Retinitis – may be focal (solitary) or multifocal; active lesions are whitish retinal opacities with indistinct borders (*Fig. 14.10*).

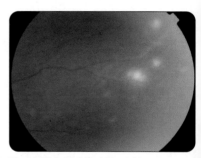

Fig. 14.10 Multifocal retinitis

3. Choroiditis – may be focal, multifocal or geographic; active lesions are round, yellow nodules (*Fig. 14.11*).

4. Vasculitis – patchy perivascular cuffing (*Fig. 14.12*).

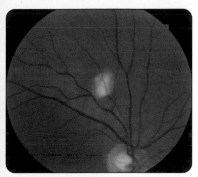

Fig. 14.11 Choroiditis

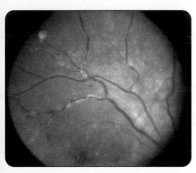

Fig. 14.12 Retinal vasculitis

Treatment

Mydriatics

Preparations

1. Short-acting
  a. *Tropicamide* (0.5% and 1%) – duration 6 hours.
  b. *Cyclopentolate* (0.5% and 1%) – duration 24 hours.
  c. *Phenylephrine* (2.5% and 10%) – duration 3 hours but no cycloplegia.

2. Long-acting
  a. *Homatropine 2%* – duration up to 2 days.
  b. *Atropine 1%* – duration of up to 2 weeks.

Indications

1. **To promote comfort** – by relieving ciliary and pupillary spasm with atropine or homatropine.
2. **To break down recently formed posterior synechiae**
   • Intensive topical mydriatics (atropine, phenylephrine).
   • Subconjunctival injections of mydricaine (adrenaline, atropine and procaine).
3. **To prevent formation of posterior synechiae** – with a short-acting mydriatic that allows some mobility of the pupil.

Topical steroids

1. **Treatment of AAU**
   • Initial used either hourly or every minute for the first 5 minutes of every hour.
   • Tapered to 2-hourly, followed by 3-hourly, then four times a day, and eventually reduced by one drop/week.
   • Usually discontinued by 5–6 weeks.
2. **Treatment of CAU**
   • Exacerbations are treated in the same way as AAU.
   • If the inflammation is controlled the rate of instillation can be further reduced by one drop/month.

3. Complications – elevation of IOP, cataract, microbial keratitis, and occasionally systemic side-effects.

Periocular steroids

1. Anterior subconjunctival
- Short-acting steroids (prednisolone) in severe AAU.
- Long-acting steroids (triamcinolone acetonide, methylprednisolone acetate) in severe CAU.

2. Posterior sub-Tenon long-acting steroids (*Fig. 14.13*) – in intermediate uveitis and selected cases of posterior uveitis.

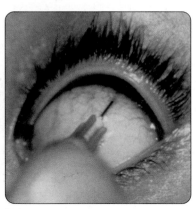

Fig. 14.13 Posterior sub-Tenon steroid injection

3. Complications – globe penetration, elevation of IOP, sub-dermal fat atrophy, ptosis, optic nerve injury, and extraocular muscle paresis.

Intraocular steroids

1. Injection (triamcinolone acetonide) – for posterior uveitis and CMO unresponsive to other forms of therapy.

2. Slow-release implants (fluocinolone acetonide) – for posterior uveitis unresponsive or intolerant to conventional treatment.

Systemic steroids

1. Preparations
- **a.** *Oral prednisolone* (5 mg or 25 mg tablets).
- **b.** *Intravenous methylprednisolone* (1 g/day).

2. Indications
- Intermediate uveitis unresponsive to posterior sub-Tenon injections.
- Sight-threatening posterior or panuveitis, particularly when bilateral.

3. Contraindications
- Poorly controlled diabetes – relative contraindication.
- Peptic ulceration.
- Osteoporosis.
- Active systemic infection.
- Psychosis on previous exposure to steroids.

4. General rules of administration
- Starting dose of prednisolone is 1–2 mg/kg/day.
- Followed by a slow taper over several weeks.
- Doses of 40 mg or less for 3 weeks or less do not require gradual reduction.
- Doses of more than 15 mg/day are unacceptable long-term.

5. Side-effects
- **a.** *Of short-term therapy* – dyspepsia, mental changes, electrolyte imbalance, aseptic necrosis of the head of the femur and, very rarely, hyperosmolar hyperglycaemic non-ketotic coma.
- **b.** *Of long-term therapy* – Cushingoid state, osteoporosis, limitation of growth in children, reactivation of

infections such as TB, cataract, and exacerbation of diabetes.

Antimetabolites

1. Indications
   a. *Sight-threatening uveitis* – usually bilateral, non-infectious, and steroid resistant.
   b. *Steroid-sparing therapy* – in patients with intolerable side-effects from systemic steroids.
2. Agents – azathioprine, methotrexate, and mycophenolate mofetil.
3. Side-effects – bone marrow suppression, gastrointestinal upset, and hepatotoxicity.

Immune modulators

Ciclosporin
1. Indications – Behçet disease, intermediate uveitis, birdshot retinochoroidopathy, Vogt–Koyanagi–Harada syndrome, sympathetic ophthalmitis, and idiopathic retinal vasculitis.
2. Side-effects – nephrotoxicity, hyperlipidaemia, hepatotoxicity, hypertension, hirsutism, and gingival hyperplasia.

Tacrolimus
1. Indications – alternative to ciclosporin in intolerant or unresponsive patients.
2. Side-effects – hyperglycaemia, neurotoxicity and nephrotoxicity.

Intermediate uveitis

1. Introduction
   • Intermediate uveitis (IU) – idiopathic or associated with a systemic disease.
   • Pars planitis (PP) – subset of idiopathic IU in which there is snowbanking or snowball formation.
2. Presentation – insidious onset of blurred vision often accompanied by vitreous floaters.
3. Anterior uveitis
   • Mild in PP.
   • May be severe in the other forms of IU.
4. Vitreous
   • Predominantly anterior vitreous cells.
   • Condensation (*Fig. 14.14*).
   • Snowball opacities most numerous inferiorly (*Fig. 14.15*).

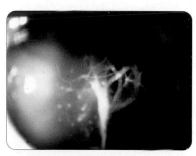

Fig. 14.14 Vitreous condensations

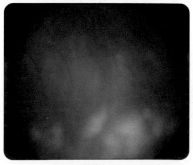

Fig. 14.15 Vitreous snow balls

5. Posterior segment
- Peripheral periphlebitis, particularly in MS.
- Inferior snowbanking (*Fig. 14.16*).
- Neovascularization on the snowbank or optic nerve head.

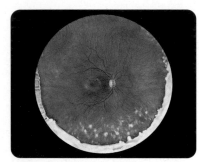

Fig. 14.16 Snowbanking

6. **Course** – ranges from short and benign with spontaneous resolution, to severe and prolonged with episodes of exacerbations.
7. **Complications** – CMO in 30%, macular epiretinal membrane, cataract, vasoproliferative tumour, RD, and vitreous haemorrhage.
8. **Treatment of CMO**
   - Initial posterior sub-Tenon injections of triamcinolone.
   - Further options – systemic steroids, vitrectomy, and antimetabolites.
9. **Systemic associations** – multiple sclerosis, sarcoidosis, and Lyme disease.

Uveitis in spondyloarthropathies

HLA-B27 and spondyloarthropathies

A strong association exists between HLA-B27 and spondyloarthropathies; the prevalence of HLA-B27 is as follows:
- 6–8% of the Caucasian population of the USA.
- 50% of patients with AAU who are otherwise fit and well.
- 90% of patients with AAU who have an associated spondyloarthropathy, most notably ankylosing spondylitis.

Ankylosing spondylitis

1. **AAU**
   - Affects 25% of patients with AS.
   - Conversely, 25% of males with AAU will have AS.
   - Typically unilateral, severe, recurrent, and associated with a fibrinous exudate.
2. **Other manifestation** – conjunctivitis.

Reiter syndrome

1. **AAU**
   - Occurs in up to 12% of patients.
   - Prevalence is higher in carriers of HLA-B27.
2. **Other manifestations** – conjunctivitis (very common), nummular keratitis, scleritis and episcleritis.

Psoriatic arthritis

1. **AAU** – affects about 7% of patients.
2. **Other manifestations** – conjunctivitis, marginal corneal infiltrates, and KCS.

Uveitis in juvenile arthritis

Juvenile idiopathic arthritis (JIA)

1. **Definition** – inflammatory arthritis of at least 6 weeks' duration occurring before the age of 16 years.
2. **Classification** – based on the onset and the extent of joint involvement during the first 6 months as follows:
   a. *Pauciarticular onset* (60% of cases)
   - Four or fewer joints.
   - Uveitis in about 20% of patients.
   - Risk factors for uveitis – early-onset JIA, and positive findings for ANA and HLA-DR5.
   b. *Polyarticular onset* (20% of cases)
   - Five or more joints.
   - Uveitis in about 5% of patients.
   c. *Systemic onset* – accounts for about 20% of patients but is not associated with uveitis.
3. **Presentation of uveitis** – frequently detected on routine slit-lamp examination or when complications such as band keratopathy and cataract have occurred (*Fig. 14.17*).

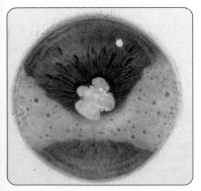

Fig. 14.17 Band keratopathy and cataract

4. **Signs** – non-granulomatous CAU in a white eye, which is bilateral in 70% of cases.
5. **Screening for uveitis** – for at least 7 years from the onset of arthritis or until the age of 12 years. The frequency is governed by the following risk factors:
   - Systemic onset = not required.
   - Polyarticular onset = every 9 months.
   - Polyarticular onset + ANA = every 6 months.
   - Pauciarticular onset = every 3 months.
   - Pauciarticular onset + ANA = every 2 months.

Familial juvenile systemic granulomatosis syndrome (Blau syndrome, Jabs disease)

1. **Inheritance** – AD.
2. **Definition** – childhood onset of granulomatous disease of skin, eyes and joints but absence of pulmonary disease.
3. **Uveitis** – panuveitis and multifocal choroiditis.
4. **Differential diagnosis** – sarcoidosis and JIA.

Uveitis in bowel disease

1. **Ulcerative colitis**
   - AAU occurs in about 5% – more common if associated with ankylosing spondylitis.
   - Other manifestations – peripheral corneal infiltrates, conjunctivitis, episcleritis, scleritis, and retinal vasculitis.

2. Crohn disease
- AAU occurs in about 3%.
- Other manifestations – conjunctivitis, episcleritis, peripheral corneal infiltrates and retinal periphlebitis.
3. Whipple disease – vitritis, retinitis, multifocal choroiditis, retinal haemorrhages and cotton-wool spots.

Uveitis in renal disease

Tubulointerstitial nephritis and uveitis (TINU)

1. **Definition** – uncommon disorder characterized by a combination of idiopathic acute tubulointerstitial nephritis and uveitis.
2. **Presentation** – in late childhood with proteinuria, anaemia, hypertension, and renal failure.
3. **Uveitis** – anterior, bilateral, and non-granulomatous.

IgA glomerulonephritis

1. **Definition** – common disease in which IgA is found in the glomerular mesangium.
2. **Presentation** – 3rd–5th decade with recurrent macroscopic haematuria and upper respiratory tract infection.
3. **Ocular manifestations** – anterior uveitis, keratoconjunctivitis, and scleritis.

Sarcoidosis

1. **Anterior uveitis**
   - AAU in acute-onset sarcoid.
   - Granulomatous CAU in patients with chronic pulmonary disease.
2. **Intermediate uveitis** – may antedate systemic disease.

3. **Periphlebitis** – 'candlewax drippings' (*en taches de bougie* – *Fig. 14.18*).

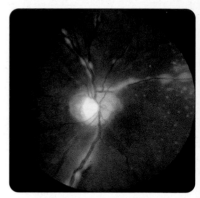

Fig. 14.18 Candlewax drippings

4. **Choroiditis**
   - Multifocal choroiditis (*Fig. 14.19*).
   - Multiple, small, pale-yellow, infiltrates, which may have a 'punched-out' appearance.
   - Large, confluent, infiltrates which may have amoeboid margins (*Fig. 14.20*).
   - Solitary choroidal granulomas are uncommon.

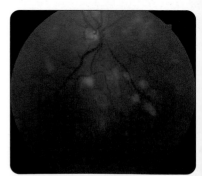

Fig. 14.19 Multifocal choroiditis

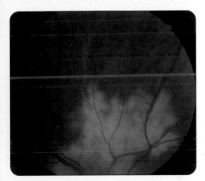

Fig. 14.20 Amoeboid Infiltration

5. **Retinal granulomas** – small, discrete, yellow lesions (*Fig. 14.21*).

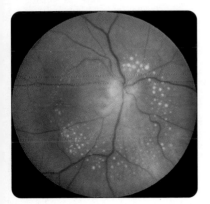

Fig. 14.21 Retinal granulomas

6. **Peripheral retinal neovascularization** – secondary to retinal capillary dropout (*Fig. 14.22*).

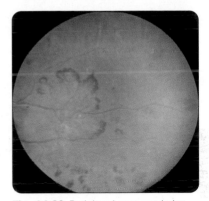

Fig. 14.22 Peripheral neovascularization

7. **Optic nerve** – granulomas (*Fig. 14.23*) and persistent disc oedema.

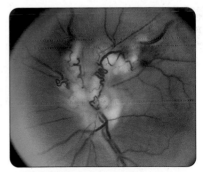

Fig. 14.23 Disc granuloma

8. **Investigations** – biopsy of conjunctiva or lacrimal gland, chest x-ray, angiotensin-converting enzyme (ACE) and lysozyme assay.
9. **Treatment of posterior uveitis** – posterior sub-Tenon steroid injections or systemic steroids; rarely ciclosporin or methotrexate.

Behçet syndrome

1. **Incidence of uveitis**
   - 95% of men and 70% of women within 2 years of oral ulceration.
   - Presenting manifestation in about 10% of cases.
2. **AAU** – associated with transient mobile hypopyon in a white eye.
3. **Transient retinal infiltrates** – during the acute stage of the systemic disease (see *Fig. 14.10*).
4. **Retinal vasculitis**
   - May involve both veins and arteries (*Fig. 14.24*).
   - May result in vascular occlusion and optic atrophy (*Fig. 14.25*).

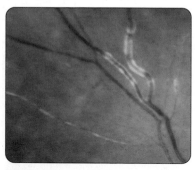

Fig. 14.24 Vasculitis

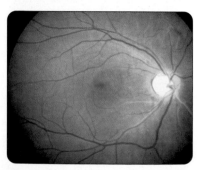

Fig. 14.25 End-stage disease

5. **Vitritis** – universal in eyes with active disease (*Fig. 14.26*).

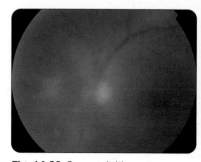

Fig. 14.26 Severe vitritis

6. **Other manifestations** – conjunctivitis, conjunctival ulcers, episcleritis, scleritis, and ophthalmoplegia.
7. **Treatment of posterior uveitis**
   - Systemic steroids short-term and azathioprine long-term.
   - Other options – ciclosporin, subcutaneous interferon alfa-2a, and biological blockers.
8. **Prognosis** – guarded – 20% blindness despite treatment.

Vogt–Koyanagi–Harada syndrome

1. **Anterior uveitis** – non-granulomatous during the acute phase but shows granulomatous features during recurrences.
2. **Posterior uveitis** in chronological order:
   - Diffuse choroidal infiltration.
   - Multifocal serous retinal detachments and disc oedema (*Fig. 14.27*).
   - Exudative RD.

- Diffuse RPE atrophy (sunset-glow fundus) which may be associated with small, peripheral, discrete atrophic spots (*Fig. 14.28*).

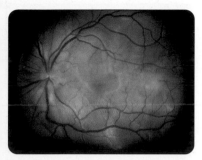

Fig. 14.27 Multifocal serous RDs

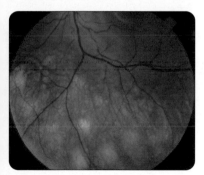

Fig. 14.28 Sunset glow fundus

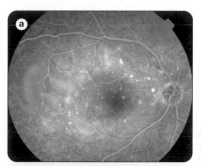

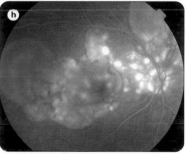

Fig. 14.29 (a) Early hyperfluorescent spots; (b) late accumulation of subretinal dye

3. FA
- Early phase – multifocal hyperfluorescent spots (*Fig. 14.29a*).
- Late phase – accumulation of dye in the subretinal space (*Fig. 14.29b*).

4. ICG – hypofluorescent dark spots, delayed or patchy filling, indistinct choroidal vessels in the early phase.

5. Treatment of posterior uveitis – intravenous or high-dose oral steroids; ciclosporin for non-responders.

Parasitic uveitis

Toxoplasma retinitis

1. Pathogenesis
- Infestation with *Toxoplasma gondii*, an obligate intracellular protozoan.

- The cat is the definitive host and other animals including humans are intermediate hosts (Fig. 14.30).

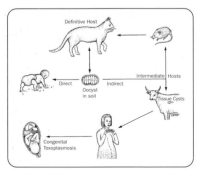

Fig. 14.30 Life cycle of *Toxoplasma gondii*

2. Signs
- 'Spill-over' anterior uveitis, often granulomatous.
- Focal retinitis near an old pigmented scar ('satellite lesion' – Fig. 14.31).
- Severe vitritis (headlight in the fog – Fig. 14.32).
- Inactive lesions – atrophic scar with a hyperpigmented border (Fig. 14.33).

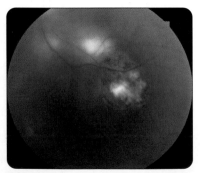

Fig. 14.31 Acute toxoplasma retinitis

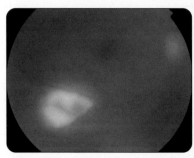

Fig. 14.32 Headlight in fog appearance

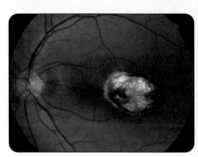

Fig. 14.33 Inactive lesion

3. Investigations – dye test (Sabin–Feldman), immunofluorescent antibody, haemagglutination, and ELISA.

4. Treatment of vision threatening lesions.
   a. *Oral prednisolone + anti-toxoplasma agent.*
   b. *Clindamycin 300 mg q.i.d. for 3–4 weeks + a sulfonamide.*
   c. *Sulfadiazine 1 g q.i.d. for 3–4 weeks + pyrimethamine.*
   d. *Pyrimethamine 25–50 mg daily for 4 weeks + folinic acid 5 mg three times weekly.*
   e. *Co-trimoxazole (Septrin) 960 mg b.d. for 4–6 weeks as monotherapy or in combination with clindamycin.*

f. *Atovaquone* 750 mg t.i.d.
g. *Azithromycin* 500 mg daily a good alternative to sulfadiazine.

Toxocariasis

Toxocariasis is caused by an infestation with a common intestinal ascarid (roundworm) of dogs called *Toxocara canis*.

Chronic endophthalmitis

1. Presentation – 2–9 years with leukocoria (*Fig. 14.34*), strabismus or unilateral visual loss.

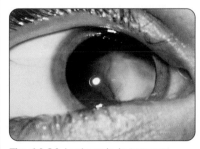

Fig. 14.34 Leukocoria in toxocara endophthalmitis

2. Signs
- CAU and vitritis.
- Peripheral granuloma in some cases.
- Peripheral dense greyish-white exudate.

3. Treatment – steroids may be used to reduce the inflammatory activity.

4. Prognosis – very poor.

Posterior pole granuloma

1. Presentation – 6–14 years with unilateral visual impairment.
2. Signs
- Absence of intraocular inflammation.

- Granuloma in the posterior fundus (*Fig. 14.35*).
- Vitreoretinal traction bands and localized tractional RD.

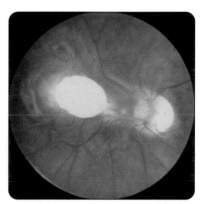

Fig. 14.35 Posterior pole granuloma

Peripheral granuloma

1. Presentation – adolescence or adult life with visual impairment or detected by chance.
2. Signs
- Absence of intraocular inflammation.
- White hemispherical peripheral granuloma (*Fig. 14.36*).
- 'Dragging' of the disc and macula.

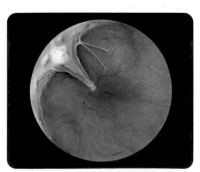

Fig. 14.36 Peripheral granuloma

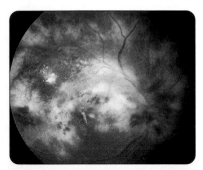

Fig. 14.42 Fulminating CMV retinitis

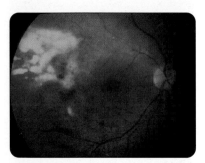

Fig. 14.43 Inactive CMV retinitis

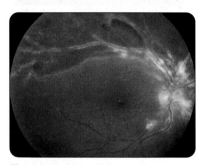

Fig. 14.44 RD in CMV retinitis

Systemic treatment

1. Ganciclovir
- Induction – intravenously every 12 hours for 2–3 weeks and then every 24 hours.
- Oral maintenance.

2. Valganciclovir – as effective as intravenous ganciclovir for treatment and prophylaxis.

3. Intravenous foscarnet – may also improve life expectancy.

4. Intravenous cidofovir – where other agents are unsuitable.

Intravitreal treatment

1. Ganciclovir slow-release device (Vitrasert) – duration of 8 months.

2. Intravitreal injections
- **a.** *Ganciclovir* – may be performed prior to implantation of a slow-release implant to determine the likely response to the drug.
- **b.** *Fomivirsen* – different mechanism of action from other agents.
- **c.** *Cidofovir* – may occasionally cause severe uveitis.

Progressive outer retinal necrosis

1. Definition – necrotizing retinitis caused by VZV that affects patients with profound immunosuppression as in AIDS.

2. Presentation – rapidly progressive visual loss which is initially unilateral in 75% of cases.

3. Signs in chronological order:
- Minimal anterior uveitis.
- Multifocal, yellow-white, retinal infiltrates with minimal vitritis.
- Early macular involvement (*Fig. 14.45*).
- Rapid confluence and full-thickness retinal necrosis.

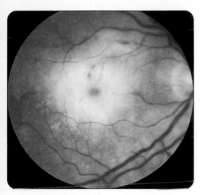

Fig. 14.45 Macular involvement in PORN

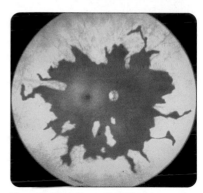

Fig. 14.46 Advanced ARN with macular sparing

4. Treatment – ganciclovir and foscarnet.
5. Prognosis – very poor.

Acute retinal necrosis

1. Definition – necrotizing retinitis that affects healthy individuals which tends to be caused by herpes simple (HSV) in younger patients and VZV in older individuals.
2. Presentation – initially unilateral and varies according to severity.
3. Signs
- Anterior granulomatous uveitis and vitritis.
- Peripheral periarteritis associated with retinal infiltrates.
- Progressive full-thickness retinal necrosis with macular sparing until late (*Fig. 14.46*).
- Acute lesions resolve within 6–12 weeks, leaving behind a transparent necrotic retina with hyperpigmented borders.

4. Treatment – aciclovir.
5. Prognosis – guarded.

Herpes simplex anterior uveitis

1. Granulomatous CAU
- May occur with or without active corneal disease.
- Patchy iris atrophy is uncommon.
- Spontaneous hyphaema is uncommon.
2. Treatment – topical steroids (in the absence of active corneal epithelial disease) and oral aciclovir.

Varicella zoster anterior uveitis

1. Granulomatous CAU
- Affects nearly 50% of the patients with HZO particularly when the rash involves the side of the nose (Hutchinson sign – see *Fig. 9.14*).
- Sectoral iris atrophy is common (*Fig. 14.47*).
2. Treatment – topical steroids.

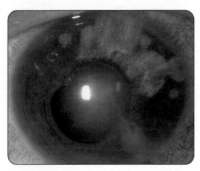

Fig. 14.47 Sectoral iris atrophy in zoster

Congenital rubella

1. **Anterior uveitis** – may result in diffuse iris atrophy (*Fig. 14.48*).

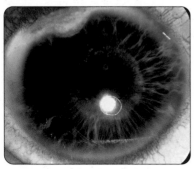

Fig. 14.48 Diffuse iris atrophy in rubella

2. **Retinopathy**
   - Diffuse 'salt and pepper' pigmentary disturbance (*Fig. 14.49*).
   - A few eyes later develop CNV.

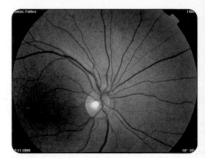

Fig. 14.49 Rubella retinopathy

3. **Other manifestations** – cataract, microphthalmos, glaucoma, keratitis, and extreme refractive errors.

Subacute sclerosing panencephalitis

1. **Definition** – chronic, progressive, neurodegenerative and usually fatal disease of children caused by the measles virus.
2. **Posterior uveitis** – papillitis, macular oedema, whitish retinal infiltrates, and choroiditis (*Fig. 14.50*).

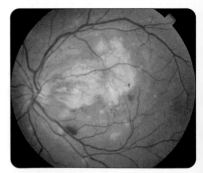

Fig. 14.50 Retinopathy in subacute sclerosing panencephalitis

Fungal uveitis

Presumed ocular histoplasmosis syndrome

1. **Pathogenesis** – immunologic mediated response in individuals previously exposed to *Histoplasma capsulatum*.
2. **HLA association** – HLA-B7 and HLA-DR2.
3. **Absence of intraocular inflammation**.
4. **Atrophic 'histo' spots** – roundish, slightly irregular, yellowish-white lesions often associated with pigment clumps scattered in the mid-retinal periphery and posterior fundus (*Fig. 14.51*).

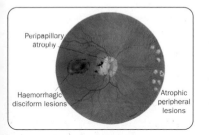

Peripapillary atrophy

Haemorrhagic disciform lesions

Atrophic peripheral lesions

Fig. 14.51 Signs in POHS

5. **Peripapillary atrophy.**
6. **Exudative (wet) maculopathy**
   - CNV develops between the ages of 20 and 45 years in about 5% of eyes.
   - Treatment options include argon laser photocoagulation, photodynamic therapy (PDT), and surgical removal.

Cryptococcosis

1. **Pathogenesis** – associated with cell-mediated immune dysfunction and affects 5–10% of patients with AIDS; ocular involvement is present in approximately 6% of patients with cryptococcal meningitis.
2. **Signs**
   - Meningitis-associated manifestations – papilloedema, ophthalmoplegia, ptosis, optic neuropathy and 6th nerve palsy.
   - Multifocal choroiditis (*Fig. 14.52*).

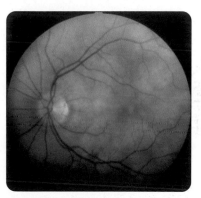

Fig. 14.52 Cryptococcal choroiditis

3. **Treatment** – intravenous amphotericin, oral fluconazole and itraconazole.

Endogenous fungal endophthalmitis

1. **Pathogenesis**
   - Metastatic spread from a septic focus associated with catheters, intravenous drug abuse, parenteral nutrition, and chronic lung disease.

- Pathogens – *Candida* spp.; less common *Cryptococcus* spp., *Sporothrix schenckii*, and *Blastomyces* spp.

2. Signs

- Creamy white chorioretinal lesions with overlying vitritis (*Fig. 14.53*).
- Extension into the vitreous (*Fig. 14.54*).
- Vitritis and floating cotton-ball colonies (*Fig. 14.55*).
- Chronic endophthalmitis.

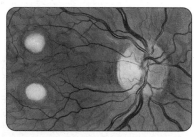

Fig. 14.53 Fungal chorioretinitis

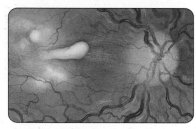

Fig. 14.54 Vitreous extension

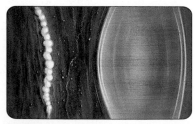

Fig. 14.55 Cotton-ball colonies

3. Course
— chronic and may result in retinal necrosis and RD.

4. Investigations
– vitreous biopsy, and smears and cultures.

5. Treatment

a. *Medical* – for systemic disease and ocular disease without vitreous involvement.
- Intravenous amphotericin.
- Oral fluconazole for 3–6 weeks.
- Oral voriconazole for cases resistant to fluconazole.

b. *Vitrectomy + intravitreal amphotericin* – for vitreous involvement.

Bacterial uveitis

Tuberculosis

1. CAU
– usually granulomatous.

2. Choroiditis

- Unilateral focal or less frequently multifocal.
- Large solitary granulomas.
- Extensive diffuse choroiditis in patients with AIDS (*Fig. 14.56*).

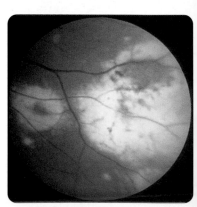

Fig. 14.56 Diffuse TB choroiditis in AIDS

- Occasionally may resemble serpiginous choroidopathy.

3. Periphlebitis – may be occlusive (*Fig. 14.57*).

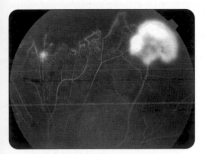

Fig. 14.57 FA showing capillary non-perfusion and neovascularization in occlusive TB vasculitis

4. Treatment – initially with at least three drugs (isoniazid, rifampicin, pyrazinamide or cthambutol) and then with isoniazid and rifampicin.

Syphilis

1. AAU – uncommon and bilateral in 50%, and may be associated with dilated iris capillaries (roseolae – *Fig. 14.58*), papules and nodules.

2. Chorioretinitis
- Multifocal disease which is frequently bilateral and results in scarring (*Fig. 14.59*).
- Acute posterior placoid chorioretinitis in AIDS (*Fig. 14.60*).

3. Neuroretinitis.

4. Periphlebitis – may be occlusive.

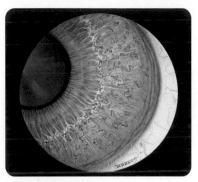

Fig. 14.58 Roseolae

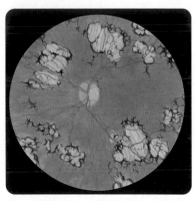

Fig. 14.59 Old syphilitic chorioretinitis

5. Treatment involves one of the following regimens:
   a. *Intravenous* aqueous penicillin G for 10–15 days.
   b. *Intramuscular* procaine penicillin, supplemented with oral proben-ecid for 10–15 days.
   c. *Oral* amoxicillin for 28 days.

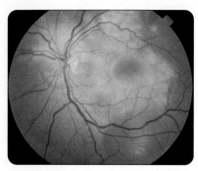

Fig. 14.60 Placoid syphilitic chorioretinitis in AIDS

Lyme disease (borreliosis)

1. **Pathogen** – flagellated spirochaete *Borrelia burgdorferi*.
2. **Uveitis** – anterior, intermediate, peripheral multifocal choroiditis, retinal periphlebitis and neuroretinitis; all are uncommon.
3. **Other manifestations** – follicular conjunctivitis, episcleritis, keratitis, scleritis, orbital myositis, optic neuritis, ocular motor nerve palsies and reversible Horner syndrome.
4. **Treatment** – steroids for uveitis.

Brucellosis

1. **Pathogens** – zoonotic disease caused by the Gram-negative bacteria *Brucella melitensis* or *Brucella abortus*.
2. **Uveitis** – CAU, multifocal choroiditis, and rarely, endogenous endophthalmitis.
3. **Other manifestations** – dacryoadenitis, episcleritis, nummular keratitis and optic neuritis.

4. **Treatment** – tetracycline for 6 weeks and streptomycin for 2 weeks; doxycycline and rifampicin are alternatives.

Endogenous bacterial endophthalmitis

1. **Pathogenesis**
   - Organisms enter the eye through the blood–eye barrier from the bloodstream.
   - *Klebsiella* spp. – most common although a wide variety or organisms may be responsible.
2. **Risk factors** – diabetes, cardiac disease, malignancy, indwelling catheters, intravenous drug abuse, liver abscess, pneumonia, endocarditis, cellulitis, urinary tract infection (*E. coli*), meningitis, septic arthritis, and abdominal surgery.
3. **Anterior segment**
   - Proptosis, chemosis, swollen lids, and corneal oedema.
   - Discrete iris nodules or plaques, anterior fibrinous uveitis and hypopyon.
4. **Posterior segment**
   - White or yellow retinal infiltrates (*Fig. 14.61*).
   - Vitreous haze and abscess.
   - Retinal necrosis in severe cases.
5. **Investigations**
   a. *Systemic*
   - Search for septic foci (skin, joints).
   - Blood and urine cultures.
   - Appropriate cultures from other sites depending on the clinical features.
   - Investigations for endocarditis.
   - Abdominal ultrasound.
   b. *Ocular* – aqueous and vitreous samples.

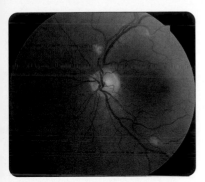

Fig. 14.61 Retinal infiltrates in early endogenous endophthalmitis

6. **Treatment** – intravenous antibiotics for systemic infection and oral ciprofloxacin and intravitreal antibiotics for endophthalmitis.

Cat-scratch disease

1. **Pathogenesis** – subacute infection caused by *Bartonella henselae* a Gram-negative rod.
2. **Ocular manifestations** – neuroretinitis (see Chapter 21), Parinaud oculoglandular syndrome, focal choroiditis, intermediate uveitis, exudative maculopathy, retinal vascular occlusion, and panuveitis.
3. **Treatment** – oral doxycycline or erythromycin, with or without rifampicin.

Leprosy

1. **Pathogenesis** – direct invasion of the iris by *Mycobacterium leprae*.

2. **Signs**
   - Low-grade uveitis associated with synechiae.
   - Iris pearls that enlarge and coalesce, and drop into the anterior chamber (*Fig. 14.62*).
   - Eventual miosis and iris atrophy (*Fig. 14.63*).
3. **Treatment** – systemic antibiotics and topical steroids.

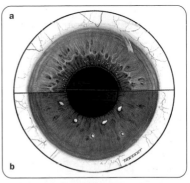

Fig. 14.62 Iris pearls

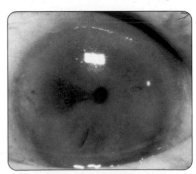

Fig. 14.63 Miosis and iris atrophy

Primary idiopathic inflammatory choriocapillaropathies (white dot syndromes)

Acute posterior multifocal placoid pigment epitheliopathy

1. **Definition** – usually bilateral idiopathic condition which presents in the 3rd–6th decade.
2. **HLA association** – HLA-B7 and HLA-DR2.
3. **Presentation** – subacute visual impairment in one eye and then the other within a few days or weeks.
4. **Signs** in chronological order:
   - Mild vitritis.
   - Multiple, cream or greyish-white, placoid lesions at the posterior pole and post-equatorial fundus (*Fig. 14.64a*).
   - After 2 weeks the majority are replaced by RPE changes.
   - Vision recovers within a few weeks although scotomas may persist.
5. **FA** – early dense hypofluorescence (*Fig. 14.64b*) and late hyperfluorescence (*Fig. 14.64c*).
6. **EOG** – may be subnormal.
7. **Treatment** – not appropriate.
8. **Prognosis** – very good.

Birdshot retinochoroidopathy

1. **Definition** – chronic, recurrent, bilateral disease which presents in the 5th–7th decade; predominantly affects females.
2. **HLA association** – HLA-A29 in 95% of cases.
3. **Signs** in chronological order:
   - Vitritis and retinal vasculitis.

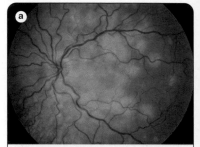

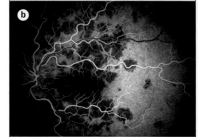

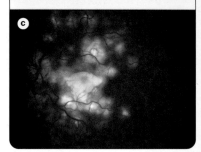

Fig. 14.64 APMPPE

- Multiple, small, cream, choroidal spots in the posterior pole and mid-periphery (*Fig. 14.65*).
- Inactive lesions – well delineated, atrophic spots.
- End-stage disease – vascular attenuation, retinal degeneration, and optic atrophy (*Fig. 14.66*).

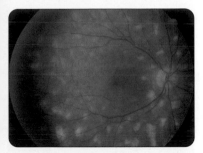

Fig. 14.65 Active birdshot

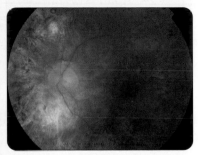

Fig. 14.66 End-stage birdshot

4. **ICG** – well defined hypofluorescent spots in the early phases (*Fig. 14.67*) that later become hyperfluorescent.

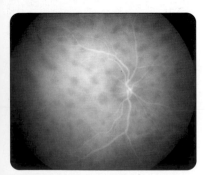

Fig. 14.67 ICG of birdshot

5. **ERG** – with time the b-wave amplitude and then oscillatory potential become decreased; delay in implicit time of the 30 Hz flicker ERG is the most sensitive change.

6. **Treatment** – based on ERG abnormalities; involves systemic steroids, azathioprine or mycophenolate mofetil.

7. **Prognosis** – guarded.

Punctate inner choroidopathy

1. **Definition** – chronic, bilateral disease that typically affects young myopic women.

2. **Signs** in chronological order:
   - Absent or minimal intraocular inflammation.
   - Multiple, small, deep, spots with fuzzy borders at the posterior pole (*Fig. 14.68a*).
   - Residual atrophic scars after a few weeks.
   - CNV develops in up to 40% of eyes.

3. **FA** – early hyperfluorescence (*Fig. 14.68b*) and late staining of the PIC lesions as well as CNV (*Fig. 14.68c*).

4. **ERG** – normal.

5. **Treatment of CNV** – PDT or surgical excision.

6. **Prognosis** – guarded.

Serpiginous choroidopathy

1. **Definition** – chronic, bilateral, recurrent disease which presents in the 4th–6th decade; affects men more frequently than women.

2. **HLA association** – HLA-B7.

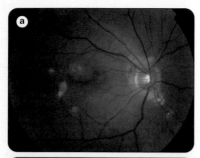

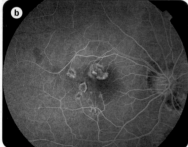

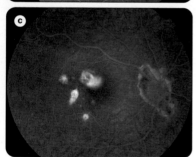

Fig. 14.68 (a) PIC; (b) FA early phase; (c) FA late phase

3. Signs

- Mild vitritis.
- Grey-white to yellow deep peripapillary lesions (*Fig. 14.69*).

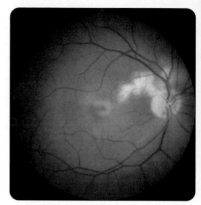

Fig. 14.69 Early serpiginous

- Gradual spread in a serpentine manner towards the macula and periphery.
- Residual scalloped, atrophic 'punched-out' areas (*Fig. 14.70*).
- Subretinal fibrosis and CNV may occur.

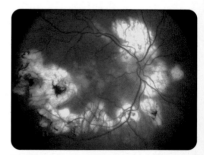

Fig. 14.70 Late serpiginous

4. FA – early hypofluorescence and late hyperfluorescence.

5. ICG – marked hypofluorescence throughout all phases.

6. Treatment – systemic steroids, azathioprine and ciclosporin.

7. Prognosis – poor.

Multifocal choroiditis with panuveitis

1. Definition – usually bilateral, chronic, recurrent, frequently asymmetrical disease that presents in the 3rd–4th decade; predominantly affects myopic females.

2. Signs
- Vitritis is universal and anterior uveitis common.
- Bilateral, multiple, deep, discrete, ovoid, spots at the posterior pole and/or periphery (*Fig. 14.71*).
- Residual 'punched-out' lesions with pigmented borders (*Fig. 14.72*).
- Subretinal fibrosis is uncommon.

3. FA – early hypofluorescence and late hyperfluorescence.

4. ICG – hypofluorescence of acute lesions which may not be clinically apparent.

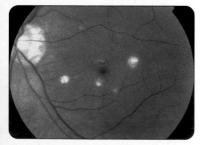

Fig. 14.71 Active central multifocal choroiditis

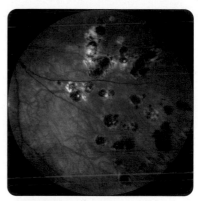

Fig. 14.72 Old peripheral multifocal choroiditis

5. Large visual field defects – may appear acutely.

6. Treatment – systemic and periocular steroids.

7. Prognosis – variable because the disease has a wide spectrum.

Progressive subretinal fibrosis and uveitis syndrome

1. Definition – chronic, bilateral disease which typically affects myopic young females.

2. Signs
- Mild anterior uveitis and vitritis.
- Indistinct subretinal lesions which coalesce into dirty-yellow mounds at the posterior pole and midperiphery.
- Eventually large areas of subretinal fibrosis (*Fig. 14.73*).

3. FA – early mottled hyperfluorescence and window defects with late hyperfluorescence along the edges of the lesions.

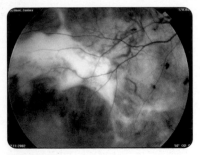

Fig. 14.73 Subretinal fibrosis

4. **ERG** – may be decreased.
5. **Treatment** – systemic immunosuppressive agents.
6. **Prognosis** – poor.

Multiple evanescent white dot syndrome

1. **Definition** – usually unilateral, self-limiting disease which presents in the 3rd–4th decade and predominantly affects females.
2. **Signs**
   - Mild afferent pupillary defect and vitritis.
   - Numerous, very small, subtle, ill-defined, deep, white dots at the posterior pole and mid-periphery (*Fig. 14.74*).
   - Macula is spared but has a granular appearance.
   - Disc oedema and blind spot enlargement.
   - Resolution over several weeks to months but foveal granularity may remain.

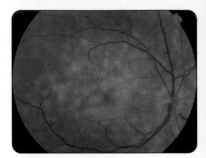

Fig. 14.74 MEWDS

3. **ICG** – shows more numerous hypofluorescent spots (*Fig. 14.75b–d*) than are apparent clinically and on FA (*Fig. 14.75a*).

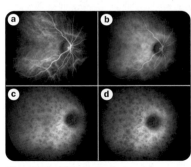

Fig. 14.75 ICG (b–d) shows more numerous lesions than FA (a)

4. **ERG** – decrease in a-wave amplitude.
5. **Treatment** – not appropriate.
6. **Prognosis** – excellent.

Acute idiopathic blind spot enlargement syndrome

1. **Definition** – rare condition which exclusively affects females in the 3rd–6th decade.
2. **Presentation** – mild blurred vision and photopsia.

3. Signs
- Visual acuity – normal or reduced.
- Afferent pupillary defect may be present.
- Blind spot enlargement of variable extent.
- Mild disc swelling or hyperaemia with peripapillary subretinal pigmentary changes in 50% of cases.
- Resolution after several weeks.

4. FA – late staining of the optic nerve head.

5. Treatment – not appropriate.

6. Prognosis – good although the blind spot may remain enlarged.

Fuchs uveitis syndrome

1. Definition – idiopathic CAU that typically affects one eye of a young adult.

2. Presentation
- Chronic floaters.
- Cataract formation.
- Colour difference between the two eyes.
- Incidental detection.

3. General signs
- Mild CAU but absence of posterior synechiae.
- KP – small, round or stellate, scattered throughout the endothelium frequently associated with feathery fibrin filaments (Fig. 14.76).
- Small nodules at the pupillary border and iris stroma (see Fig. 14.80).
- Vitritis and stringy opacities (Fig. 14.77).

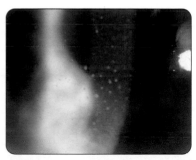

Fig. 14.76 KP in Fuchs

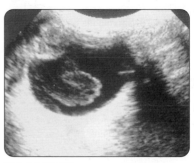

Fig. 14.77 Vitreous opacities

4. Diffuse iris atrophy
- Stromal atrophy particularly in the pupillary zone (Fig. 14.78).
- Posterior pigment layer iris atrophy best detected by retroillumination (Fig. 14.79).

5. Heterochromia iridis – most frequently the affected eye is hypochromic (Fig. 14.80).

6. Gonioscopy – may be normal or may show fine radial twig-like vessels in the angle.

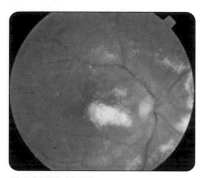

Fig. 14.88 IRVAN

3. **Treatment** – laser photocoagulation in eyes with extensive peripheral ischaemia and retinal neovascularization.
4. **Prognosis** – guarded.

Chapter 15

Ocular Tumours and Related Conditions

Benign conjunctival tumours

Naevus

1. Signs
- Solitary, flat or slightly elevated, lesion most frequently in the juxtalimbal area (*Fig. 15.1*), and less commonly on the plica or caruncle.
- Cystic spaces within the naevus are frequent.
- Around puberty the naevus may enlarge and become more pigmented (*Fig. 15.2*).

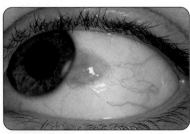

Fig. 15.1 Lightly pigmented naevus

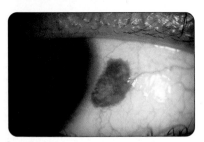

Fig. 15.2 Pigmented naevus

2. Signs of potential malignancy
- An unusual site such as palpebral or forniceal conjunctiva.
- Corneal extension.
- Sudden increase in pigmentation or growth.
- Development of vascularity except in a child.

3. Treatment – excision for cosmetic reasons, irritation, and suspicion of malignant transformation.

Pedunculated papilloma

1. **Pathogenesis** – infection with human papillomavirus.
2. **Presentation** – any age.
3. **Signs** – single or multiple, occasionally bilateral lesions most frequent juxtalimbal, on the caruncle or fornix (*Fig. 15.3*).

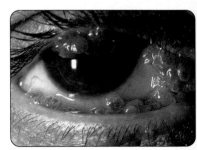

Fig. 15.3 Multiple pedunculated papillomas

4. **Treatment**
   a. *Small lesions* – may resolve spontaneously.
   b. *Large lesions* – excision or cryotherapy.
   c. *Recurrences* – subconjunctival alpha-interferon, topical mitomycin C or oral cimetidine (Tagamet).

Sessile papilloma

1. **Presentation** – middle-age.
2. **Signs** – single, unilateral bulbar or juxtalimbal (*Fig. 15.4*).

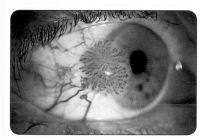

Fig. 15.4 Sessile papilloma

3. **Treatment** – excision.

Solid dermoid

1. **Presentation** – early childhood.
2. **Signs** – smooth, soft, yellowish mass most frequently at the infero-temporal limbus (*Fig. 15.5*).

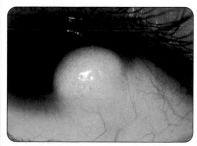

Fig. 15.5 Solid dermoid

3. **Treatment** – small lesions can be excised although the removal of large lesions may require lamellar corneal or scleral grafting.

4. **Systemic associations** – Goldenhar syndrome, Treacher Collins syndrome, and naevus sebaceus of Jadassohn.

Dermolipoma

1. **Presentation** – adult life.
2. **Signs** – soft, movable, subconjunctival mass at the outer canthus (*Fig. 15.6*).

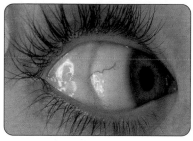

Fig. 15.6 Lipodermoid

3. **Treatment** – should be avoided.

Pyogenic granuloma

1. **Pathogenesis** – proliferation of granulation tissue that develops after procedures that involve conjunctival incisions.
2. **Presentation** – few weeks after surgery.
3. **Signs** – fast growing, fleshy, vascularized mass near the conjunctival wound (*Fig. 15.7*).

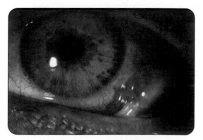

Fig. 15.7 Pyogenic granuloma

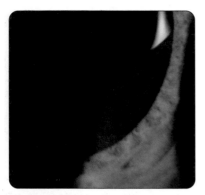

Fig. 15.30 Primary epithelial cyst

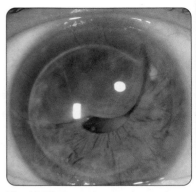

Fig. 15.32 Secondary serous cyst following keratoplasty

Secondary cysts

1. **Implantation** – originate by deposition of surface epithelial cells from the conjunctiva or cornea onto the iris after penetrating injury or surgery.
   a. *Pearly* – white, stromal lesion with opaque walls not connected to the wound (*Fig. 15.31*).
   b. *Serous* – translucent, fluid-filled lesion that may be connected to the wound (*Fig. 15.32*).

2. **Prolonged use of long-acting miotics** – multiple small cysts along the pupillary border (*Fig. 15.33*); prevented by using topical phenylephrine 2.5%.

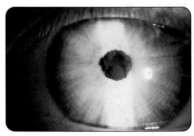

Fig. 15.33 Cysts due to miotics

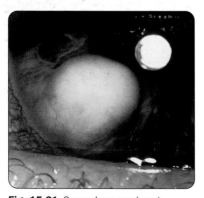

Fig. 15.31 Secondary pearl cyst

3. Parasitic – very rare (*Fig. 15.34*).

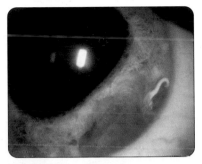

Fig. 15.34 Parasitic cyst

Ciliary body tumours

Ciliary body melanoma

1. **Presentation** – 6th decade with visual symptoms but occasionally discovered incidentally.
2. **Signs** depend on the size and location of the tumour:
   - Sentinel vessels in the same quadrant (*Fig. 15.35*).
   - Erosion through the iris root (*Fig. 15.36*).
   - Extraocular extension (*Fig. 15.37*).
   - Pressure on the lens – astigmatism, subluxation or cataract formation (*Fig. 15.38*).
   - Large tumour may be visible on ophthalmoscopy (*Fig. 15.39*).
   - Exudative RD from posterior extension.
   - Circumferential growth for 360° is uncommon and difficult to diagnose.

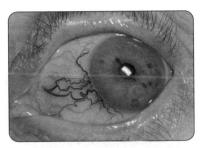

Fig. 15.35 Sentinel vessels

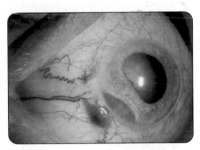

Fig. 15.36 Sentinel vessels, erosion through iris root and early extraocular extension

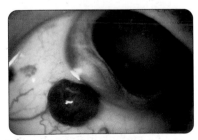

Fig. 15.37 Extensive extraocular extension

2. **Chromosomal abnormalities** – loss of chromosome 3 and gains in chromosome 8.
3. **Large tumour.**
4. **Extrascleral extension.**
5. **Anterior location.**
6. **Local tumour recurrence**.

Diagnosis

1. **Presentation** – around the age of 60 years with visual impairment, metamorphopsia, visual field loss, floaters, or photopsia.
2. **Signs**
   - Elevated, subretinal, dome-shaped mass, which may be pigmented (*Fig. 15.45*) or amelanotic (*Fig. 15.46*).
   - Collar-stud or mushroom-like appearance (*Fig. 15.47*).
   - Exudative RD initially confined to the surface of the tumour which later shifts inferiorly and becomes bullous (*Fig. 15.48*).

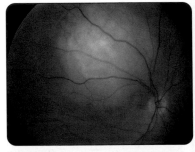

Fig. 15.46 Amelanotic melanoma

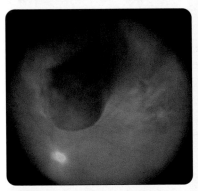

Fig. 15.47 Collar stud melanoma

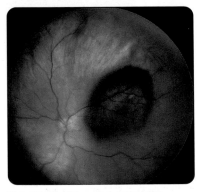

Fig. 15.45 Pigmented melanoma

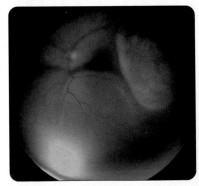

Fig. 15.48 Bullous exudative RD

3. US

- Acoustic hollow lesion with choroidal excavation and orbital shadowing (*Fig. 15.49*).
- Collar stud configuration is almost pathognomonic (*Fig. 15.50*).

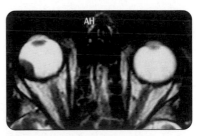

Fig. 15.51 T2-weighted axial MR of a right melanoma

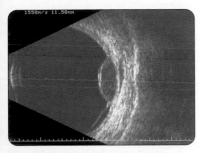

Fig. 15.49 Dome-shaped tumour

Treatment

1. **Brachytherapy** – ruthenium-106 or iodine-125 plaques (*Fig. 15.52*) if less than 20 mm in basal diameter.

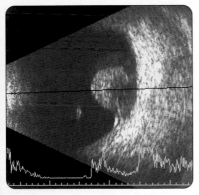

Fig. 15.50 Collar stud tumour

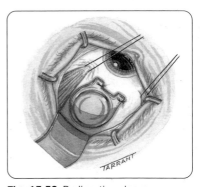

Fig. 15.52 Radioactive plaque

4. **MR** – hyperintensity on T1-weighted and hypointensity on T2-weighted images (*Fig. 15.51*).

2. **Charged particle irradiation** – if unsuitable for brachytherapy.
3. **Stereotactic radiosurgery** (gamma knife).
4. **Transpupillary thermotherapy** (TTT) – for some small tumours or as an adjunct to radiotherapy.
5. **Choroidectomy** – if too thick for radiotherapy and less than 16 mm in diameter (*Fig. 15.53*).

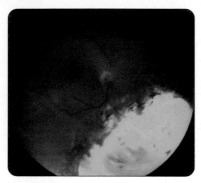

Fig. 15.53 Appearance following choroidectomy

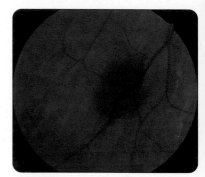

Fig. 15.54 Small naevus

6. **Enucleation** – for large tumours, optic disc invasion, extensive involvement of the ciliary body or angle, and irreversible loss of useful vision.
7. **Exenteration** – when orbital disease cannot be controlled by surgery and radiotherapy.
8. **Metastatic disease** – systemic chemotherapy and/or immunotherapy. Liver metastases may be treated with intra-hepatic chemotherapy or partial hepatectomy.

Other choroidal tumours

Choroidal naevus

1. **Signs**
   - Oval, slate-blue lesion with slightly blurred outline (*Fig. 15.54*).
   - Dimensions are <5 mm in basal diameter (i.e. 3 disc diameters) and <1 mm thickness.
   - Surface drusen over a large lesion (*Fig. 15.55*).

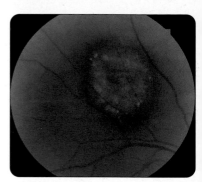

Fig. 15.55 Large naevus with surface drusen

2. **Suspicious naevus** – the following features may suggest that a melanocytic lesion is not naevus but a small melanoma:
   - Blurred vision, metamorphopsia, and photopsia.
   - Dimensions >5 mm in diameter and >1 mm in thickness.
   - Traces of surface orange pigment (lipofuscin – *Fig. 15.56*).
   - Absence of surface drusen on a large lesion.
   - Margin at or near the optic disc.

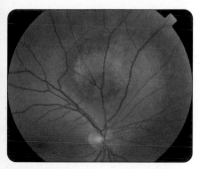

Fig. 15.56 Suspicious naevus with lipofuscin pigment

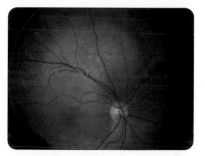

Fig. 15.57 Circumscribed choroidal haemangioma

3. Management
   a. *Typical naevi* – do not require follow-up.
   b. *Suspicious naevi* – baseline fundus photography and ultrasonography, and then indefinite follow-up.
4. Systemic associations – NF 1 and dysplastic naevus syndrome.

Circumscribed choroidal haemangioma

1. Presentation – 4th–5th decade with blurring of central vision, visual field defect, or metamorphopsia.
2. Signs – oval orange-red mass with indistinct margins posterior to the equator (*Fig. 15.57*).
3. FA – early spotty hyperfluorescence and late diffuse intense hyperfluorescence.

4. US – acoustically solid lesion with a sharp anterior surface but lacking choroidal excavation and orbital shadowing (*Fig. 15.58*).

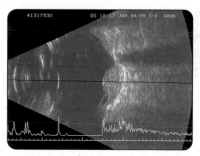

Fig. 15.58 US of circumscribed choroidal melanoma

5. **Complications** – fibrous metaplasia, cystoid retinal degeneration, and serous RD.
6. **Treatment** – photodynamic therapy (PDT), if vision is threatened.

Diffuse choroidal haemangioma

1. **Systemic association** – Sturge–Weber syndrome in the majority of cases.
2. **Signs** – deep-red 'tomato ketchup' colour most marked at the posterior pole (*Fig. 15.59*).

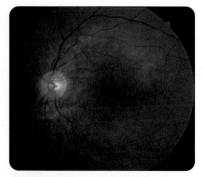

Fig. 15.59 Diffuse choroidal haemangioma

3. **US** – diffuse choroidal thickening.
4. **Complications** – cystoid retinal degeneration and exudative RD.
5. **Treatment** – external beam radiotherapy, if vision is threatened.

Melanocytoma

1. **Definition** – non-progressive, heavily pigmented tumour which is seen most frequently in the optic nerve head but which can arise anywhere in the uvea.

2. **Signs** – dark brown or black lesion with feathery edges within the NFL that extends over the edge of the disc (*Fig. 15.60*).

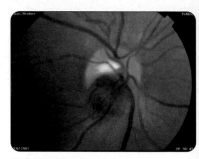

Fig. 15.60 Melanocytoma

3. **Treatment** – not required.

Osseous choristoma

1. **Definition** – benign, slow-growing, ossifying tumour which is more common in females; affects both eyes in 25% of cases but not usually simultaneously.
2. **Presentation** – 2nd–3rd decade with gradual visual impairment if the macula is involved by the tumour itself or by CNV.
3. **Signs**
   - Orange-yellow lesion with well-defined, scalloped borders in the posterior fundus (*Fig. 15.61*).
   - Overlying RPE changes in longstanding cases (*Fig. 15.62*).
4. **US** – highly reflective anterior surface and orbital shadowing (*Fig. 15.63*).

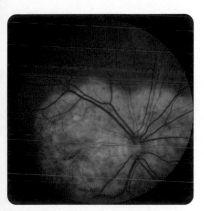

Fig. 15.61 Choroidal osteoma

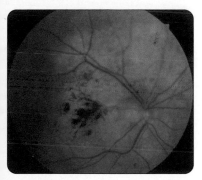

Fig. 15.62 Choroidal osteoma with RPE changes

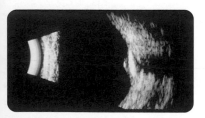

Fig. 15.63 US of osteoma

5. CT – bone-like features (*Fig. 15.64*).

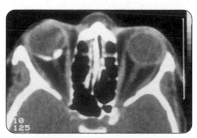

Fig. 15.64 Axial CT of a right osteoma

6. Treatment – not possible.

Metastatic choroidal tumour

1. **Primary sites** – breast in women and the bronchus in both sexes; less commonly gastrointestinal tract, kidney, and skin melanoma.
2. **Signs**
   - Fast-growing, creamy-white, placoid lesion most frequently at the posterior pole (*Fig. 15.65*).
   - Secondary exudative RD.
   - Deposits are multifocal in 30% and bilateral in 10–30% (*Fig. 15.66*).

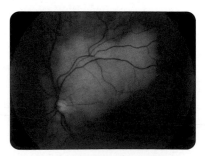

Fig. 15.65 Metastasis from breast carcinoma

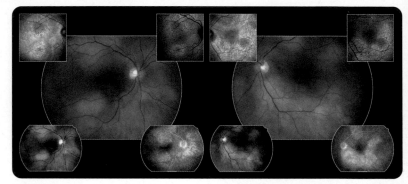

Fig. 15.66 Bilateral multifocal metastases

3. Treatment
   a. *Observation* – for asymptomatic patients or those receiving systemic chemotherapy.
   b. *Radiotherapy* – external beam or brachytherapy.
   c. *TTT* – for small tumours with minimal subretinal fluid.
   d. *Systemic therapy* – for the primary tumour may be beneficial.

Retinoblastoma

Histology

The tumour is composed of small basophilic cells (retinoblasts) with large hyperchromatic nuclei and scanty cytoplasm. Many tumours are undifferentiated (*Fig. 15.67*) but varying degrees of differentiation are characterized by the formation of rosettes, of which there are three types:

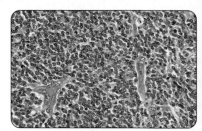

Fig. 15.67 Undifferentiated retinoblastoma

1. Flexner–Wintersteiner – central lumen surrounded by tall columnar cells the nuclei of which lie away from the lumen (*Fig. 15.68*).

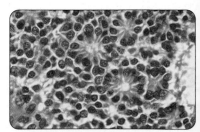

Fig. 15.68 Flexner–Wintersteiner rosettes

2. **Homer–Wright** – cells form around a tangled mass of eosinophilic processes without a lumen (*Fig. 15.69*).

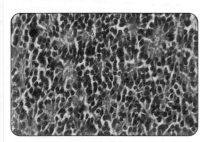

Fig. 15.69 Homer–Wright rosettes

3. **Fleurettes** – clusters of cells with long cytoplasmic processes project through a fenestrated membrane resembling a bouquet of flowers (*Fig. 15.70*).

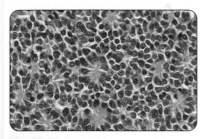

Fig. 15.70 Fleurettes

Patterns of tumour spread

1. **Growth pattern** – endophytic (into the vitreous – *Fig. 15.71*) or exophytic (into the subretinal space) causing RD (*Fig. 15.72*).

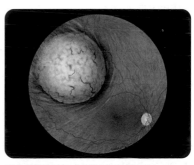

Fig. 15.71 Endophytic tumour

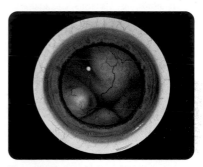

Fig. 15.72 Exophytic tumour

2. **Optic nerve invasion** – then spread of tumour along the subarachnoid space to the brain.
3. **Diffuse retinal infiltration**.
4. **Metastatic spread** – to regional nodes, lung, brain and bone.

Genetics

Retinoblastoma results from malignant transformation of primitive retinal cells before final differentiation and may be heritable or non-heritable. The predisposing gene (RB1) is at 13q14.

2. Signs
- Peripheral, yellowish plaque or nodule (*Fig. 15.79*).
- Peripapillary mulberry-like lesion (*Fig. 15.80*).
- Longstanding lesions may become calcified (*Fig. 15.81*).

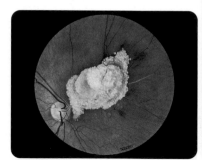

Fig. 15.81 Giant calcified astrocytoma

- Prevalence of retinal tumours in VHL is approximately 60%.
2. Presentation – in adult life with visual loss.
3. Signs
- Peripheral orange-red mass with dilatation and tortuosity of the supplying artery and draining vein (*Fig. 15.82*).
- Optic nerve head involvement is less common (*Fig. 15.83*).

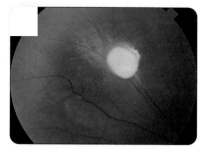

Fig. 15.79 Nodular astrocytoma

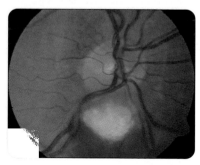

Fig. 15.80 Mulberry-like astrocytoma

3. Treatment – not required.

Retinal haemangioblastoma

1. Systemic association
- About 50% of patients with solitary lesions and virtually all patients with multiple lesions have von Hippel–Lindau disease (VHL).

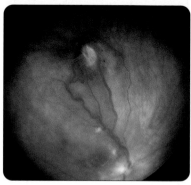

Fig. 15.82 Haemangioblastoma

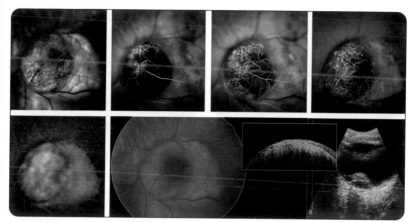

Fig. 15.83 Optic disc haemangioblastoma; FA shows early filling and late leakage

4. **FA** – early hyperfluorescence and late leakage (*Fig. 15.83*).
5. **Complications** – hard exudate formation (*Fig. 15.84*), macular oedema, RD, and vitreous haemorrhage.

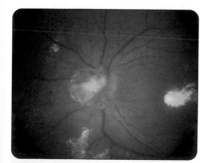

Fig. 15.84 Exudation from disc haemangioblastoma

6. **Treatment** – laser photocoagulation, cryotherapy, PDT, and anti-VEGF therapy.

Cavernous haemangioma

1. **Systemic associations** – the tumour is usually sporadic but occasionally AD and associated with lesions of the skin and CNS ('neuro-oculo-cutaneous phacomatosis').
2. **Signs**
   * Peripheral clusters of saccular aneurysms resembling a 'bunch of grapes' (*Fig. 15.85*).
   * Optic nerve head involvement is less common (*Fig. 15.86*).
   * Erythrocytes may sediment and separate from plasma giving rise to 'menisci' best seen on fluorescein angiography (*Fig. 15.87*).

Chapter 16

Retinal Vascular Disease

Diabetic retinopathy

Risk factors

1. **Type 1 diabetes**.
2. **Duration of diabetes** – most important.
3. **Poor metabolic control** – less important than duration.
4. **Pregnancy** – occasionally associated with rapid progression of DR.
5. **Hypertension** – should be rigorously controlled (<140/80 mmHg).
6. **Nephropathy** – if severe is associated with worsening of DR.
7. **Other** – obesity, hyperlipidaemia, and anaemia.

Pathogenesis

DR is a microangiopathy that exhibits features of occlusion (*Fig. 16.1*) and leakage.

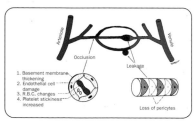

Fig. 16.1 Pathogenesis of microvascular occlusion

1. **Capillaropathy** – degeneration and loss of pericytes, proliferation of endothelial cells, thickening of the basement membrane and occlusion.
2. **Haematological changes** that predispose to decreased capillary blood flow:
   - Deformation of erythrocytes and rouleaux formation.
   - Activation and reduced deformability of white cells.
   - Increased platelet stickiness and aggregation.
   - Increased plasma viscosity.
3. **Occlusion** and retinal hypoxia which may cause (*Fig. 16.2*):
   a. *Arteriovenous shunts* – intraretinal microvascular abnormalities (IRMA).
   b. *Neovascularization* – on the retina and optic disc (proliferative retinopathy), and occasionally rubeosis iridis.

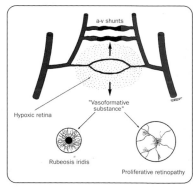

Fig. 16.2 Consequences of microvascular occlusion

4. **Leakage** (*Fig. 16.3*)
   - Extensive capillary leakage causes diffuse retinal oedema.
   - Focal leakage from microaneurysms gives rise to localized retinal oedema and hard exudate formation.

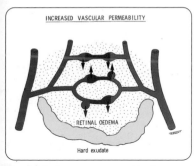

Fig. 16.3 Consequences of leakage

Background diabetic retinopathy

Diagnosis (*Fig. 16.4*)

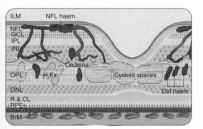

Fig. 16.4 Location of lesions in BDR

1. Microaneurysms
a. *Signs* – tiny, red dots, initially temporal to the fovea are the earliest signs of DR (*Fig. 16.5*).
b. *FA* – hyperfluorescent dots followed by diffuse hyperfluorescence.

2. Hard exudates
a. *Signs* – waxy, yellow lesions often arranged in clumps and/or rings at the posterior pole (*Fig. 16.6*).
b. *FA* – hypofluorescence due to blockage of background choroidal fluorescence.

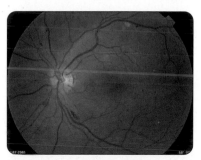

Fig. 16.5 Mild BDR

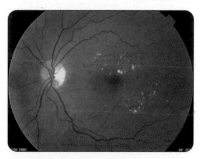

Fig. 16.6 Moderate BDR

3. Retinal haemorrhages
a. *Intraretinal haemorrhages* – 'dot-blot' configuration (*Fig. 16.7*).
b. *Flame-shaped haemorrhages* – along the NFL.

4. Macular oedema
a. *Signs* – retinal thickening at the macula.
b. *FA* – late hyperfluorescence.
c. *OCT* – retinal thickening.

Management
1. Mild BDR – no treatment and annual review.
2. Severe BDR – assess for clinically significant macular oedema.

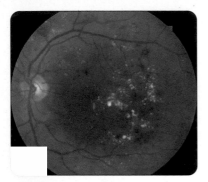

Fig. 16.7 Severe BDR

Diabetic maculopathy

Diagnosis

1. Focal
   a. *Signs* – well-circumscribed retinal thickening associated rings of hard exudates (*Fig. 16.8a*).

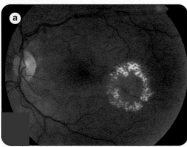

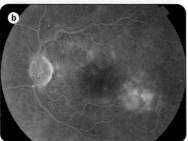

Fig. 16.8 Focal maculopathy

   b. *FA* – late, focal hyperfluorescence due to leakage and good macular perfusion (*Fig. 16.8b*).

2. Diffuse
   a. *Signs* – diffuse retinal thickening, which may be associated with CMO (*Fig. 16.9a*).
   b. *FA* – late diffuse hyperfluorescence (*Fig. 16.9b*).

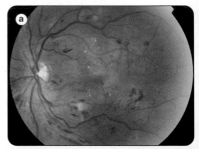

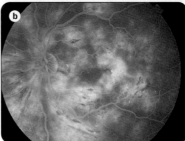

Fig. 16.9 Diffuse maculopathy

3. Ischaemic
   a. *Signs* – pre-proliferative signs may be present (*Fig. 16.10a*).
   b. *FA* – capillary non-perfusion at the fovea (*Fig. 16.10b*).

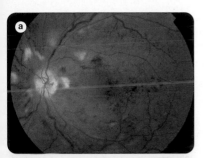

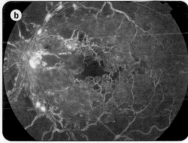

Fig. 16.10 Ischaemic maculopathy

4. Clinically significant macular oedema (CSMO – *Fig. 16.11*) definition:

- Retinal oedema within 500 µm of the centre of the fovea (*Fig. 16.11a*).
- Hard exudates within 500 µm of the centre of the fovea, if associated with retinal thickening (which may be outside the 500 µm – *Fig. 16.11b*).
- Retinal oedema one disc area (1500 µm) or larger, any part of which is within one disc diameter of the centre of the fovea (*Fig. 16.11c*).

Argon laser photocoagulation

1. Indications – all eyes with CSMO should be considered for treatment irrespective of the level of visual acuity as this reduces the risk of visual loss by 50%.

2. Focal treatment

- To microaneurysms and microvascular lesions in the centre of rings of hard exudates located 500–3000 µm from the centre of the fovea.
- Spot size is 50–100 µm and exposure 0.10 sec with sufficient power to obtain gentle whitening or darkening of the microaneurysm.

3. Grid treatment

- To areas of diffuse retinal thickening more than 500 µm from the centre of the fovea and 500 µm from the temporal margin of the optic disc.
- Spot size is 100 µm and exposure 0.10 sec giving a very light intensity burn.

4. Results – 70% achieve stable visual acuity, 15% show improvement, and 15% subsequently deteriorate.

5. Poor ocular prognostic factors

- Hard exudates involving the centre of the fovea.
- Diffuse macular oedema.
- CMO.
- Mixed exudative–ischaemic maculopathy.

6. Poor systemic prognostic factors

- Uncontrolled hypertension.
- Renal disease.
- Elevated glycosylated haemoglobin levels.

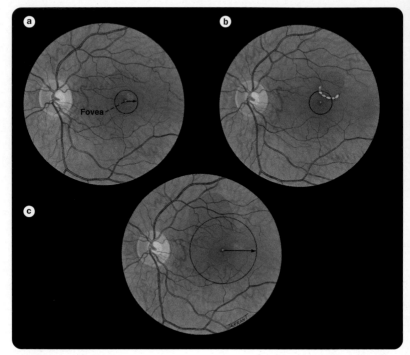

Fig. 16.11 CSMO

Other forms of treatment

1. **Low energy Nd:YAG** (532 nm) – green laser in which the energy employed is the lowest capable of producing barely visible burns.
2. **Subthreshold micropulse diode laser** (810 nm) – microseconds burns applied to the RPE without significantly affecting the outer retina and choriocapillaris.
3. **Pars plana vitrectomy** – for macular oedema associated with tangential traction from a thickened and taut posterior hyaloid.
4. **Intravitreal triamcinolone acetonide** – for diffuse macular oedema that fails to respond to conventional laser.
5. **Anti-VEGF** – for CMO.
6. **Oral atorvastatin** – in type 2 diabetes with dyslipidaemia reduces hard exudates and subfoveal lipid migration in eyes with CSMO.

Preproliferative diabetic retinopathy

Definition

BDR that exhibits signs of imminent proliferative disease is termed PPDR. The clinical signs (*Fig. 16.12*) indicate progressive retinal ischaemia, seen on FA as extensive hypofluorescent areas representing capillary non-perfusion (dropout – *Fig. 16.13*).

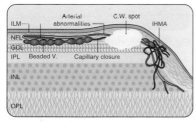

Fig. 16.12 Lesions in PPDR

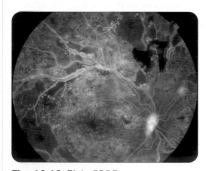

Fig. 16.13 FA in PPDR

Diagnosis (*Fig. 16.14*)

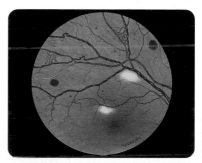

Fig. 16.14 PPDR

1. **Cotton-wool spots**
   a. *Signs* – small, whitish, fluffy, superficial lesions.
   b. *FA* – focal hypofluorescence frequently associated with adjacent capillary dropout.
2. **IRMA**
   a. *Signs* – fine, irregular, red lines that run from arterioles to venules.
   b. *FA* – focal hyperfluorescence associated with adjacent capillary dropout.
3. **Venous changes** – dilatation, tortuosity, looping, beading and 'sausage-like' segmentation.
4. **Arterial changes** – peripheral narrowing, silver-wiring and obliteration.
5. **Dark blot haemorrhages** – haemorrhagic retinal infarcts.

Management

Patients with PPDR should be watched closely because of the risk of PDR. Laser treatment is usually not appropriate unless regular follow-up is not possible, or vision in the fellow eye has been lost due to proliferative disease.

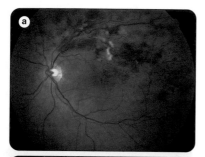

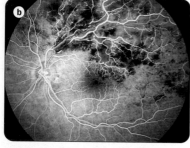

Fig. 16.20 (a) Acute BRVO; (b) FA

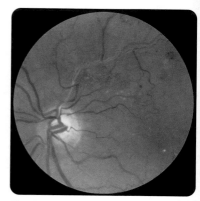

Fig. 16.21 Old BRVO

2. **FA** – hypofluorescence due to blockage by blood and capillary dropout, staining of the vessel wall and 'pruning' of vessels (*Fig. 16.20b*).
3. **Chronic signs** (*Fig. 16.21*)
   - Hard exudates, venous sheathing and sclerosis.
   - Collaterals which may be local or develop across the horizontal raphe.
4. **Prognosis** – within 6 months about 50% of eyes have a visual acuity to 6/12 or better; main vision-threatening complications are chronic macular oedema and neovascularization.

Treatment
1. **Macular oedema**
   a. *Grid laser photocoagulation* – to the area of leakage identified on FA.
   b. *Intravitreal triamcinolone acetonide* – may improve visual acuity for up to 12 months.
   c. *Arteriovenous sheathotomy* – experimental treatment.
2. **Neovascularization** – not normally treated unless vitreous haemorrhage occurs.

Non-ischaemic central retinal vein occlusion

1. **VA** – moderate to severe reduction.
2. **Afferent pupillary defect** (APD) – absent or mild.
3. **Acute signs** (*Fig. 16.22b*)
   - Tortuosity and dilatation of all branches of the central retinal vein.

- Dot-blot and flame-shaped haemorrhages, disc and macular oedema, and variable cotton-wool spots.

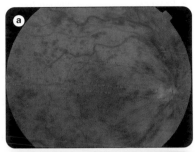

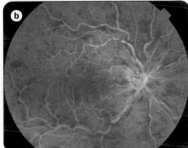

Fig. 16.22 (a) Acute non-ischaemic CRVO; (b) FA

4. **FA** – blockage by haemorrhages, good retinal capillary perfusion (*Fig. 16.22b*), and late leakage.
5. **Chronic signs**
   - Disc collaterals, and macular epiretinal gliosis and pigmentary changes.
   - Conversion to ischaemic CRVO in 15% of cases within 4 months and 34% within 3 years.
6. **Prognosis** – return of vision to normal or near normal in about 50%.

7. **Treatment** – currently inadequate but the following experimental therapies require further evaluation: laser-induced chorioretinal venous anastomosis, infusion of tissue plasminogen activator (t-PA) into the vein, intravitreal triamcinolone acetonide, and optic nerve sheathotomy.

Ischaemic central retinal vein occlusion

1. **VA** – CF or worse.
2. **APD** – marked.
3. **Acute signs** (*Fig. 16.23a*)
   - Severe tortuosity and dilatation of all branches of the central retinal vein.

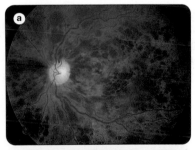

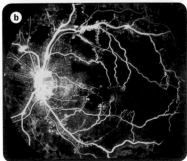

Fig. 16.23 (a) Acute ischaemic CRVO; (b) FA

5. **Periarteritis** – in dermatomyositis, systemic lupus erythematosus, polyarteritis nodosa, Wegener granulomatosis, and Behçet disease.
6. **Thrombophilic disorders** – hyperhomocysteinaemia, antiphospholipid antibody syndrome and inherited defects of natural anticoagulants.
7. **Sickling haemoglobinopathies.**
8. **Retinal migraine** – rarely responsible for retinal artery occlusion in young individuals.
9. **Susac syndrome** – triad of retinal artery occlusion, sensorineural deafness, and encephalopathy.

Branch retinal artery occlusion

1. **Presentation** – sudden profound altitudinal or sectoral visual field loss.
2. **VA** – variable.
3. **Fundus** (*Fig. 16.27a*)
   - Attenuated arteries and veins with sludging and segmentation of the blood column (cattle trucking).
   - Cloudy white retina that corresponds to the area of ischaemia.
4. **FA** – delayed arterial filling and hypofluorescence of the involved segment (*Fig. 16.27b*).

5. **Prognosis** – poor unless the obstruction is relieved within a few hours.

Central retinal artery occlusion

1. **Presentation** – sudden profound loss of vision.
2. **VA** – severely reduced.
3. **APD** – severe or total.
4. **Fundus**
   - Similar to BRAO but more extensive with a 'cherry-red spot' at the macula (*Fig. 16.28*).
   - In eyes with a cilioretinal artery part of the macula is normal colour (*Fig. 16.29*).

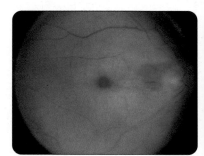

Fig. 16.28 CRAO

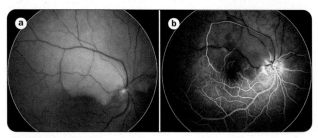

Fig. 16.27 (a) BRAO; (b) FA

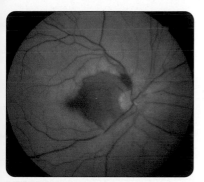

Fig. 16.29 CRAO with patent cilio-retinal artery

5. FA – similar to BRAO but more extensive.
6. Prognosis – poor.

Cilioretinal artery occlusion

1. **Isolated** – young patients with associated systemic vasculitis.
2. **Combined with CRVO** (*Fig. 16.30*) – similar prognosis to non-ischaemic CRVO.

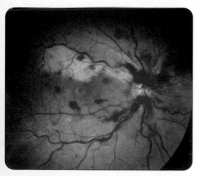

Fig. 16.30 Cilioretinal artery occlusion and CRVO

3. **Combined with anterior ischaemic optic neuropathy** (*Fig. 16.31*) – in giant cell arteritis.

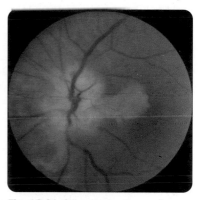

Fig. 16.31 Cilioretinal artery occlusion and anterior ischaemic optic neuropathy

4. **FA** – corresponding filling defect (*Fig. 16.32*).

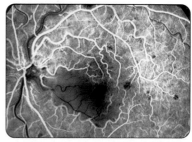

Fig. 16.32 FA of cilioretinal artery occlusion

Treatment of acute retinal artery occlusion

The following treatment may be tried in patients with occlusions of less than 48 hours' duration at presentation.

1. **Ocular massage** – using a three-mirror contact lens for approximately 10 seconds, to obtain central retinal artery pulsation or cessation of flow (for BRAO), followed by 5 seconds of release.
2. **Anterior chamber paracentesis.**
3. **Intravenous acetazolamide** – to obtain a more prolonged lowering of intraocular pressure than with repeated paracentesis, if this was initially successful but flow has ceased.

Ocular ischaemic syndrome

1. **Pathogenesis** – chronic ocular hypoperfusion secondary to severe ipsilateral atherosclerotic carotid stenosis of more than 90% resulting in 50% reduction of ipsilateral perfusion pressure.
2. **Anterior segment signs**
   - Diffuse episcleral injection and corneal oedema.
   - Aqueous flare with few if any cells (ischaemic pseudo-iritis).
   - Iris atrophy and mid-dilated and poorly reacting pupil.
   - Rubeosis iridis.
3. **Fundus**
   - Venous dilatation, arteriolar narrowing, and haemorrhages.
   - Proliferative retinopathy.

4. **Treatment** – topical steroids for anterior segment disease; PRP for proliferative retinopathy.
5. **Prognosis** – poor.

Hypertensive disease

Retinopathy (*Fig. 16.33*)

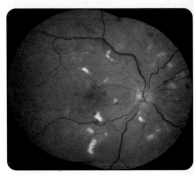

Fig. 16.33 Severe hypertensive retinopathy

1. **Vasoconstriction** – focal or generalized.
2. **Ischaemia** – cotton-wool spots.
3. **Leakage**
   - Flame-shaped haemorrhages and oedema.
   - Hard exudates with a macular star configuration and disc swelling in malignant (accelerated) hypertension (*Fig. 16.34*).
4. **Grading of arteriolosclerosis** (*Fig. 16.35*)
   - *Grade 1* – subtle broadening of the arteriolar light reflex, mild generalized arteriolar attenuation, and vein concealment.

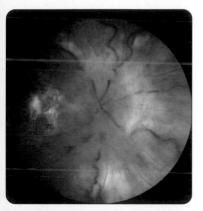

Fig. 16.34 Malignant hypertension

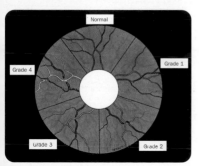

Fig. 16.35 Grading of arteriolosclerosis

- *Grade 2* – obvious broadening of the arteriolar light reflex and deflection of veins at arteriovenous crossings (Salus sign)
- *Grade 3* – copper-wiring of arterioles, banking of veins distal to arteriovenous crossings (Bonnet sign), and tapering of veins on both sides of the crossings (Gunn sign) and right-angled deflection of veins.
- *Grade 4* – silver-wiring of arterioles associated with grade 3 changes.

Choroidopathy

Choroidopathy may occur as the result of an acute hypertensive crisis in young adults.

1. **Elschnig spots** – small, black spots surrounded by yellow halos.
2. **Siegrist streaks** – flecks arranged linearly along choroidal vessels.
3. **Exudative RD** – sometimes bilateral (*Fig. 16.36*), may occur in severe acute hypertension as in toxaemia of pregnancy.

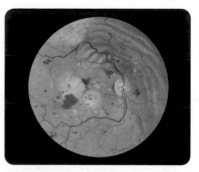

Fig. 16.36 Exudative RD

Sickle-cell retinopathy

Sickling haemoglobinopathies

- Sickling haemoglobinopathies are caused by abnormal haemoglobins which cause the red blood cell to adopt an anomalous shape under conditions of hypoxia and acidosis.
- The sickling disorders in which the mutant haemoglobins S and C are inherited as alleles of normal haemoglobin A have important ocular manifestations.

- Retinopathy is most severe in patients with SC (sickle cell C disease) and SThal (sickle cell thalassaemia).

Proliferative retinopathy

1. **Staging** (*Fig. 16.37*)
   a. *Stage 1* – arteriolar occlusion.
   b. *Stage 2* – arteriovenous anastomoses.
   c. *Stage 3* – sprouting of new vessels from the anastomoses ('sea-fans').
   d. *Stage 4* – neovascular tufts may continue to proliferate and bleed.
   e. *Stage 5* – fibrovascular proliferation and RD.

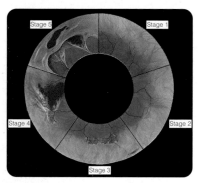

Fig. 16.37 Staging of proliferative retinopathy

2. **FA** – stage 3 shows filling of 'sea-fans' and peripheral capillary dropout (*Fig. 16.38*)
3. **Treatment** – not required in most cases; RD and vitreous haemorrhage may require vitrectomy.

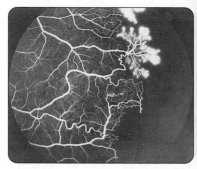

Fig. 16.38 FA in proliferative retinopathy

Non-proliferative retinopathy

1. **Venous tortuosity** – due to peripheral arteriovenous shunts.
2. **Silver-wiring of arterioles** – represents previously occluded vessels.
3. **Salmon patches** – peripheral, preretinal (*Fig. 16.39*) or superficial intraretinal haemorrhages.

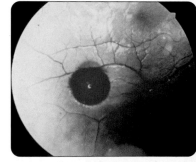

Fig. 16.39 Salmon patch

4. **Black sunbursts** – patches of peripheral RPE hyperplasia (*Fig. 16.40*).

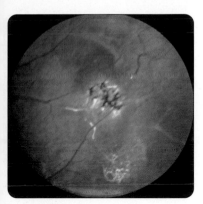

Fig. 16.40 Black sunburst

5. Macular depression sign – oval depression of the bright central macular reflex.
6. Macular arteriolar occlusion – in about 30% of patients.
7. Acute CRAO – rare.
8. Retinal vein occlusion – uncommon.
9. Angioid streaks – rare.

Anterior segment features

1. Conjunctival – isolated dark red vascular anomalies shaped like commas or corkscrews.
2. Iris – circumscribed areas of ischaemic atrophy, usually at the pupillary edge and extending to the collarettes.

Retinopathy of prematurity

Pathogenesis

- Retinopathy of prematurity (ROP) is a proliferative retinopathy affecting premature infants of very low birth weight, who have usually been exposed to high ambient oxygen concentrations.
- Incompletely vascularized temporal retina is particularly susceptible to oxygen damage in the premature infant.

Active disease

1. Location (*Fig. 16.41*)
- *Zone 1* – bounded by an imaginary circle the radius of which is twice the distance from the disc to the macula.
- *Zone 2* – extends concentrically from the edge of zone 1.
- *Zone 3* – residual temporal crescent anterior to zone 2.

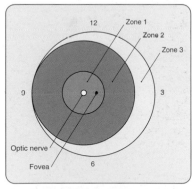

Fig. 16.41 Grading of ROP according to location

2. Extent of involvement – number of clock hours of retina involved or as 30° sectors.

3. **Staging** (*Fig. 16.42*)
   - *Stage 1* – demarcation line associated (*Fig. 16.42a*).
   - *Stage 2* – ridge associated with blood vessels (*Fig. 16.42b*).
   - *Stage 3* – extraretinal fibrovascular proliferation extends from the ridge into the vitreous (*Fig. 16.42c*).
   - *Stage 4* – partial RD; extrafoveal (stage 4a – *Fig. 16.42c*); foveal (stage 4b).
   - *Stage 5* – total RD.
4. **Plus disease** – failure of the pupil to dilate, vascular iris engorgement, vitreous haze, dilated veins and tortuous arteries involving at least two quadrants of the posterior fundus, and increasing preretinal and vitreous haemorrhage.
5. **Pre-plus disease** – dilatation and tortuosity that is insufficient to be designated as plus disease.
6. **Threshold disease** – five contiguous clock hours or eight cumulative clock hours of extraretinal neovascularization (stage 3 disease) in zone 1 or zone 2, associated with plus disease, is an indication for treatment.
7. **Aggressive posterior (rush disease)** – prominence of plus disease and ill-defined nature of the retinopathy. It is most

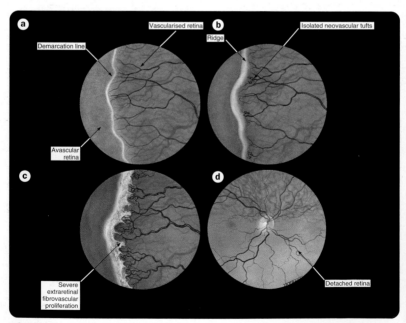

Fig. 16.42 Staging of ROP

commonly observed in zone 1 and does not usually progress through the classical stages 1 to 3.

8. Regression – in about 80% of cases.

9. Screening
- Babies born at or before 31 weeks gestational age, or weighing 1500 g or less, should be screened at 4–7 weeks postnatally to detect the onset of threshold disease.
- Subsequent review should be one- to two-weekly intervals, depending on the severity of the disease until retinal vascularization reaches zone.

10. Treatment
- **a.** *Laser photocoagulation* – in threshold disease (*Fig. 16.43*) is successful in 85% of cases, but the remainder progress to RD in spite of treatment.
- **b.** *Lens-sparing pars plana vitrectomy* – for stage 4a.

Cicatricial disease

1. Staging
- Peripheral retinal pigmentary disturbance and haze at the vitreous base.
- Temporal vitreoretinal fibrosis and straightening of vascular arcades (*Fig. 16.44*).
- 'Dragging' of the disc and macula (*Fig. 16.45*).

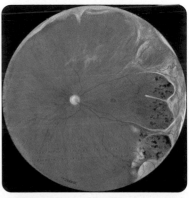

Fig. 16.44 Cicatricial ROP

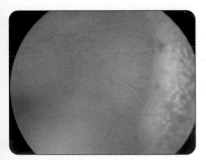

Fig. 16.43 Appearance following laser

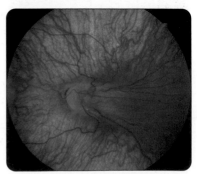

Fig. 16.45 Dragging of disc and macula

- Severe peripheral fibrosis and a falciform retinal fold (*Fig. 16.46*).
- Partial ring of retrolental fibrovascular tissue with partial RD.
- Complete ring of retrolental fibrovascular tissue with total RD (*Fig. 16.47*).

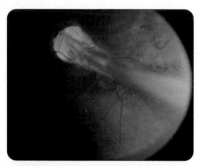

Fig. 16.46 Falciform fold

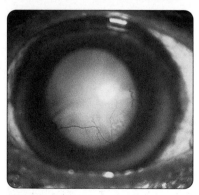

Fig. 16.47 End-stage disease

2. **Secondary angle-closure glaucoma** – progressive shallowing of the anterior chamber caused by a forward movement of the iris-lens diaphragm and the development of anterior synechiae.

Retinal artery macroaneurysm

1. **Definition** – localized dilatation of a retinal arteriole which has a predilection for elderly hypertensive women and involves one eye in 90% of cases.
2. **Signs** – saccular or fusiform arteriolar dilatation, most frequently at a bifurcation or an arteriovenous crossing along the temporal vascular arcades and often associated with retinal haemorrhage (*Fig. 16.48a*).
3. **FA** – immediate uniform filling (*Fig. 16.48b*) with late leakage (*Fig. 16.48c*) provided the lesion is patent.
4. **Course**
   a. *Chronic leakage* – hard exudate formation (*Fig. 16.49*).
   b. *Rupture* – haemorrhage (subretinal, intraretinal, preretinal or vitreous).
   c. *Spontaneous involution* – following thrombosis and fibrosis is common.
5. **Treatment** – laser photocoagulation if oedema or hard exudates threaten or involve the fovea.

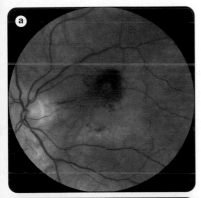

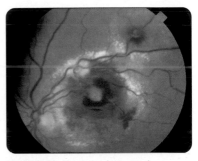

Fig. 16.49 Hard exudates and haemorrhage

Primary retinal telangiectasia

Idiopathic juxtafoveolar retinal telangiectasia (JFRT)

1A. Unilateral congenital

1. **Presentation** – in a middle-aged man with mild to moderate blurring of vision.
2. **Signs** – telangiectasia involving an area about 1.5 disc diameters temporal to the fovea (*Fig. 16.50a*) associated with leakage (*Fig. 16.50b*) and frequently hard exudates.
3. **Treatment** – laser photocoagulation may occasionally be beneficial.

1B. Unilateral idiopathic focal

1. **Presentation** – similar to type 1A.
2. **Signs** – telangiectasia confined to one clock hour at the edge of the foveal avascular zone without leakage.
3. **Treatment** – is not appropriate and the prognosis good.

2A. Bilateral idiopathic acquired

1. **Presentation** – 6th decade with mild, slowly progressive disturbance of

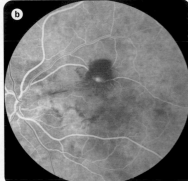

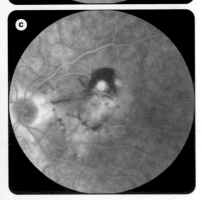

Fig. 16.48 (a) Retinal artery macro-aneurysm; (b, c) FA

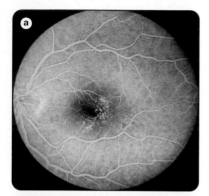

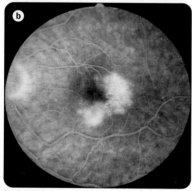

Fig. 16.50 JFRT group 1A

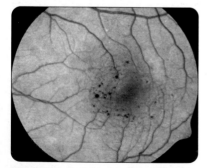

Fig. 16.51 Red free image of JFRT group 2A

central vision in one or both eyes. Both sexes are affected equally.

2. **Signs**
   - Symmetrical telangiectasia, one disc area or less, involving all or a part of the parafoveal area without hard exudates (*Fig. 16.51*).
   - Stellate pigmented plaques of RPE hyperplasia.
   - Multiple refractile white juxtafoveolar dots and solitary small yellow central deposits may be present.
   - Subretinal CNV may develop in advanced cases.
3. **FA** – telangiectasia outside the FAZ and late leakage.
4. **Prognosis** – guarded, although intravitreal anti-VEGF therapy or PDT may be beneficial for subfoveal CNV.

2B. Bilateral familial occult

This is similar to 2A but presents earlier and is associated with neither superficial retinal refractile deposits nor stellate pigmented plaques.

3. Idiopathic occlusive

1. **Systemic associations** – polycythaemia, multiple myeloma, chronic lymphatic leukaemia, and neurological disease.
2. **Presentation** – 6th decade with slowly progressive loss of central vision.
3. **Signs**
   - Marked aneurysmal dilatation of terminal capillaries and progressive occlusion of parafoveal capillaries.
   - Optic atrophy may be present.
4. **FA** – widening of the FAZ but absence of leakage (*Fig. 16.52*).
5. **Prognosis** – poor as there is no effective treatment.

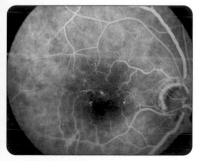

Fig. 16.52 JFRT group 3

Coats disease

1. **Definition** – idiopathic, non-hereditary, retinal telangiectasia that typically affects one eye of a young boy.
2. **Presentation** – 1st decade of life (average 5 years) with unilateral visual loss, strabismus or leukocoria.
3. **Signs** – telangiectasia (*Fig. 16.53*), progressive intraretinal and subretinal exudate formation (*Figs 16.54 & 16.55*), and exudative RD (*Fig. 16.56*).
4. **FA** – early hyperfluorescence of the telangiectasia, and late staining and leakage (*Fig. 16.57*).

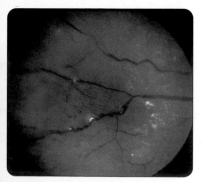

Fig. 16.53 Telangiectasia in Coats disease

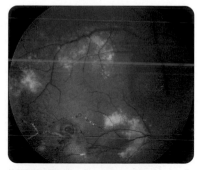

Fig. 16.54 Early exudate formation

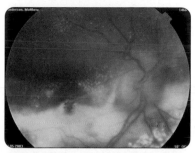

Fig. 16.55 Severe exudation

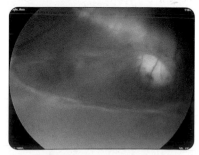

Fig. 16.56 RD

5. **Complications** – rubeosis iridis, glaucoma, uveitis, cataract, and phthisis bulbi.

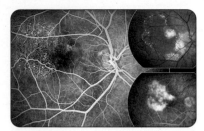

Fig. 16.57 FA in early Coats disease

6. Association – atypical PR is rare.
7. Treatment
   a. *Laser photocoagulation* – for progressive exudation.
   b. *Cryotherapy* – for extensive exudation or subtotal RD.
   c. *Vitreoretinal surgery* – for total RD.

Eales disease

1. Definition – bilateral, peripheral occlusive vasculitis particularly affecting Asian men.
2. Presentation – 3rd–5th decade with vitreous haemorrhage.
3. Signs
   • Vascular sheathing associated with capillary non-perfusion.
   • Peripheral neovascularization at the junction of perfused and non-perfused retina (*Fig. 16.58*).

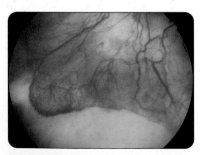

Fig. 16.58 Peripheral neovascularization in Eales disease

4. Complications – recurrent vitreous haemorrhage, tractional RD, rubeosis iridis, glaucoma, and cataract.
5. Treatment – systemic and intravitreal steroids, PRP to non-perfused retina, and vitrectomy for vitreous haemorrhage and RD.

Radiation retinopathy

1. Causes – treatment of intraocular tumours by plaque therapy (brachytherapy) or external beam irradiation of sinus, orbital or nasopharyngeal malignancies
2. Signs
   • Capillary dropout with the development of collateral channels and microaneurysms, best seen on FA (*Fig. 16.59*).
   • Cotton-wool spots and retinal haemorrhages.
   • Macular oedema and hard exudates.
   • Papillopathy and proliferative retinopathy.
3. Treatment – laser photocoagulation.
4. Prognosis – guarded.

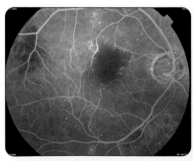

Fig. 16.59 FA of radiation retinopathy

Purtscher retinopathy

1. **Pathogenesis** – microvascular occlusion associated with severe trauma, embolism, acute pancreatitis, connective tissue diseases, thrombotic thrombocytopenic purpura, and bone marrow transplantation.
2. **Signs** – multiple, unilateral or bilateral, superficial, white retinal patches, resembling large cotton-wool spots, often associated with superficial peripapillary haemorrhages (*Fig. 16.60*).

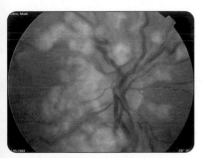

Fig. 16.60 Purtscher retinopathy

3. **Treatment** – of the underlying cause is desirable but not always possible.
4. **Prognosis** – guarded.

Benign idiopathic haemorrhagic retinopathy

1. **Presentation** – in adult life with acute unilateral visual impairment.
2. **Signs** – multiple, large, intraretinal haemorrhages at the posterior pole and around the optic disc (*Fig. 16.61*).

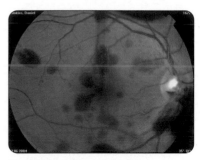

Fig. 16.61 Benign idiopathic haemorrhagic retinopathy

3. **Course** – vision recovers within 4 months and no treatment is required.

Valsalva retinopathy

1. **Pathogenesis** – sudden elevation of retinal venous pressure caused by forcible exhalation against a closed glottis creates a sudden increase in intrathoracic and intra-abdominal pressure, results in rupture of perifoveal capillaries.
2. **Signs** – unilateral or bilateral premacular haemorrhage (*Fig. 16.62*).

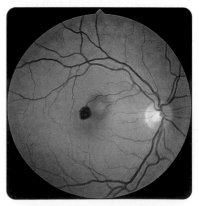

Fig. 16.62 Valsalva retinopathy

3. **Treatment** – not appropriate as spontaneous resorption is the rule.

Lipaemia retinalis

1. **Cause** – hypertriglyceridaemia.
2. **Signs** – creamy white retinal blood vessels due to the visualization of high levels of chylomicrons (*Fig. 16.63*).

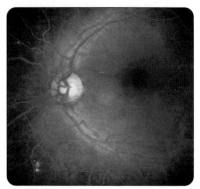

Fig. 16.63 Lipaemia retinalis

Takayasu disease

1. **Definition** – obstructive vascular disease affecting the major branches of the aorta.
2. **Anterior segment** – corneal oedema, anterior chamber cells and rubeosis iridis.
3. **Fundus** – arteriolar attenuation, cotton-wool spots, retinal haemorrhages, microaneurysms, arteriovenous malformations, ischaemic optic neuropathy, and neovascularization.
4. **Treatment** – systemic steroids and cytotoxic agents.

High-altitude retinopathy

1. **Systemic features** – progressive severe headache, followed by impaired cortical function and judgement, irrationality, projectile vomiting, diplopia, ataxia and coma.
2. **Ocular features** in chronological order:
   - Mild venous dilatation and a few small retinal haemorrhages.
   - Progression of venous dilatation and large retinal haemorrhages.
   - Severe venous dilatation and multiple large retinal haemorrhages.
   - Venous engorgement, vitreous haemorrhage and papilloedema.

Retinopathy in blood disorders

Leukaemia

1. **Fundus**
   - Cotton-wool spots and deep and superficial retinal haemorrhages, some of which may have white centres (Roth spots – *Fig. 16.64*).

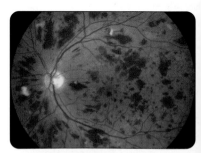

Fig. 16.64 Leukaemic retinopathy

- Peripheral retinal neovascularization is an occasional feature of chronic myeloid leukaemia.
- Choroidal deposits in chronic leukaemia may give rise to a 'leopard skin' appearance (*Fig. 16.65*).

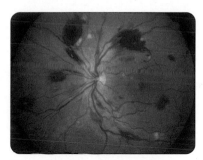

Fig. 16.66 Retinopathy in aplastic anaemia

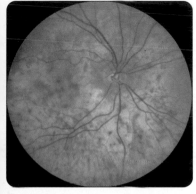

Fig. 16.65 Leopard spot fundus

2. Optic neuropathy – may occur in patients with pernicious anaemia.

Hyperviscosity

1. **Causes** – polycythaemia or abnormal plasma proteins as in Waldenström macroglobulinaemia and myeloma.
2. **Fundus** – retinal haemorrhages, and venous dilatation, segmentation and tortuosity (*Fig. 16.67*).

2. Other manifestations
- Orbital involvement, particularly in children.
- Iris thickening, iritis and pseudo-hypopyon.
- Spontaneous subconjunctival haemorrhage and hyphaema.

Anaemia

1. Retinopathy
- Retinal venous tortuosity is usually related to the severity of anaemia.
- Deep and flame-shaped haemorrhages, Roth spots, and cotton-wool spots are more common with coexisting thrombocytopenia in aplastic anaemia (*Fig. 16.66*).

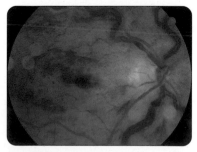

Fig. 16.67 Retinopathy in hyperviscosity

Acquired Macular Disorders

Age-related macular degeneration

Drusen

1. Histopathology (*Fig. 17.1*)
- Discrete deposits of the abnormal material located between the basal lamina of the RPE and the inner collagenous layer of Bruch membrane.
- Thickening of Bruch membrane compounded by excessive production of basement membrane deposit by the RPE.

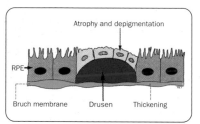

Fig. 17.1 Histopathology of drusen

2. Signs – yellow sub-RPE excrescences distributed symmetrically at both posterior poles.
- **a.** *Small hard drusen* – less than half a vein width in diameter with discrete margins (*Fig. 17.2*).
- **b.** *Large soft drusen* – vein width or more in diameter with indistinct margins (*Fig. 17.3a*).
- **c.** *Calcified drusen* – may be hard or soft (*Fig. 17.4*).

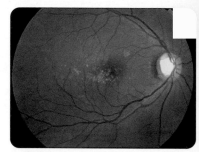

Fig. 17.2 Hard drusen

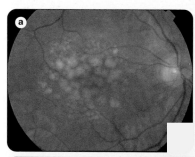

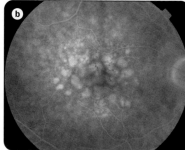

Fig. 17.3 (a) Soft drusen; (b) FA

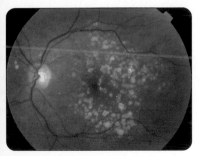

Fig. 17.4 Calcified drusen

3. FA

    a. *Hyperfluorescence* – window defect due to atrophy of the overlying RPE and late staining (see *Fig. 17.3b*).

    b. *Hypofluorescence* – of hydrophobic (high lipid content) drusen.

4. Drusen and AMD – features associated with an increased risk of subsequent visual loss include large soft and/or confluent drusen, and focal RPE hyperpigmentation (*Fig. 17.5*), particularly if the other eye has AMD.

5. Prophylactic treatment – high-dose multivitamins and antioxidants can decrease the risk of progression of AMD in eyes with the following high risk characteristics: visual loss in the contralateral eye from pre-existing dry or wet AMD, and confluent soft drusen even in the absence of visual loss.

Atrophic (dry) age-related macular degeneration

1. Pathogenesis – slowly progressive atrophy of the photoreceptors, RPE, and choriocapillaris.

2. Presentation – gradual impairment of vision over months or years.

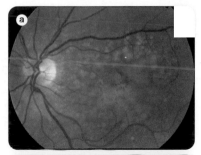

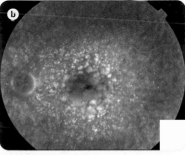

Fig. 17.5 (a) Confluent soft drusen with RPE changes; (b) FA

3. Signs in chronological order:

- Focal hyperpigmentation or atrophy of the RPE associated with drusen.
- Sharply circumscribed, areas of RPE atrophy associated with variable loss of the choriocapillaris (*Fig. 17.6*).
- Enlargement of the atrophic areas (*Fig. 17.7*).

4. FA – hyperfluorescence due to an RPE window defect (*Fig. 17.8*).

5. Treatment – not possible.

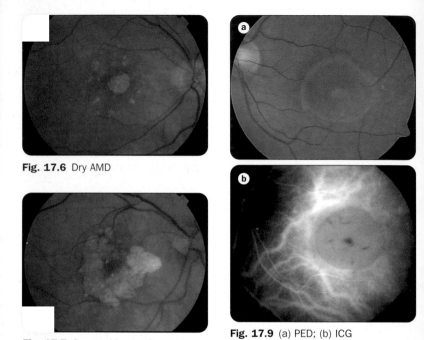

Fig. 17.6 Dry AMD

Fig. 17.7 Geographic atrophy

Fig. 17.9 (a) PED; (b) ICG

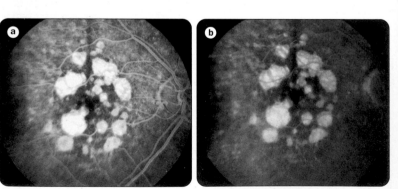

Fig. 17.8 Window defect in dry AMD

Retinal pigment epithelial detachment

1. **Pathogenesis** – reduction of hydraulic conductivity of the thickened Bruch membrane impeding movement of fluid from the RPE towards the choroid.
2. **Presentation** – metamorphopsia and impairment of central vision.
3. **Signs** – circumscribed, dome-shaped elevation at the posterior pole (*Fig. 17.9a*).
4. **ICG** – oval hypofluorescence with a faint ring of surrounding hyperfluorescence (*Fig. 17.9b*).
5. **OCT** – separation of the RPE from Bruch membrane (*Fig. 17.10*).

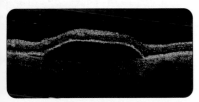

Fig. 17.10 OCT of PED

6. **FA** – well demarcated oval area of hyperfluorescence which increases in density but not in size (*Fig. 17.11*).
7. **Course** – may follow one of the following patterns:
   a. *Spontaneous resolution* – without residua.
   b. *Geographic atrophy* – following spontaneous resolution.
   c. *Detachment of the sensory retina.*
   d. *RPE tear formation.*

Retinal pigment epithelial tear

1. **Pathogenesis** – tearing of the RPE at the junction of attached and detached RPE due to tangential stress – may be spontaneous, or more commonly, follows laser photocoagulation, PDT or anti-VEGF therapy of CNV.
2. **Presentation** – sudden worsening of central vision.
3. **Signs** – crescent shaped RPE dehiscence with a retracted and folded flap (*Fig. 17.12a*).
4. **FA** – relative hypofluorescence over the flap with adjacent hyperfluorescence due to the exposed choriocapillaris (*Fig. 17.12b–d*).

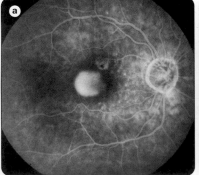
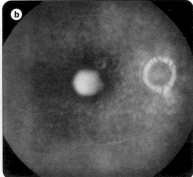

Fig. 17.11 FA of PED

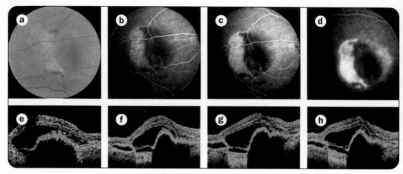

Fig. 17.12 RPE tear

5. OCT – loss of the normal dome-shaped profile of the RPE in the PED, with hyper-reflectivity adjacent to the folded RPE (*Fig. 17.12e–h*).

6. Prognosis – poor for subfoveal tears.

Neovascular (wet) age-related macular degeneration

Pathogenesis

- CNV originating from the choriocapillaris grows through defects in Bruch membrane (*Fig. 17.13*).
- Initial visual loss is caused by leakage from CNV under the sensory retina and under the RPE.
- This is followed by bleeding from CNV.
- Permanent visual loss is caused by subretinal (disciform) scarring.

Clinical features

1. Presentation – metamorphopsia, positive scotoma, and blurring of central vision.

2. Signs – serous retinal elevation, foveal thickening, CMO, subretinal haemorrhage, and hard exudate formation (*Fig. 17.14a*).

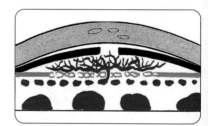

Fig. 17.13 CNV in wet AMD

Fluorescein angiography

1. Classic CNV

- Well-defined membrane which fills with dye in a 'lacy' pattern during the very early phase of dye transit (*Fig. 17.14b*), fluoresces brightly during peak dye transit (*Fig. 17.14c*), and then leaks into the subretinal space and around the CNV within 1–2 min.
- Late staining of fibrous tissue within the CNV (*Fig. 17.14d*).
- Classic CNV is classified according to its relation to the centre of FAZ as extrafoveal, subfoveal, and juxtafoveal.

- CNV can be further subdivided into wholly classic and predominantly classic in which 50% or less of the lesion has a classic component.
2. **Occult CNV** – poorly defined with less precise features on the early frames (*Fig. 17.15b*) and gives rise to late, diffuse or multifocal leakage (*Fig. 17.15c,d*).
3. **Fibrovascular PED** – combination of CNV and PED in which the CNV fluoresces brighter (hot spot) than the detachment; in other cases, the CNV may be obscured by blood or turbid fluid.

Course

The course of untreated CNV is often relentless and the prognosis very poor due to the following complications.
1. **Haemorrhagic PED**
   - Initially, the blood is confined to the sub-RPE space and appears as a dark elevated mound (*Fig. 17.16*).
   - The blood may then break into the subretinal space and assumes a more diffuse outline and a lighter red colour (*Fig. 17.17*).
2. **Vitreous haemorrhage** – when subretinal blood breaks through into the vitreous cavity; rare.
3. **Subretinal (disciform) scarring** – causes permanent loss of central vision (*Fig. 17.18*).

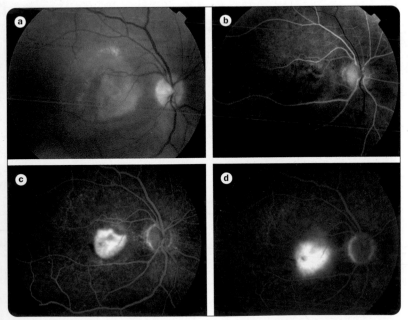

Fig. 17.14 FA of classic subfoveal CNV

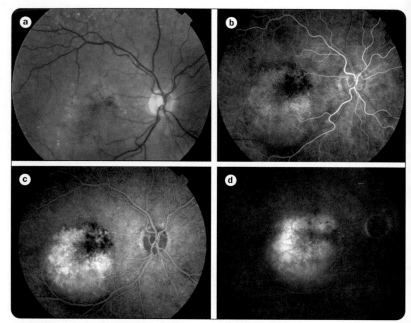

Fig. 17.15 FA of occult CNV

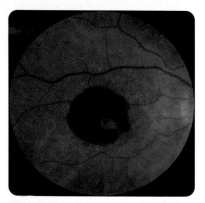

Fig. 17.16 Sub-RPE haemorrhage

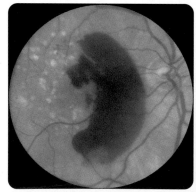

Fig. 17.17 Subretinal haemorrhage

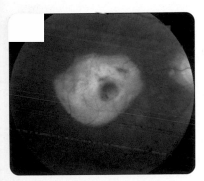

Fig. 17.18 Disciform scar

4. Massive subretinal exudation – due to chronic leakage from CNV (*Fig. 17.19*).

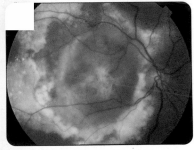

Fig. 17.19 Massive exudation

Treatment

1. **Photodynamic therapy (PDT)** – for subfoveal, predominantly classic CNV not larger than 5400 μm in eyes with a visual acuity of 6/60 or better.
2. **Anti-vascular endothelium growth factor (anti-VEGF) agents** – intravitreal bevacizumab (Avastin), ranibizumab (Lucentis) and pegaptanib (Macugen) are used to treat any type of CNV.

Retinal angiomatous proliferation

1. **Definition** – uncommon type of wet AMD in which neovascularization originates from the retinal vasculature and not the choriocapillaris.
2. **Signs**
   - Intraretinal and subretinal neovascularization often accompanied by haemorrhage and oedema.
   - CNV associated with fibrovascular PED and retinochoroidal anastomoses.
3. **FA** – similar to purely occult or minimally classic CNV.
4. **ICG** – hot spot in mid or late frames.
5. **Treatment** – PDT with adjunctive intravitreal triamcinolone.

Polypoidal choroidal vasculopathy

1. **Definition** – bilateral, choroidal vascular disease in which the inner choroidal vessels consist of a dilated network with multiple terminal aneurysmal protuberances that have a polypoidal configuration.
2. **Signs**
   a. *Exudative* – multiple PED, serous RD, and lipid deposits (*Fig. 17.20a*).
   b. *Haemorrhagic* – haemorrhagic PED and subretinal haemorrhage (*Fig. 17.21a*).
3. **ICG** – polypoidal dilatations beneath the RPE that fill slowly and then leak intensely (*Figs 17.20b & 17.21b*).
4. **Course**
   - Spontaneous resolution in 50%.
   - In the remainder occasional repeated bleeding and leakage, resulting in macular damage and visual loss.
5. **Treatment** – PDT.

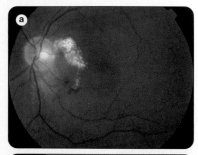

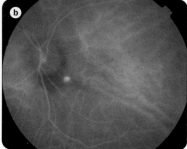

Fig. 17.20 (a) Exudative polypoidal; (b) ICG

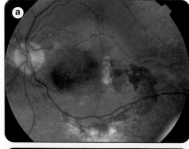

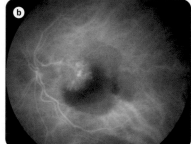

Fig. 17.21 (a) Haemorrhagic polypoidal; (b) ICG

Age-related macular hole

1. **Pathogenesis** – abnormal vitreo-foveolar attachment, with resultant antero-posterior and tangential traction.
2. **Presentation** – in old age.
3. **Staging** (*Fig. 17.22*)
   - *Stage 1a* (impending) – flat umbo, yellow foveolar spot 100–200 μm in diameter with loss of the foveolar reflex.
   - *Stage 1b* (occult) – yellow ring with a bridging interface of vitreous cortex.
   - *Stage 2* (early hole) – full-thickness defect, less than 300 μm in diameter with or without an overlying pseudo-operculum.
   - *Stage 3* (established hole) – full-thickness defect more than 400 μm in diameter with an attached posterior vitreous face with or without an overlying pseudo-operculum.
   - *Stage 4* – round defect more than 400 μm in diameter surrounded by a cuff of subretinal fluid and tiny yellowish deposits within its crater, and completely detached vitreous cortex (*Fig. 17.23*).

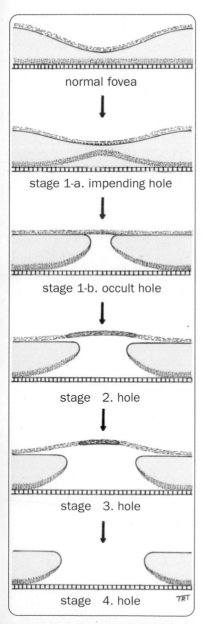

normal fovea

↓

stage 1-a. impending hole

↓

stage 1-b. occult hole

↓

stage 2. hole

↓

stage 3. hole

↓

stage 4. hole

TRT

Fig. 17.22 Staging of macular hole

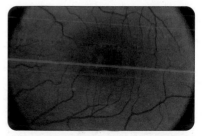

Fig. 17.23 Full-thickness macular hole

4. **OCT** – useful in the diagnosis and staging of macular holes (*Fig. 17.24*).

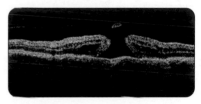

Fig. 17.24 Macular hole with operculum

5. **FA** – corresponding area of hyper-fluorescence.
6. **Surgery** (*Fig. 17.25*)
   - Indicated for stage 2 and above, associated with a visual acuity worse than 6/9.
   - Following successful surgery, visual improvement is achieved in 80–90% of eyes, with a final visual acuity of 6/12 or better in up to 65%.

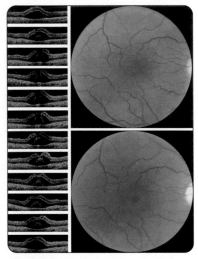

Fig. 17.25 Unsuccessful surgery for macular hole. Pre-operative appearance (above); postoperative appearance (below)

Macular microhole

1. **Presentation** – central scotoma or reduced reading vision.
2. **Signs** – very small, red, well demarcated intraretinal foveal or juxtafoveal defect that remains stationary with long-term follow-up.
3. **OCT** – well localized subtle defect that probably indicates the presence of a gap in the photoreceptors, and/ or the RPE.

Central serous retinopathy

1. **Pathogenesis** – localized detachment of the sensory retina at the macula secondary to focal RPE defects.

2. **Presentation** – unilateral relative positive scotoma, micropsia, metamorphopsia, and occasionally macropsia.
3. **Signs** – round detachment of the sensory retina at the macula that may be associated with small precipitates on its posterior surface (*Fig. 17.26*)

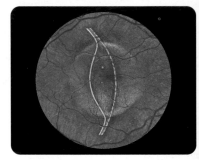

Fig. 17.26 CSR

4. **OCT** – elevation of the sensory retinal layer from the highly reflective RPE layer by an optically empty zone (*Fig. 17.27*)

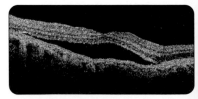

Fig. 17.27 OCT of CSR

5. **FA**
   • Small hyperfluorescent spot that enlarges and ascends vertically and laterally until the entire area

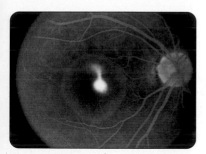

Fig. 17.28 FA of CSR

is filled with dye (smoke stack appearance – *Fig. 17.28*)
- Less frequently the hyperfluorescent spot enlarges centrifugally (ink-spot appearance).

6. ICG – early phase shows dilated choroidal vessels, mid phases show multiple areas of hyperfluorescence due to choroidal hyperpermeability.

7. Course
- Spontaneous resolution within 3–12 months is the rule.
- Occasionally the course is protracted and results in progressive widespread RPE changes (chronic retinal pigment epitheliopathy).

8. Treatment
- **a.** *Not required* – in majority.
- **b.** *Argon laser photocoagulation* – in eyes with extrafoveal leaks achieves speedier resolution and lowers the recurrence rate but does not influence the final visual outcome.
- **c.** *PDT* – in acute CSR with subfoveal leaks and in chronic disease.

Cystoid macular oedema

1. Definition
- Accumulation of fluid in the outer plexiform and inner nuclear layers with the formation of fluid-filled cyst-like changes (*Fig. 17.29a*).
- Lamellar hole formation in longstanding cases (*Fig. 17.29b*).

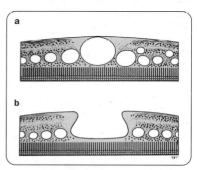

Fig. 17.29 (a) CMO; (b) lamellar hole

2. Signs – loss of the foveal depression, retinal thickening, and multiple cystoid areas in the sensory retina (*Fig. 17.30*).

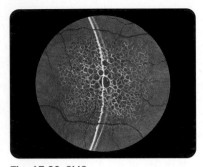

Fig. 17.30 CMO

3. OCT – collection of hyporeflective spaces within the retina, with overall macular thickening and loss of the foveal depression (*Fig. 17.31*).

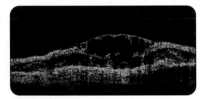

Fig. 17.31 OCT of CMO

4. FA – late phase shows a 'flower-petal' pattern of hyperfluorescence (*Fig. 17.32*).

5. Vascular causes
- Diabetic retinopathy, retinal vein occlusion, hypertensive retinopathy, idiopathic retinal telangiectasis, retinal artery macroaneurysm, and radiation retinopathy.
- Treatment – laser photocoagulation in selected cases.

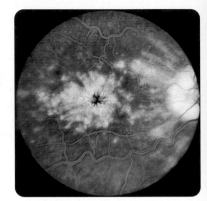

Fig. 17.32 FA of CMO

6. Inflammatory causes
- Chronic anterior uveitis, intermediate uveitis, and certain forms of posterior uveitis.
- Treatment – control of uveitis with anti-inflammatory agents; systemic carbonic anhydrase inhibitors may be beneficial in CMO associated with intermediate uveitis.

7. Following cataract surgery
- Risk factors – posterior capsular rupture, vitreous loss and incarceration into the incision site, anterior chamber and secondary IOL implantation, diabetes, and CMO in the other eye.
- Treatment – correction of the underlying cause, if possible; persistent cases may require systemic carbonic anhydrase inhibitors, topical and periocular steroids, topical NSAIDs, intravitreal triamcinolone, and pars plana vitrectomy.

8. Drug-induced – topical adrenaline 2% (especially in the aphakic eye), topical latanoprost, and systemic nicotinic acid.

9. Retinal dystrophies
- RP, gyrate atrophy, and dominantly inherited CMO.
- Treatment – systemic carbonic anhydrase inhibitors in RP.

10. Vitreomacular traction syndrome (see below).

11. Macular epiretinal membranes (see below).

12. CNV – CMO is an adverse prognostic factor.

13. Tumours – retinal haemangioblastoma and choroidal haemangioma.

Macular epiretinal membrane

Pathogenesis

- Proliferation of retinal glial cells at the vitreoretinal interface that have gained access to the retinal surface through breaks in the internal limiting membrane.
- May be idiopathic or secondary to RD surgery and cryotherapy, retinal vascular disease, intraocular inflammation, and trauma.

Cellophane maculopathy

1. Presentation – mild metamorphopsia although frequently the condition is asymptomatic and is discovered by chance.

2. Signs
- Irregular light reflex or sheen at the macula.

- The membrane is translucent and best detected with 'red-free' light (*Fig. 17.33*).

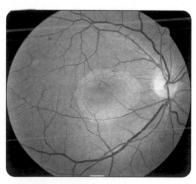

Fig. 17.33 Cellophane maculopathy

3. Treatment – not appropriate.

Macular pucker

1. Presentation – metamorphopsia and blurring of central vision.

2. VA – 6/12 or worse.

3. Signs
- Severe vascular distortion, retinal wrinkling and white striae (*Fig. 17.34*).
- Macular pseudo-hole (*Fig. 17.35*) and occasionally CMO.

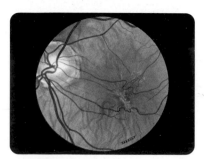

Fig. 17.34 Macular pucker

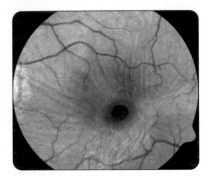

Fig. 17.35 Macular pseudohole

4. OCT – highly reflective (red) layer on the retinal surface associated with thickening (*Fig. 17.36*).

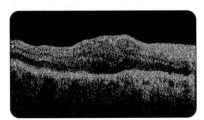

Fig. 17.36 OCT of macular pucker

5. FA – highlights the vascular tortuosity and may show hyperfluorescence if leakage is present (*Fig. 17.37*).
6. Treatment – removal of the membrane improves or eliminates distortion, and improves visual acuity in about 50% of cases.

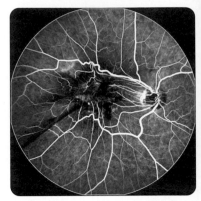

Fig. 17.37 FA of macular pucker

Degenerative myopia

1. Definition
- Refractive error > –6 D and axial length >26 mm.
- Affects approximately 0.5% of the general population and 30% of myopic eyes.

2. Signs
- Pale tessellate (tigroid) fundus with visibility of large choroidal vessels (*Fig. 17.38*).

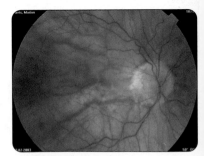

Fig. 17.38 Tessellate fundus

- 'Lacquer cracks' consist of ruptures in the RPE–Bruch membrane–choriocapillaris complex (*Fig. 17.39*).
- Focal chorioretinal atrophy with visibility of the sclera (*Fig. 17.40*).
- Staphylomas due to expansion of the globe and scleral thinning.

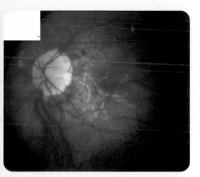

Fig. 17.39 Lacquer cracks

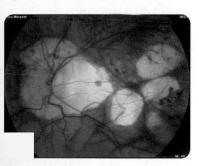

Fig. 17.40 Chorioretinal atrophy

3. Maculopathy
- CNV associated with 'lacquer cracks'.
- Subretinal 'coin' haemorrhages from lacquer cracks without CNV (*Fig. 17.41*).
- Fuchs spot – pigmented lesion after absorption of a macular haemorrhage (*Fig. 17.42*).

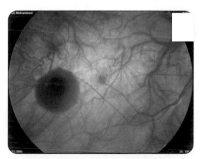

Fig. 17.41 Coin haemorrhage

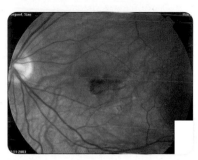

Fig. 17.42 Fuchs spot

4. **FA** – filling of large choroidal vessels but not of the choriocapillaris (*Fig. 17.43*).

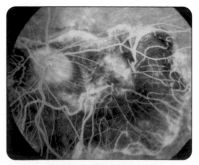

Fig. 17.43 FA in high myopia

5. Ocular complications
- Rhegmatogenous RD.
- Cataract, which may be posterior subcapsular or early-onset nuclear sclerosis.
- Increased prevalence of primary open-angle glaucoma, pigmentary glaucoma, and steroid responsiveness.

6. Systemic associations
- Stickler syndrome.
- Marfan syndrome.
- Ehlers–Danlos syndrome.
- Pierre–Robin syndrome.

Angioid streaks

1. Definition – crack-like dehiscences in thickened, calcified and abnormally brittle collagenous and elastic portions of Bruch membrane.

2. Signs
- Mottled pigmentation ('peau d'orange').
- Grey or dark-red linear lesions with irregular serrated edges intercommunicate around the optic disc and then radiate outwards (*Fig. 17.44*).
- Associated RPE hyperplasia in longstanding cases (*Fig. 17.45*).

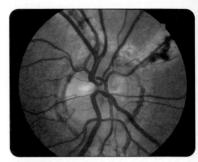

Fig. 17.45 Angioid streaks with RPE hyperplasia

3. FA – hyperfluorescence over the streaks associated with variable hypofluorescence corresponding to RPE hyperplasia.

4. Prognosis – visual loss in 70% of cases due to CNV (*Fig. 17.46*), traumatic choroidal rupture, or foveal involvement by a streak.

5. Systemic associations – in 50% of patients:

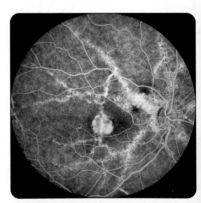

Fig. 17.46 FA in angioid streaks with CNV

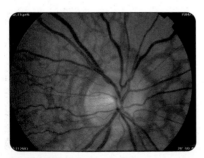

Fig. 17.44 Angioid streaks

a. *Pseudoxanthoma elasticum* – most common (Groenblad–Strandberg syndrome).

b. *Ehlers–Danlos syndrome type 6* (ocular sclerotic) – occasional.

c. *Paget disease* – uncommon.

d. *Haemoglobinopathies* – occasional.

Choroidal folds

1. **Definition** – parallel grooves or striae involving the inner choroid, Bruch membrane, RPE, and sometimes the outer sensory retina.
2. **Causes**
   a. *Idiopathic* – affect both eyes of healthy hypermetropic patients.
   b. *Orbital disease* – retrobulbar tumours and thyroid ophthalmopathy.
   c. *Miscellaneous* – choroidal tumours, chronic papilloedema, posterior scleritis, and scleral buckle for RD.
3. **Signs** – horizontal parallel grooves at the posterior pole in which the crest is yellow and less pigmented than the darker trough (*Fig. 17.47a*).
4. **FA** – alternating hyperfluorescent and hypofluorescent streaks (17.47b).

Hypotony maculopathy

1. **Causes** – very low IOP (usually <6 mmHg) following filtration surgery, particularly when adjunctive antimetabolites are used, trauma and chronic anterior uveitis.
2. **Signs** – irregular chorioretinal folds (*Fig. 17.48*).
3. **Treatment** – depends on the cause.

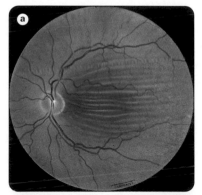

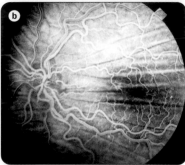

Fig. 17.47 (a) Choroidal folds; (b) FA

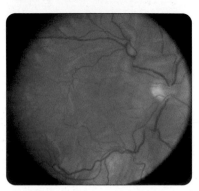

Fig. 17.48 Hypotony maculopathy

Vitreomacular traction syndrome

1. **Pathogenesis**
   - Vitreous cortex is attached to the fovea and the optic disc but detached temporal to the fovea and the area of the papillomacular bundle.
   - This incomplete posterior vitreous detachment exerts persistent anterior traction on the fovea, which leads to macular changes, notably CMO.

2. **Signs**
   - Partial posterior vitreous detachment with persistent attachment of vitreous to the macula.
   - The macula may show retinal surface wrinkling, distortion, an epiretinal membrane or CMO.

3. **OCT** – is used to confirm the diagnosis (*Fig. 17.49*).

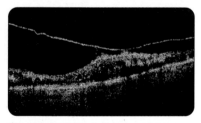

Fig. 17.49 OCT of vitreomacular traction syndrome

4. **Treatment** – pars plana vitrectomy.

Solar maculopathy

1. **Pathogenesis** – retinal injury caused by photochemical effects of solar radiation is caused by directly or indirectly viewing the sun (eclipse retinopathy).

2. **Presentation** – within 1–4 hours of solar exposure with unilateral or bilateral impairment of central vision and a small central scotoma.

3. **Fundus**
   - Small yellow or red foveolar spot which fades within a few weeks.
   - The spot is replaced by a sharply defined foveolar defect with irregular borders or a lamellar hole (*Fig. 17.50*).

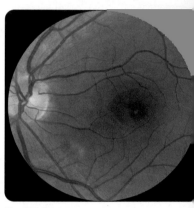

Fig. 17.50 Late solar maculopathy

4. **Treatment** – not possible.
5. **Prognosis** – good with improvement of vision within 6 months.

Idiopathic choroidal neovascularization

Idiopathic CNV is an uncommon condition which affects patients under the age of 50 years. It carries a better visual prognosis than that associated with AMD and in some cases spontaneous revolution may occur. The CNV is of type 2 and lies predominantly above the RPE.

Chapter 18

Fundus Dystrophies

Retinal dystrophies

Retinitis pigmentosa

1. **Definition** – clinically and genetically diverse group of diffuse retinal dystrophies initially predominantly affecting the rod photoreceptor cells with subsequent degeneration of cones.
2. **Inheritance**
   - Sporadic or AD, AR or X-L.
   - Many cases are due to mutation of the rhodopsin gene.
   - Associated systemic disorders are usually AR.
3. **Classic clinical triad** – arteriolar attenuation, retinal bone-spicule pigmentation, and waxy disc pallor.
4. **Presentation** – nyctalopia, often during the 3rd decade, but may be sooner depending on pedigree.
5. **Signs** in chronological order:
   - Arteriolar narrowing and sparse pigmentary changes (*Fig. 18.1*).
   - Coarse, mid-peripheral, perivascular 'bone-spicule' pigmentation and optic atrophy (*Fig. 18.2*).
   - Gradual increase in pigmentary density with anterior and posterior spread (*Fig. 18.3*).

Fig. 18.2 Advanced RP

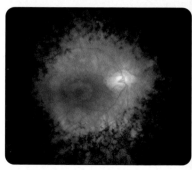

Fig. 18.3 End-stage RP

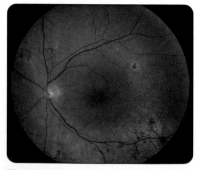

Fig. 18.1 Early RP

6. **Maculopathy** – atrophy, cellophane, and CMO.
7. **ERG** (*Fig. 18.4*)
   - Reduced scotopic rod and combined responses during the early stages when fundus changes are mild.
   - Later photopic responses become reduced and eventually the ERG becomes extinguished.
8. **DA** (adaptation) – prolonged.
9. **CV** – normal.
10. **VF** – annular mid-peripheral scotoma which expands peripherally and centrally.

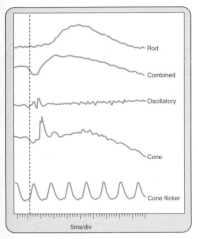

Fig. 18.4 ERG in RP

11. **Prognosis** – poor with visual loss of central vision due to direct involvement of the fovea by RP itself or maculopathy.
12. **Ocular associations** – cataract, open-angle glaucoma, myopia, keratoconus, intermediate uveitis, and optic disc drusen.
13. **Systemic associations** – Bassen–Kornzweig syndrome, Refsum syndrome, Kearns–Sayre syndrome, Bardet–Biedl Syndrome, Usher syndrome, and Friedreich ataxia.

Atypical RP

1. **Retinitis punctata albescens** – subtle, scattered white dots, usually sparing the macula, associated with vascular attenuation (*Fig. 18.5*).
2. **Sector RP** – involvement of one quadrant (usually nasal – *Fig. 18.6*) or one half (usually inferior).

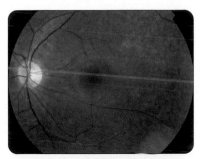

Fig. 18.5 Retinitis punctata albescens

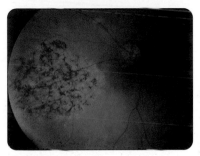

Fig. 18.6 Sector RP

3. **Pericentral RP** – pigmentary abnormalities emanate from the disc and extend along the temporal arcades and nasally.
4. **RP with exudative vasculopathy** – Coats disease-like appearance (*Fig. 18.7*).

Progressive cone dystrophy

1. **Definition** – a heterogeneous group of rare disorders characterized by initially only cone dysfunction but in many cases rod system subsequently becomes affected; the term 'cone–rod dystrophy' is therefore more appropriate.

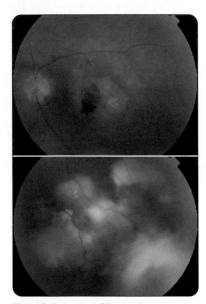

Fig. 18.7 Atypical RP with Coats disease

2. **Inheritance** – most are sporadic; of the remainder most are AD, and rarely AR or X-L.
3. **Presentation** – 1st–2nd decade with gradual impairment of central and colour vision.
4. **Signs** in chronological order:
   - Fovea may be normal or exhibit non-specific granularity.
   - Golden sheen may be seen in X-L disease.
   - Bull's-eye maculopathy is common (Fig. 18.8a).
   - Progressive RPE atrophy at the macula with eventual geographic atrophy.
5. **FA** – of bull's eye maculopathy shows an oval window defect with central hypofluorescence (Fig. 18.8b).

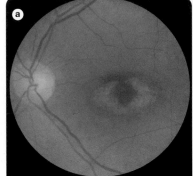
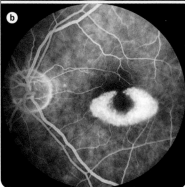

Fig. 18.8 (a) Bull's eye maculopathy; (b) FA

6. **ERG** (Fig. 18.9)
   - Photopic – subnormal or non-recordable.
   - Flicker fusion – reduced.
   - Rod responses – preserved till late.
7. **CV** – severe deuteran-tritan defect out of proportion to visual acuity.

Albinism

Definition

- A genetically determined, heterogeneous group of disorders of melanin synthesis in which the eyes alone

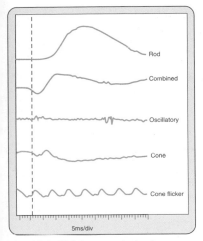

Fig. 18.9 ERG in cone dystrophy

5ms/div

Rod

Combined

Oscillatory

Cone

Cone flicker

2. Inheritance – AR (gene locus on 15p11-q13).
3. VA – <6/60 due to foveal hypoplasia.
4. Nystagmus – increases in bright illumination.
5. Iris – diaphanous and translucent (*Fig. 18.11*).

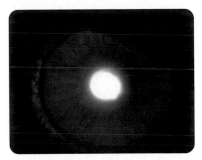

Fig. 18.11 Marked iris translucency

6. Fundus – lack of pigment, foveal hypoplasia with absence of the foveal pit and lack of vessels forming the perimacular arcades (*Fig. 18.12*).

(ocular albinism) or the eyes, skin and hair (oculocutaneous albinism) may be affected.

• The latter may be either tyrosinase-negative (complete) or tyrosinase-positive (incomplete).

Tyrosinase-negative oculocutaneous

1. Pigment – white hair and very pale skin (*Fig. 18.10*).

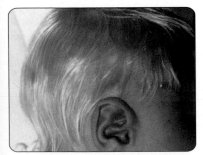

Fig. 18.10 Tyrosinase-negative albino

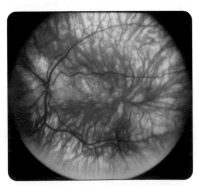

Fig. 18.12 Severe fundus hypopigmentation

7. **Optic chiasm** – fewer than normal uncrossed nerve fibres so that the majority from each eye cross to the contralateral hemisphere.

8. **Other features** – optic nerve hypoplasia, high refractive errors, positive angle kappa, and squint.

Tyrosinase-positive oculocutaneous

1. **Pigment** – hair may be white, yellow or red and darkens with age.
2. **Inheritance** – AR (gene locus on 15p11-q13).
3. **VA** – impaired due to foveal hypoplasia.
4. **Iris** – blue or dark-brown with variable translucency (*Fig. 18.13*).

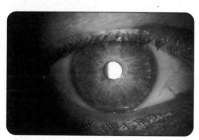

Fig. 18.13 Mild iris translucency

5. **Fundus** – variable hypopigmentation (*Fig. 18.14*).
6. **Associated syndromes** – Chediak–Higashi and Hermansky–Pudlak.

Ocular albinism

1. **Pigment** – normal hair and skin.
2. **Inheritance** – usually X-L, occasionally AR (gene locus on Xp22.2-22.3).
3. **Female carriers** – are asymptomatic although they may show partial iris

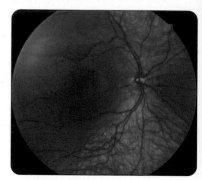

Fig. 18.14 Mild fundus hypopigmentation

translucency, macular stippling, and mid-peripheral areas of depigmentation and granularity (*Fig. 18.15*).

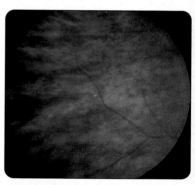

Fig. 18.15 Albino carrier

4. **Affected males** – hypopigmented fundi and irides.

Fundus flavimaculatus

1. **Inheritance** – AR (gene locus on 1p21-22).
2. **Presentation** – adult life.

3. Signs
- Ill-defined, yellow, fish-shaped flecks confined to the posterior pole (*Fig. 18.16*) or extending to the midperiphery (*Fig. 18.17*).
- Vermilion colour fundus in 50%.

4. ERG – photopic is normal to subnormal; scotopic is normal.

5. EOG – subnormal.

6. FA
- 'Dark choroid' due to lipofuscin deposits in the RPE.
- Fresh flecks show early hypofluorescence and late hyperfluorescence.
- Old flecks show RPE window defects (*Fig. 18.18*).

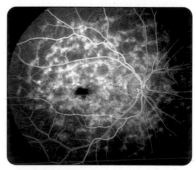

Fig. 18.18 FA of old flecks

7. Fundus autofluorescence – may be present (*Fig. 18.19*).

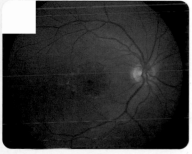

Fig. 18.16 Central flecks

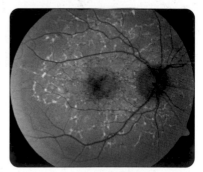

Fig. 18.19 Autofluorescence

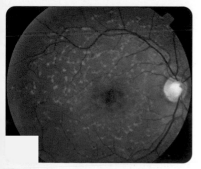

Fig. 18.17 Central and peripheral flecks

8. Prognosis – relatively good unless a fleck involves the foveola or geographic atrophy develops (*Fig. 18.20*).

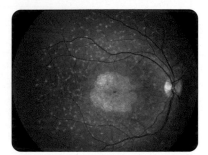

Fig. 18.20 Geographic atrophy

Stargardt disease

1. **Inheritance** – AR (gene locus on 1p21-22).
2. **Presentation** – 1st–2nd decade with gradual impairment of central vision.
3. **Signs** in chronological order:
   - Fovea – normal or shows non-specific mottling.
   - Oval, 'snail-slime' or 'beaten-bronze' fovea, which may be surrounded by flecks (*Fig. 18.21*).
   - Geographic atrophy which may have bull's eye configuration.

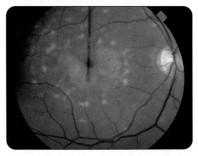

Fig. 18.21 Stargardt disease

4. **ERG** – photopic is normal to subnormal; scotopic is normal.
5. **EOG** – subnormal in advanced cases.
6. **FA** – 'dark choroid' and a window defect if geographic atrophy is present (*Fig. 18.22*).

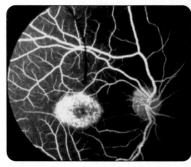

Fig. 18.22 FA in Stargardt disease

7. **Prognosis** – poor.

Juvenile Best macular dystrophy

1. **Inheritance** – AD (gene locus on 11q13).
2. **Signs**
   a. *Stage 0* (pre-vitelliform) – subnormal EOG and normal fundus.
   b. *Stage 1* – pigment mottling at the macula.
   c. *Stage 2* (vitelliform) – round egg-yolk ('sunny side up') macular lesion in infancy or early childhood (*Fig. 18.23*).
   d. *Stage 3* (pseudo-hypopyon) – at puberty when part of the lesion becomes absorbed (*Fig. 18.24*).
   e. *Stage 4* (vitelliruptive) – 'scrambled egg' and visual acuity drops (*Fig. 18.25*).

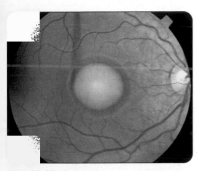

Fig. 18.23 Egg yolk

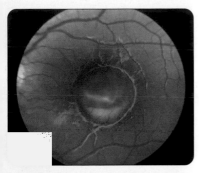

Fig. 18.24 Pseudo-hypopyon

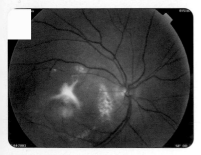

Fig. 18.25 Scrambled egg

3. **EOG** – subnormal during all stages and in carriers with normal fundi.
4. **Prognosis** – reasonably good until 5th decade.

Familial dominant drusen

Familial drusen (Doyne honeycomb choroiditis, malattia levantinese) is thought to represent an early manifestation of AMD.

1. **Inheritance** – AD (gene locus on 2p16-21).
2. **Mild disease** – few small, discrete, innocuous, hard drusen confined to the macula.
3. **Moderate disease** – large, soft drusen at the posterior pole and peripapillary region.
4. **Advanced disease** – uncommon and presents after the 5th decade with CNV or geographic atrophy.
5. **Malattia levantinese**
   • Numerous, small, elongated, basal laminar drusen with a spoke-like or radial distribution centered on the fovea and peripapillary area (*Fig. 18.26*).
   • May be accompanied by subretinal fibrosis and RPE changes (*Fig. 18.27*).
   • Most patients are asymptomatic until the 4th or 5th decade when they develop CNV or geographic atrophy.
6. **ERG** – normal.
7. **EOG** – subnormal in advanced disease.

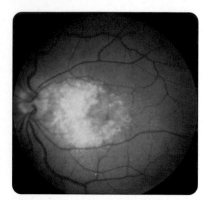

Fig. 18.26 Malattia levantinese

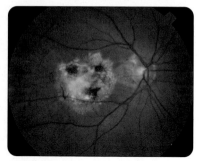

Fig. 18.27 Malattia levantinese with RPE changes

Leber congenital amaurosis

1. **Inheritance** – AR (gene locus on 17p).
2. **Presentation** – perinatal blindness.
3. **Signs** are variable and include the following:
   - Pupillary light reflexes – absent or diminished.
   - Fundi – may be initially normal despite very poor vision.

- Patches of peripheral chorioretinal atrophy and granularity are common.
- Macular coloboma-like atrophy (*Fig. 18.28*).
- Other findings include disc elevation, salt-and-pepper changes, diffuse white spots, macular pigmentation, and bull's eye maculopathy.
- Oculodigital syndrome (*Fig. 18.29*)

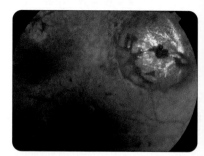

Fig. 18.28 Leber amaurosis

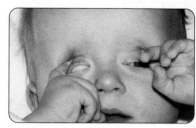

Fig. 18.29 Oculodigital syndrome

4. **Prognosis** – very poor.
5. **Ocular associations** – strabismus, hypermetropia, keratoconus, keratoglobus and cataract.
6. **ERG** – non-recordable.

7. **Systemic associations** – mental handicap, deafness, epilepsy, CNS and renal anomalies, skeletal malformations, and endocrine dysfunction.

Sorsby pseudo-inflammatory dystrophy

1. **Inheritance** – AD (gene locus on 22q12.13).
2. **Presentation** – 3rd decade with nyctalopia or sudden visual loss due to wet maculopathy in the 5th decade.
3. **Signs** in chronological order:
   - Confluent, drusen-like deposits along the arcades, nasal to the disc and mid-periphery (Fig. 18.30).
   - Wet maculopathy (Fig. 18.31) and subretinal scarring.
   - Peripheral chorioretinal atrophy may occur by the 7th decade and result in loss of ambulatory vision.

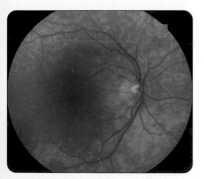

Fig. 18.30 Early Sorsby pseudo-inflammatory dystrophy

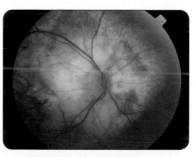

Fig. 18.31 Wet maculopathy in Sorsby

4. **ERG** – subnormal in late disease.
5. **Prognosis** – poor with severe visual loss in the 5th decade.

North Carolina macular dystrophy

1. **Inheritance** – AD (gene locus on 6q14-q16.2).
2. **Grading and prognosis**
   a. *Grade 1* – yellow-white, drusen-like peripheral (Fig. 18.32) and macular deposits develop during the 1st decade and may remain asymptomatic.
   b. *Grade 2* – deep, confluent macular deposits (Fig. 18.33) that may be later associated with CNV.
   c. *Grade 3* – coloboma-like atrophic macular lesions (Fig. 18.34) with impairment of visual acuity.

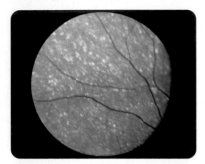

Fig. 18.32 Peripheral flecks in North Carolina

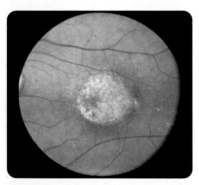

Fig. 18.33 Macular flecks

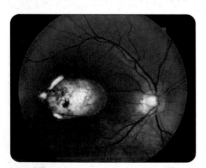

Fig. 18.34 Coloboma-like lesion

Adult-onset foveomacular vitelliform dystrophy

1. **Inheritance** – AR.
2. **Presentation** – 4th–6th decade with mild to moderate decrease of visual acuity and sometimes metamorphopsia although often the condition is discovered by chance.
3. **Signs** – small, round, slightly elevated, yellowish subfoveal deposit (*Fig. 18.35a*).
4. **FA** – central hypofluorescence surrounded by a small irregular hyperfluorescent ring (*Fig. 18.35b*).

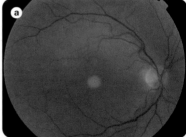

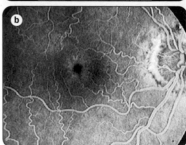

Fig. 18.35 (a) Adult vitelliform; (b) FA

5. ERG – normal.

6. Prognosis – good.

Butterfly-shaped macular dystrophy

1. **Inheritance** – AR
2. **Presentation** – 2nd–3rd decade usually by chance and occasionally with mild impairment of central vision.
3. **Signs**
   - Yellow pigment at the fovea arranged in a triradiate manner (*Fig. 18.36a*).
   - Atrophic maculopathy may occasionally develop with time.

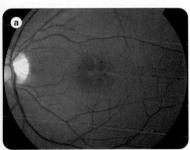

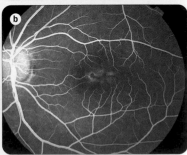

Fig. 18.36 (a) Butterfly dystrophy; (b) FA

4. **FA** – non-fluorescence of the lesions outlined by hyperfluorescence (*Fig. 18.36b*).
5. **ERG** – normal.
6. **Prognosis** – usually good.

Alport syndrome

1. **Pathogenesis** – abnormality of glomerular basement membrane caused by mutations in several different genes, all of which encode particular forms of type IV collagen.
2. **Inheritance** – X LD.
3. **Signs**
   - Yellowish, punctate flecks in the perimacular area with normal visual acuity (*Fig. 18.37*).
   - Larger peripheral flecks (*Fig. 18.38*).

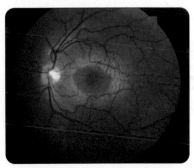

Fig. 18.37 Macular flecks in Alport

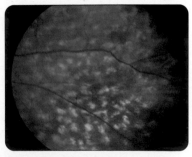

Fig. 18.38 Peripheral flecks in Alport

4. **ERG** – normal.
5. **Ocular associations** – anterior lenticonus and occasionally posterior polymorphous corneal dystrophy.
6. **Systemic manifestations** – chronic renal failure and sensorineural deafness.
7. **Prognosis** – excellent.

Benign familial flecked retina

1. **Inheritance** – AR.
2. **Presentation** – by chance.
3. **Signs** – discrete, yellow-white, polymorphous flecks that spare the macula and extend to the far periphery (*Fig. 18.39*).

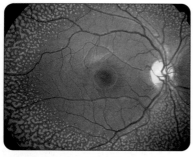

Fig. 18.39 Benign familial flecked retina

4. **ERG** – normal.
5. **Prognosis** – excellent.

Benign concentric annular macular dystrophy

1. **Inheritance** – AD.
2. **Presentation** – adult life with mild impairment of central vision.
3. **Signs** – bull's-eye maculopathy associated with slight vascular attenuation but a normal disc.
4. **VF** – paracentral ring scotoma.

5. **FA** – annular RPE window defect.
6. **Prognosis** – usually good.

Dominant macular oedema

1. **Inheritance** – AD (gene locus on 7q).
2. **Presentation** – 1st–2nd decade with gradual impairment of central vision.
3. **Signs** – bilateral CMO followed by geographic atrophy.
4. **FA** – flower-petal pattern of hyperfluorescence at the fovea.
5. **Prognosis** – poor.

Bietti crystalline dystrophy

1. **Inheritance** – AR (gene locus on 4q36).
2. **Presentation** – 3rd decade with slowly progressive visual loss.
3. **Signs** in chronological order:
   - Fine, glistening, yellow-white crystals scattered throughout the posterior fundus (*Fig. 18.40*).
   - Diffuse atrophy of the choriocapillaris with a decrease in size and number of the crystals.
   - Gradual confluence and peripheral expansion of the atrophic areas.

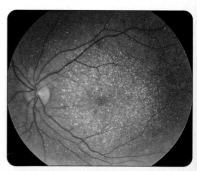

Fig. 18.40 Bietti crystalline dystrophy

4. **ERG** – subnormal.
5. **Other ocular manifestation** – crystalline keratopathy.
6. **Prognosis** – variable.

Familial internal limiting membrane dystrophy

1. **Inheritance** – AD.
2. **Presentation** – 3rd–4th decade with gradual visual loss.
3. **Signs**
   - Posterior pole manifests a glistening inner retinal surface (*Fig. 18.41*).
   - Later retinoschisis, retinal oedema, and retinal folds.

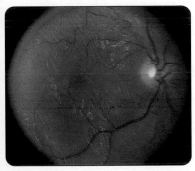

Fig. 18.41 Familial internal limiting membrane dystrophy

4. **ERG** – selective diminution of the b wave.
5. **Prognosis** – poor.

Occult macular dystrophy

1. **Presentation** – 3rd–7th decade with progressive loss of central vision.
2. **Signs** – normal fundi.
3. **ERG** – full-field is normal; focal cone and multifocal are abnormal.
4. **FA** – normal.

5. **OCT** – decreased foveal thickness.
6. **Prognosis** – poor.

Enhanced S-cone syndrome

1. **Inheritance** – AR.
2. **Presentation** – nyctalopia in childhood.
3. **Signs** – pigmentary changes along the vascular arcades and CMO without fluorescein leakage.
4. **ERG** – hyperfunction of S-cones; severe impairment of M and L cones, and non-recordable rod function.
5. **Prognosis** – guarded.

Late-onset retinal degeneration

1. **Inheritance** – AD.
2. **Presentation** – nyctalopia in the 6th decade followed by progressive loss of central and peripheral vision.
3. **Signs** – variable.
   - Normal fundus.
   - Clusters of fine yellow-white dots in the mid-periphery.
   - Pigmentary retinopathy and chorioretinal atrophy.
   - Atrophic maculopathy and optic atrophy.
4. **ERG** – initially normal; end-stage disease shows reduced amplitude.
5. **Prognosis** – very poor.

Sjögren–Larsson syndrome

1. **Definition** – neurocutaneous disorder associated with deficient activity of fatty aldehyde dehydrogenase.
2. **Inheritance** – AR.
3. **Presentation** – photophobia and poor vision in childhood.
4. **Signs** – glistening yellow-white crystalline deposits at the macula.

Cherry-red spot at macula

1. **Pathogenesis** – present in the sphingolipidoses and caused by deposition of abnormal lipids in retinal ganglion cells resulting in retinal opacification, except at the foveola where ganglion cells are absent (*Fig. 18.42*).

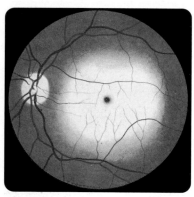

Fig. 18.42 Cherry-red spot

2. **Systemic associations** – Tay–Sachs disease, Niemann–Pick disease, Sandhoff disease, generalized gangliosidosis, and sialidosis types 1 and 2.

Congenital stationary night blindness

Definition

Congenital stationary night blindness refers to a group of disorders characterized by infantile onset nyctalopia and non-progressive retinal dysfunction. The fundus appearance may be normal or abnormal.

Normal fundus

1. **AD congenital nyctalopia** (Nougaret type) – slightly impaired cone ERG and subnormal rod ERG function.
2. **AD stationary nyctalopia without myopia** (Riggs type) – normal cone ERG.
3. **AR or X-L congenital nyctalopia with myopia** (Schubert–Bornschein type) – negative ERG in the maximal response, where there is selective loss of the b-wave.

Abnormal fundus

1. **Oguchi disease** – AR condition in which the fundus has an unusual golden-yellow colour in the light-adapted state which becomes normal after prolonged dark adaptation (Mizuo phenomenon).
2. **Fundus albipunctatus** – AR condition characterized by a multitude of tiny yellow-white spots at the posterior pole, sparing the fovea, and extending to the periphery (*Fig. 18.43*). The retinal blood vessels, optic disc, peripheral fields and visual acuity remain normal.

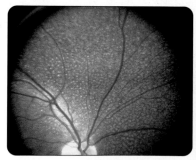

Fig. 18.43 Fundus albipunctatus

3. Kandoori flecked retina – large yellow flecks or patches of RPE atrophy between the macula and equator with macular sparing.

Congenital monochromatism

Complete rod monochromatism

1. Inheritance – AR.
2. Signs
- VA is 6/60.
- Macula is usually normal.
- Congenital nystagmus and photophobia.
3. ERG – photopic is abnormal; scotopic may be subnormal; flicker fusion <30 Hz.
4. CV – totally absent.

Incomplete rod monochromatism

1. Inheritance – AR or X-L.
2. Signs
- VA is 6/12–6/24.
- Macula is usually normal.
- Nystagmus and photophobia may be present.
3. ERG – abnormal photopic and normal scotopic.
4. CV – some colour vision may be present.

Cone monochromatism

1. Inheritance – uncertain.
2. Signs
- VA is 6/6–6/9.
- Normal macula.
- Nystagmus and photophobia are absent.
3. ERG – normal.
4. CV – totally absent.

Vitreoretinopathies

Congenital retinoschisis

1. Pathogenesis – basic defect is in the Müller cells, causing splitting of the retinal nerve fibre layer from the rest of the sensory retina.
2. Inheritance – X-L (gene locus on Xp22.2).
3. Presentation – 5–10 years with maculopathy.
4. Foveal schisis – 'bicycle-wheel' pattern of radial striae (*Fig. 18.44a*).

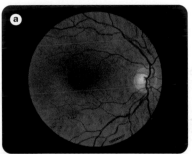

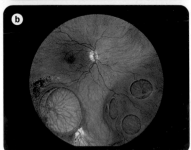

Fig. 18.44 Congenital retinoschisis. (a) Maculopathy; (b) periphery

5. Peripheral schisis – present in 50% of cases and often associated with inner layer defects (*Fig. 18.44b*).
6. Complications – haemorrhage and RD.
7. ERG – eyes with peripheral schisis show selective decrease in amplitude of the b-wave as compared with the a-wave on scotopic and photopic testing (*Fig. 18.45*).

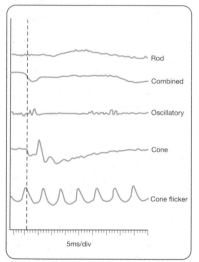

Rod
Combined
Oscillatory
Cone
Cone flicker

5ms/div

Fig. 18.45 ERG in congenital retinoschisis

8. OCT – useful in documenting progression of maculopathy (*Fig. 18.46*).

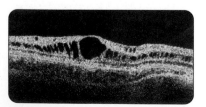

Fig. 18.46 OCT in macular schisis

9. Prognosis – poor.

Stickler syndrome

1. Inheritance – AD.
2. Signs
- Empty vitreous with circumferential equatorial membranes (*Fig. 18.47a*).
- Radial lattice-like degeneration (*Fig. 18.47b*).

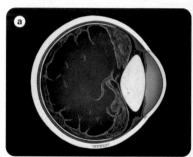

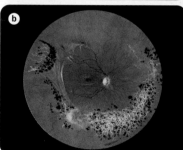

Fig. 18.47 Stickler syndrome.
(a) Vitreous; (b) retina

3. Complications – RD in 30% in the first decade of life.
4. Associations – early-onset myopia, cataract, ectopia lentis, and glaucoma.

Wagner syndrome

1. Inheritance – AD (gene locus on 5q13-14).

2. Signs
- Low myopia.
- Empty vitreous.
- Peripheral avascular membranes and progressive chorioretinal atrophy (*Fig. 18.48*).

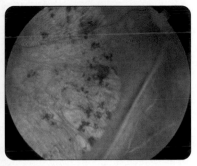

Fig. 18.48 Wagner syndrome

3. Complications – cataract and RD.

Familial exudative vitreoretinopathy (Criswick–Schepens syndrome)

1. Pathogenesis – failure of vascularization of the temporal peripheral retina.

2. Inheritance – AD, rarely X-LR.

3. Presentation – late childhood.

4. Signs
- Vitreous degeneration, and peripheral vascular tortuosity and telangiectasia.

- Fibrovascular proliferation and vitreoretinal traction resulting in ridge formation (*Fig. 18.49*).
- Vascular straightening and temporal dragging of the macula and disc (*Fig. 18.50*).

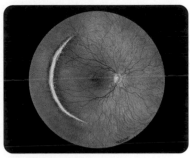

Fig. 18.49 Ridge in FEVR

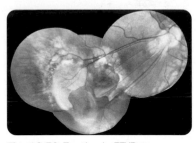

Fig. 18.50 Traction in FEVR

5. Complications – tractional RD and massive subretinal exudation.

6. FA – peripheral retinal non-perfusion (*Fig. 18.51*).

7. Prognosis – poor.

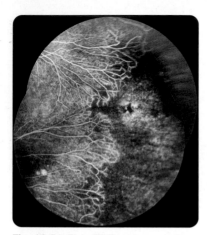

Fig. 18.51 FA in FEVR

Favre–Goldmann disease

1. **Inheritance** – AR.
2. **Presentation** – childhood with nyctalopia.
3. **Signs**
   - Vitreous liquefaction and congenital retinoschisis.
   - Peripheral RPE atrophy and pigmentation.
   - Vascular attenuation and optic atrophy.
4. **ERG** – markedly abnormal or extinguished; some exhibit enhanced S cone function.
5. **Prognosis** – poor.

Snowflake vitreoretinal degeneration

1. **Inheritance** – AD.
2. **Signs** in chronological order (*Fig. 18.52*):
   - *Stage 1* – extensive areas of 'white-without-pressure'.
   - *Stage 2* – snowflake-like spots in areas of 'white-with-pressure'.
   - *Stage 3* – vascular sheathing and pigmentation.
   - *Stage 4* – pigmentation, gross vascular attenuation, areas of chorioretinal atrophy.

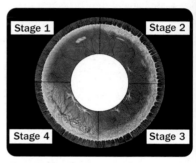

Fig. 18.52 Snowflake degeneration

3. **Associations** – myopia and vitreous degeneration.
4. **Complications** – rhegmatogenous RD and cataract.
5. **ERG** – low scotopic b-wave amplitude.
6. **Prognosis** – good.

Erosive vitreoretinopathy

1. **Inheritance** – AD (gene locus on 5q13-14).
2. **Presentation** – early childhood.
3. **Signs**
   - Vitreous liquefaction and multiple foci of vitreoretinal traction.
   - Thinning of the RPE and progressive choroidal atrophy.
   - Retinal vascular attenuation and occasionally bone spicule changes.
4. **Complications** – RD.
5. **Prognosis** – guarded.

Dominant neovascular inflammatory vitreoretinopathy

1. **Inheritance** – AD.
2. **Presentation** – 2nd–3rd decade with vitreous floaters.
3. **Signs**
   - Uveitis.
   - Pigmentary retinal degeneration.
   - Peripheral vascular closure and neovascularization.
4. **Complications** – vitreous haemorrhage, tractional RD and CMO.
5. **ERG** – selective loss of b wave amplitude.
6. **Prognosis** – guarded.

Dominant vitreoretinochoroidopathy

1. **Inheritance** – AD.
2. **Presentation** – in adult life if symptomatic, but frequently discovered by chance.
3. **Signs**
   - Encircling band of pigmentary disturbance between the ora serrata and equator with a sharply defined posterior border.
   - Within the band there is arteriolar attenuation, neovascularization, punctate white opacities and later chorioretinal atrophy.
4. **Complications** – CMO.
5. **ERG** – subnormal.
6. **Prognosis** – good.

Choroidal dystrophies

Choroideremia

1. **Inheritance** – X-LR (gene locus on Xq21).
2. **Female carriers** – mild patchy peripheral atrophy and mottling of the RPE (*Fig. 18.53*).

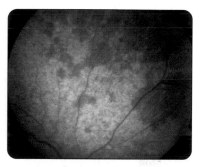

Fig. 18.53 Carrier of choroideremia

3. **Presentation** – 1st decade with nyctalopia.
4. **Signs** in chronological order:
   - Mid-peripheral diffuse atrophy of the choriocapillaris and RPE (*Fig. 18.54*).
   - Progressive atrophy of intermediate and large choroidal vessels (*Fig. 18.55*).
   - Fovea is spared until late.

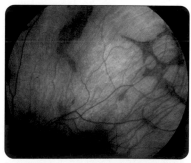

Fig. 18.54 Peripheral choroideremia

5. **ERG** – scotopic is non-recordable; photopic is severely subnormal.
6. **Prognosis** – poor.

• •

Introduction

Anatomy

Ora serrata

The ora serrata forms the junction between the retina and ciliary body and is characterized by the following (*Fig. 19.1*):

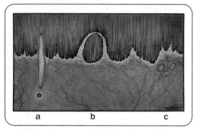

Fig. 19.1 Normal variants of the ora

1. **Dentate processes** – teeth-like extensions of retina onto the pars plana.
2. **Meridional fold** – small radial fold in line with a dentate process occasionally with a small retinal hole at its apex (*Fig. 19.1a*).
3. **Oral bays** – scalloped edges of the pars plana epithelium between dentate processes.
4. **Enclosed oral bay** – island of pars plana caused by joining of two adjacent dentate processes (*Fig. 19.1b*).
5. **Granular tissue** – multiple, white opacities within the vitreous base (*Fig. 19.1c*).

Peripheral retina

The peripheral retina extends from the equator to the ora serrata and may show the following innocuous changes (*Fig. 19.2*):

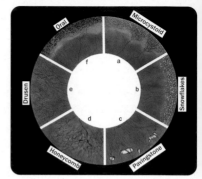

Fig. 19.2 Benign peripheral degenerations

1. **Microcystoid degeneration** – tiny vesicles with indistinct boundaries.
2. **Snowflakes** – diffuse scattering of minute glistening yellow-white dots.
3. **Pavingstone degeneration** – discrete yellow-white patches of focal chorioretinal atrophy.
4. **Honeycomb (reticular) degeneration** – fine network of perivascular pigmentation.
5. **Drusen** – clusters of small pale lesions with hyperpigmented borders.
6. **Oral pigmentary degeneration** – hyperpigmented band running adjacent to the ora serrata.

Definitions

1. **Retinal detachment (RD)** – separation of the sensory retina (SR) from the retinal pigment epithelium (RPE) by accumulation of subretinal fluid (SRF).
2. **Rhegmatogenous RD** – secondary to defect in the SR that permits fluid derived from synchytic (liquefied) vitreous to gain access to the subretinal space.

3. **Tractional RD** – SR is pulled away from the RPE in the absence of a retinal break.
4. **Exudative RD** (serous, secondary) – SRF is derived from fluid in the vessels of the SR or choroid.
5. **Vitreoretinal traction** – force exerted on the retina by structures originating in the vitreous and may be induced by eye movements (dynamic) or independent of eye movements (static).
6. **Posterior vitreous detachment (PVD)** – separation of the cortical vitreous from the internal limiting membrane (ILM) of the SR posterior to the vitreous base.

Retinal breaks

A retinal break is a full-thickness defect in the SR that can be classified according to the following characteristics:

1. **Pathogenesis**
   a. *Tear* – caused by dynamic vitreoretinal traction.
   b. *Hole* – caused by chronic atrophy of the SR.
2. **Morphology** (*Fig. 19.3*)
   a. *U-tear* (horseshoe, flap or arrowhead – *Fig. 19.3a*).
   b. *Incomplete U-tear* – linear or L-shaped (*Fig. 19.3b,c*).
   c. *Operculated tear* – flap is completely torn away (*Fig. 19.3d*).
   d. *Dialysis* – circumferential tear along the ora serrata (*Fig. 19.3e*).
   e. *Giant tear* – involves 90° or more of the circumference of the globe (*Fig. 19.4*).
3. **Location** – oral, post-oral, equatorial, post-equatorial, and macular.

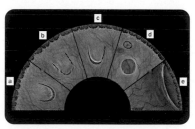

Fig. 19.3 Morphology of tears

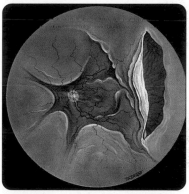

Fig. 19.4 Giant tear and total RD

Pathogenesis of rhegmatogenous RD

Vitreoretinal traction

Retinal breaks responsible for RD are caused by interplay between dynamic vitreoretinal traction and an underlying weakness in the peripheral retina (pre-disposing degeneration). The vision-threatening complications of acute PVD are dependent on the strength and extent of pre-existing vitreoretinal adhesions.

1. **No complications** – in most eyes because vitreoretinal attachments are weak (*Fig. 19.5a*).
2. **Retinal tear formation** – when attachments are strong (*Fig. 19.5b*).

Predisposing peripheral retinal degenerations

1. **Lattice degeneration**
   a. *Prevalence* – 8% of the population and 40% of eyes with RD.
   b. *Pathology* – atrophy of the SR with syneresis of overlying vitreous but strong vitreous attachments around the margins of the lesion (*Fig 19.6*).
   c. *Signs* – spindle-shaped areas of white lines (*Fig. 19.7a,c,d*).
   d. *Complications* – tears associated with acute PVD, and atrophic holes (*Fig. 19.7b,c,d*).
2. **Snailtrack degeneration**
   a. *Signs* – bands of 'snowflakes' with white frost-like appearance (*Fig. 19.8*).
   b. *Complications* – holes are common but tears are rare.

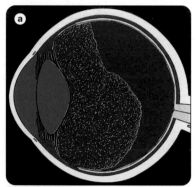

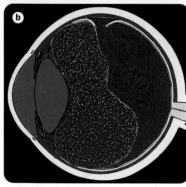

Fig. 19.5 Acute PVD

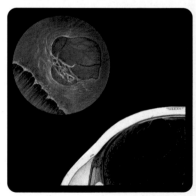

Fig. 19.6 Vitreous changes overlying lattice

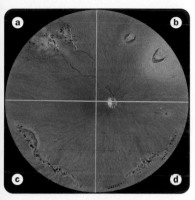

Fig. 19.7 Lattice degeneration

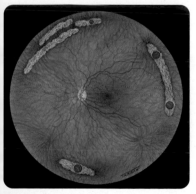

Fig. 19.8 Snailtrack degeneration

3. Degenerative retinoschisis

a. *Prevalence* – 5% of the population over the age of 20 years.

b. *Pathology*

- Splitting of the SR into an inner (vitreous) layer and outer (choroidal) layer.
- In typical retinoschisis the split is in the outer plexiform layer; in reticular retinoschisis it occurs at the level of the NFL.

c. *Signs*

- Exaggeration of microcystoid degeneration with a smooth elevation of the retina that may progress to involve the entire fundus periphery (*Fig. 19.9*).
- Surface of the inner layer may show 'snowflakes', vascular sheathing, 'white-without-pressure'; cavity may be bridged by rows of torn grey-white tissue (*Fig 19.10*).

d. Complications – RD if breaks in reticular schisis involve both layers.

4. Diffuse chorioretinal atrophy

a. *Signs* – choroidal depigmentation and thinning of the overlying retina in the equatorial area of highly myopic eyes.

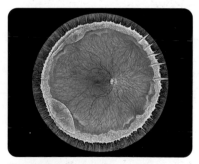

Fig. 19.9 Retinoschisis

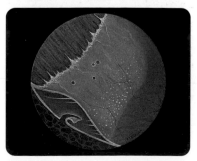

Fig. 19.10 Breaks within retinoschisis

b. *Complications* – holes (*Fig. 19.11*) may lead to RD.

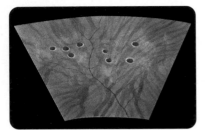

Fig. 19.11 Holes within diffuse atrophy

Pathogenesis of non-rhegmatogenous RD

1. Diabetic tractional RD

a. *Progressive* contraction of fibrovascular membranes over large areas of vitreoretinal adhesion.

b. *Static* vitreoretinal traction may be tangential, anteroposterior and bridging (trampoline – *Fig. 19.12*).

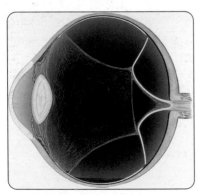

Fig. 19.12 Pathogenesis of diabetic tractional RD

2. Traumatic tractional RD

a. *Blunt trauma* – compression of the anteroposterior diameter of the globe and simultaneous expansion of the equatorial plane (*Fig. 19.13a*) that may result in dialyses associated with avulsion of the vitreous base (*Fig. 19.13b*) or equatorial tears.

b. *Penetrating trauma* – vitreous incarceration in the wound and blood in the vitreous (*Fig. 19.14a*) act as stimuli to fibroblastic proliferation and vitreoretinal traction (*Fig. 19.14b*).

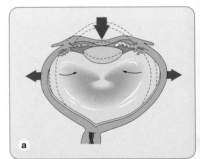

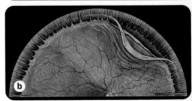

Fig. 19.13 Pathogenesis of RD due to blunt trauma

3. Exudative RD

- Occurs in a variety of vascular, inflammatory or neoplastic diseases involving the SR, RPE

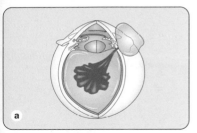

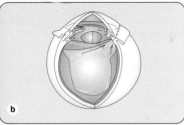

Fig. 19.14 Pathogenesis of RD due to penetration

and choroid in which fluid leaks outside the vessels and accumulates under the retina.
- Causes include choroidal tumours, posterior uveitis, posterior scleritis, bullous central serous retinopathy, iatrogenic, subretinal neovascularization, hypertensive choroidopathy, and uveal effusion syndrome.

Clinical features

Rhegmatogenous RD

1. Symptoms
- Photopsia and vitreous floaters caused by acute PVD with collapse.
- Peripheral visual field defect which may progress to involve central vision.

2. General signs
- Weiss ring (*Fig. 19.15*) and 'tobacco dust' in the anterior vitreous (*Fig 19.16*).
- RD has a convex configuration and a slightly opaque and corrugated appearance (*Fig. 19.17*).
- SRF extends up to the ora serrata.

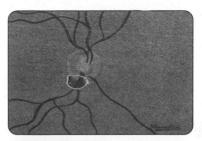

Fig. 19.15 Weiss ring

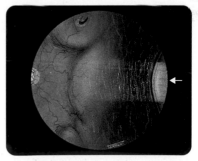

Fig. 19.16 Tobacco dust

3. Longstanding RD (*Fig. 19.18*) – thin retina with secondary cysts, and subretinal demarcation lines (high water marks).

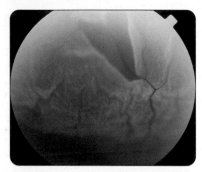

Fig. 19.17 Fresh rhegmatogenous RD

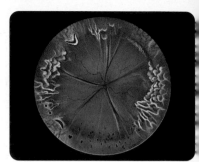

Fig. 19.19 PVR

2. Signs – RD has a concave configuration, reduced retinal mobility, shallow SRF that does not extend to the ora serrata.

Exudative RD

1. Symptoms – photopsia is absent and the visual field defect may develop suddenly and progress rapidly.

2. Signs – RD has a convex configuration and a smooth surface, SRF is deep and mobile ('shifting fluid'); the cause, such as a choroidal tumour, may be apparent (*Fig. 19.20*).

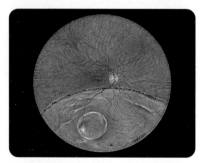

Fig. 19.18 Longstanding rhegmatogenous RD

4. Proliferative vitreoretinopathy (PVR) (*Fig. 19.19*) – stiff retina, decreased mobility of vitreous gel, rigid retinal folds, and tears with rolled edges.

Tractional RD

1. Symptoms – photopsia and floaters are absent and the visual field defect usually progresses slowly and may become stationary.

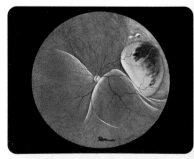

Fig. 19.20 Exudative RD

Prophylaxis of rhegmatogenous RD

Criteria to be considered in the selection of patients for prophylactic treatment can be divided into the following:

1. **Characteristics of the break** – type (hole or tear), size, presence of symptoms, location, and presence or absence of pigmentation (see below).
2. **Other adverse considerations** – myopia, family history of RD, and systemic diseases associated with increased risk of RD such as Marfan syndrome, Stickler syndrome, and Ehlers–Danlos syndrome.
3. **Predisposing degenerations** – lattice and snailtrack do not usually merit prophylaxis unless PVD has not yet occurred and the fellow has suffered a RD in the past.
4. **High risk breaks**
   - Subclinical RD associated with a large symptomatic U-tear and located in the upper temporal quadrant (*Fig. 19.21a*).
   - Large U-tear in the upper temporal quadrant associated with acute PVD (*Fig. 19.21b*).
5. **Moderate risk breaks** – operculated U-tear bridged by a patent blood vessel (*Fig. 19.21c*).
6. **Low risk breaks**
   - Operculated U-tear in the lower temporal quadrant detected by chance (*Fig. 19.21d*).
   - Pigment demarcation associated with an inferior U-tear and a dialysis detected by chance (*Fig. 19.20e*).
   - Degenerative retinoschisis with breaks in both layers (*Fig. 19.21f*).

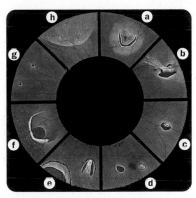

Fig. 19.21 Prophylactic treatment of retinal breaks

7. **Very low risk breaks**
   - Two small asymptomatic holes near the ora serrata (*Fig. 19.21g*).
   - Small inner layer holes in retinoschisis (*Fig. 19.21h*).
8. **Treatment modalities**
   - Laser photocoagulation (*Fig. 19.22*) using a slit lamp or indirect ophthalmoscopic delivery system.
   - Cryotherapy (*Fig. 19.23*).

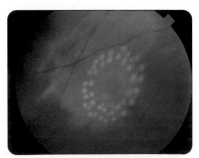

Fig. 19.22 Prophylactic laser to retinal break

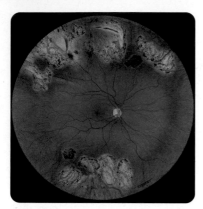

Fig. 19.23 Extensive prophylactic cryotherapy of multiple breaks

9. Causes of failure
- Failure to surround the entire lesion.
- Failure to apply contiguous treatment.
- Failure to use an explant or gas tamponade in subclinical RD.
- New break formation.

Surgery of rhegmatogenous RD

Pneumatic retinopexy

- Out-patient procedure in which an intravitreal expanding gas bubble is used to seal a retinal break without scleral buckling (*Fig. 19.24*).
- The procedure is usually reserved for treatment of uncomplicated RD with a small break or a cluster of breaks extending over an area of less than two clock hours situation in the upper two-thirds of the fundus.

Principles of scleral buckling

1. **Definition** – procedure in which material sutured onto the sclera (explant) creates an inward indentation (buckle).
2. **Purposes** – to close retinal breaks by apposing the RPE to the SR, and to reduce dynamic vitreoretinal traction at sites of local vitreoretinal adhesion
3. **Radial explants** – (*Fig. 19.25a*) for U-tears or posterior breaks.
4. **Segmental circumferential explants** – (*Figs 19.25b & 19.26*) for multiple breaks and dialyses.
5. **Encircling explants** – (*Fig. 19.27*) now seldom used unless accompanied by pars plana vitrectomy.

Drainage of subretinal fluid

1. **Indications** – deep SRF and longstanding RD with viscous SRF.
2. **Technique**
   a. *'Prang'* – perforation is made with the tip of a hypodermic needle in a single, swift but controlled fashion.
   b. *'Cut-down'* – radial sclerotomy is performed and the choroid perforated with low-heat cautery or a hypodermic needle (*Fig. 19.28*).
3. **Complications** – failure of drainage ('dry tap'), haemorrhage, retinal perforation, and retinal incarceration into the sclerotomy.

Causes of failure

1. **Missed breaks** – at the time of surgery.

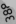

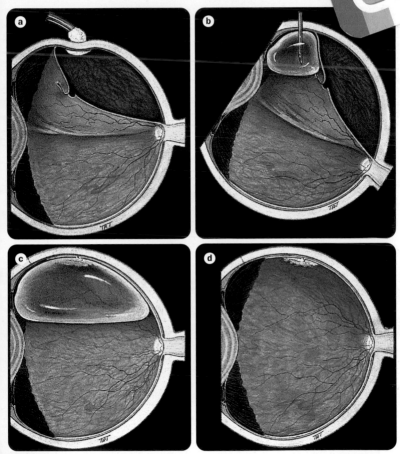

Fig. 19.24 Pneumatic retinopexy

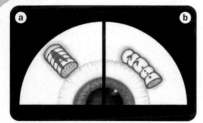

Fig. 19.25 Local explants

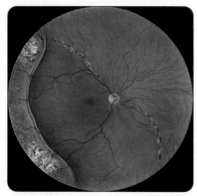

Fig. 19.26 Circumferential buckle

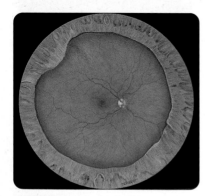

Fig. 19.27 Encircling buckle

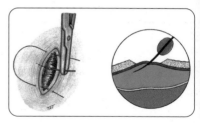

Fig. 19.28 Drainage of SRF

2. **Buckle failure** – explant of inadequate size, incorrect positioning, or inadequate height.
3. **PVR** – most common.
4. **Re-opening of a retinal break** – inadequate cryotherapy or buckling.
5. **Operative complications** – retinal incarceration and perforation.

Pars plana vitrectomy

Instrumentation

1. **Cutter** – inner guillotine blade which oscillates up to 1500 times/minute (*Fig. 19.29*).

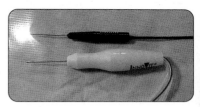

Fig. 19.29 Cutter and light pipe

2. **Intraocular illumination source** – 20-gauge light pipe (*Fig. 19.29*).
3. **Accessory instruments** – infusion cannula, scissors, forceps, flute needle, endodiathermy, and endolaser.

Tamponading agents

1. Expanding gases
- Sulphur hexafluoride (SF6) – doubles its volume and lasts 10–14 days.
- Perfluorethane (C2F6) – triples its volume and lasts 30–35 days.
- Perfluoropropane (C3F8) – quadruples its volume and lasts 55–65 days.

2. Heavy liquids (perfluorocarbons) – high specific gravity and thus remain in a dependent position.

3. Silicone oils – low specific gravity and buoyant; allow for more controlled intraoperative retinal manipulation and may also be used for prolonged postoperative tamponade.

Indications for vitrectomy

1. Rhegmatogenous RD
- Vitreous haemorrhage obscures breaks.
- Breaks cannot be closed by scleral buckling (e.g. giant tears, PVR).

2. Tractional RD
- Diabetic RD threatening or involving the macula.
- Diabetic combined tractional–rhegmatogenous RD requires urgent treatment.
- Traumatic RD.

Technique

1. Basic vitrectomy
- Infusion cannula is secured to the sclera.
- Cutter and light pipe are introduced (*Fig. 19.30*).
- Excision of central vitreous gel and posterior hyaloid face.

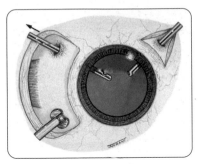

Fig. 19.30 Infusion cannula, light pipe and cutter in position

2. Closure of giant tears
- Fluid–air exchange to flatten the retina (*Fig. 19.31*).
- The flap is unrolled with heavy liquid and the tear is treated.
- Prolonged internal tamponade with gas or silicone oil.

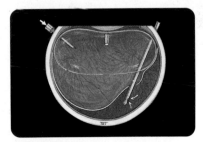

Fig. 19.31 Gas–fluid exchange

3. PVR
- Dissection and peeling of epiretinal membranes (*Fig. 19.32*) to restore retinal mobility and allow closure of breaks.
- Relieving retinotomy, if appropriate (*Fig. 19.33*).
- Prolonged internal tamponade.

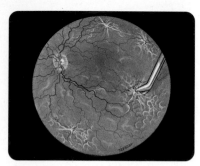

Fig. 19.32 Membrane dissection and removal

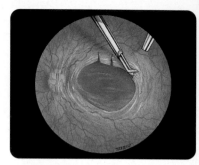

Fig. 19.34 Excision of fibrovascular membranes

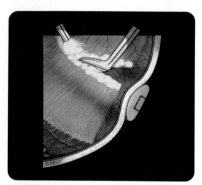

Fig. 19.33 Relieving retinotomy

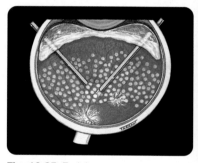

Fig. 19.35 Endolaser

Postoperative complications

4. Tractional RD

- Segmentation or delamination of fibrovascular membranes to release anteroposterior and/or circumferential vitreoretinal traction (*Fig. 19.34*).
- Endolaser photocoagulation, if appropriate (*Fig. 19.35*).

1. Elevation of IOP may be caused by the following:
- Overexpansion of intraocular gas.
- Silicone oil-associated glaucoma – may be caused by pupil block by silicone or trabecular block by emulsified oil in the anterior chamber (*Fig. 19.36*).

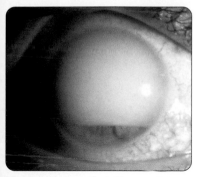

Fig. 19.36 Emulsified silicone oil

2. **Cataract** may be caused by:
   - Gas-induced opacities; usually transient.
   - Silicone-induced cataract; develops in almost all phakic eyes.
   - Delayed nuclear cataract; occurs in a large proportion of patients over 50 years of age within 1 year of surgery.
3. **Band keratopathy** due to prolonged contact between silicone oil and the corneal endothelium.

Introduction

Definitions

1. **Anatomical axis** – line passing from the posterior pole through the centre of the cornea.
2. **Visual axis** (line of vision) – passes from the fovea, through the nodal point of the eye to the point of fixation.
3. **Angle kappa** – angle subtended by the visual and anatomical axes (about 5° – *Fig. 20.1*).
4. **Orthophoria** – perfect alignment in the absence of any stimulus for fusion.
5. **Heterophoria** ('phoria') – tendency to deviation when fusion is blocked (latent squint) which may be inwards (esophoria) or outwards (exophoria).
6. **Heterotropia** ('tropia') – manifest deviation in which the visual axes do not intersect at the point of fixation.

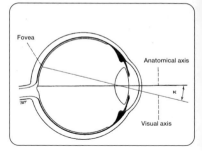

Fig. 20.1 Angle kappa

Ocular movements

1. **Monocular** – adduction, abduction, elevation, depression, intorsion, and extorsion.
2. **Binocular**
   a. *Versions* – binocular, simultaneous, conjugate movements (in the same direction – *Fig. 20.2,* top).

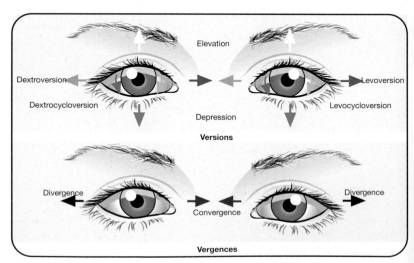

Fig. 20.2 Binocular movements

b. *Vergences* – binocular, simultaneous, disjunctive movements (in opposite directions – *Fig. 20.2*, bottom).

- Convergence – may be voluntary or reflex.
- Divergence – outward movement from a convergent position.

Positions of gaze

1. **Six cardinal** – one muscle in each eye has moved the globe into that position as follows:
   - Dextroversion (right lateral rectus and left medial rectus).
   - Laevoversion (left lateral rectus and right medial rectus).
   - Dextroelevation (right superior rectus and left inferior oblique).
   - Laevoelevation (left superior rectus and right inferior oblique).

- Dextrodepression (right inferior rectus and left superior oblique).
- Laevodepression (left inferior rectus and right superior oblique).

2. **Nine diagnostic** – in which deviations are measured. They consist of the six cardinal positions, the primary position, elevation and depression (*Fig. 20.3*).

Laws of ocular motility

1. **Agonist–antagonist pairs** – muscles of the same eye that move the eye in opposite directions.
2. **Synergists** – muscles of the same eye that move the eye in the same direction.
3. **Yoke muscles** (contralateral synergists) – pairs of muscles, one in each eye producing conjugate ocular movements.

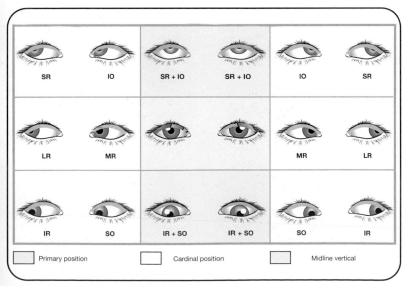

Fig. 20.3 Diagnostic positions of gaze

4. **Sherrington law of reciprocal innervation (inhibition)** – increased innervation to an extraocular muscle is accompanied by a reciprocal decrease in innervation to its antagonist.

5. **Hering law of equal innervation** – during any conjugate eye movement, equal and simultaneous innervation flows to the yoke muscles.

6. **Muscle sequelae** – effects of the interactions described by these laws. The full pattern of changes takes time to develop and can be summarized as follows:
   - Primary underaction (e.g. left superior oblique).
   - Secondary contracture of the unopposed direct antagonist (left inferior oblique).
   - Secondary contracture of the contralateral synergist or yoke muscle (right inferior rectus – Hering law).
   - Secondary inhibitional palsy (right superior rectus – Sherrington law)

Sensory adaptations to strabismus

1. **Suppression**
   - Active inhibition in the visual cortex of an image from one eye when both are open.
   - Stimuli include diplopia, confusion, and a blurred image from one eye resulting from astigmatism/anisometropia.
2. **Abnormal retinal correspondence** (ARC) – non-corresponding retinal elements acquire a common subjective visual direction (i.e. fusion occurs in the presence of a small angle manifest squint).
3. **Microtropia** – small angle squint (<10°) in which stereopsis is present

but reduced and there is a relative amblyopia of the more ametropic eye.

4. **Consequences of strabismus**
   - Fovea of the squinting eye is suppressed to avoid confusion.
   - Diplopia will occur since non-corresponding retinal elements receive the same image (*Fig. 20.4*).

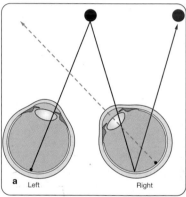

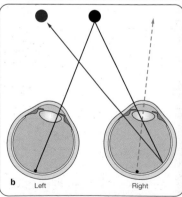

Fig. 20.4 Diplopia. (a) Homonymous (uncrossed) in right esotropia; (b) heteronymous (crossed) in right exotropia

- To avoid diplopia the patient will develop either peripheral suppression of the squinting eye or ARC.
- Constant unilateral suppression will subsequently lead to strabismic amblyopia.

Motor adaptation to strabismus

Motor adaptation involves the adoption of an abnormal head posture (AHP) and occurs primarily in children with congenitally abnormal eye movements who use the AHP to maintain BSV. AHP is analysed in terms of the following three components (*Fig. 20.5*):
- Face turn to right or left.
- Head tilt to right or left.
- Chin elevation or depression.

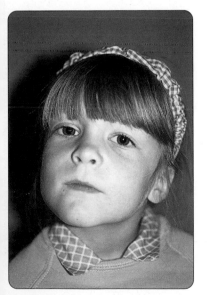

Fig. 20.5 Abnormal head posture

Amblyopia

1. **Definition** – unilateral, or (rarely) bilateral, decrease of best-corrected visual acuity caused by form vision deprivation and/or abnormal binocular interaction, for which there is no pathology of the eye or visual pathway.
2. **Classification** – strabismic, anisometropic, stimulus deprivation, bilateral ametropic, and meridional.
3. **Treatment**
   - Sensitive period during which acuity of an amblyopic eye can be improved is usually up to 7–8 years in strabismic amblyopia and may be longer (into teens) for anisometropic amblyopia where good binocular function is present.
   - The two methods of treatment are occlusion and penalization in which the normal eye is blurred with atropine.

Heterophoria

1. **Presentation** – bilateral headache, eye strain, asthenopia and transient diplopia, particularly at times of stress or poor health, when the fusional amplitudes are insufficient to maintain alignment.
2. **Treatment**
   - Orthoptic treatment for convergence weakness exophoria.
   - Correction of significant refractive errors.
   - Temporary stick-on Fresnel prisms or prisms incorporated into spectacles.
   - Surgery may be required for large deviations.

Esotropia

Early onset esotropia

1. Presentation – first 6 months of life.
2. Signs
- No significant refractive error.
- Large (>30°) and stable angle.
- Alternating fixation in the primary position, and cross fixation in side gaze (*Fig. 20.6*).
- Inferior oblique overaction (*Fig. 20.7*).
- Dissociated vertical deviation (DVD – *Fig. 20.8*) is common by the age of 3 years.

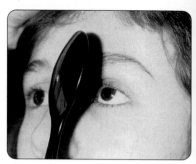

Fig. 20.8 DVD

3. Treatment – eyes should be surgically aligned by the age of 12 months, and at the very latest by the age of 2 years.

Accommodative esotropia

Refractive accommodative

AC/A ratio is normal and esotropia is a physiological response to excessive hypermetropia.

1. Fully accommodative – angle is eliminated by correction of hypermetropia (*Fig. 20.9*).

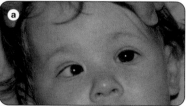

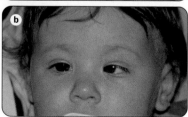

Fig. 20.6 Cross fixation. (a) Left gaze; (b) right gaze

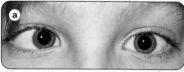

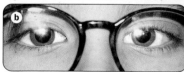

Fig. 20.9 Fully accommodative esotropia

2. Constant accommodative – angle is reduced but not eliminated by correction of hypermetropia (*Fig. 20.10*).

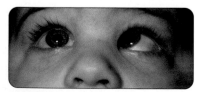

Fig. 20.7 Left inferior oblique overaction

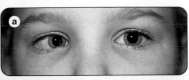

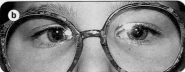

Fig. 20.10 Constant accommodative esotropia

Non-refractive accommodative

AC/A ratio is high so that a unit increase of accommodation is accompanied by a disproportionately large increase of convergence.

1. **Convergence excess** – high AC/A ratio due to increased accommodative convergence.
   - Straight eyes with BSV for distance (Fig. 20.11a).

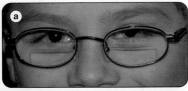

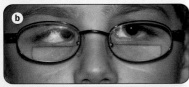

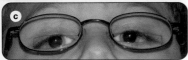

Fig. 20.11 Convergence excess esotropia

- Esotropia for near (Fig. 20.11b).
- Straight through bifocals (Fig. 20.11c).

2. **Hypoaccommodative convergence excess** – high AC/A ratio is due to weak accommodation.
   - Remote near point of accommodation.
   - Straight eyes with BSV for distance.
   - Esotropia for near, usually with suppression.

Treatment

1. **Correction of refractive error**
   - Under the age of 6 years – full cycloplegic refraction revealed on retinoscopy should be prescribed.
   - After the age of 8 years – refraction without cycloplegia and the maximal amount of 'plus' that can be tolerated (manifest hypermetropia) prescribed.
2. **Surgery** – only if spectacles do not fully correct the deviation and after every attempt has been made to treat amblyopia.

Microtropia

Microtropia may be primary or follow surgery for a large deviation.
1. **Signs**
   - Very small angle (8Δ or less).
   - Central suppression scotoma of the deviating eye.
   - ARC with reduced stereopsis and variable peripheral fusional amplitudes.
   - Anisometropia.
2. **Treatment** – correction of refractive error and occlusion for amblyopia as indicated.

Other esotropias

1. Near
- Absence of refractive error, BSV for distance, and esotropia for near but normal or low AC/A ratio.
- Treatment – bilateral medial rectus recessions.

2. Distance
- Intermittent or constant esotropia for distance, and minimal or no deviation for near.
- Treatment – prisms or surgery.

3. Acute (late onset)
- Presents at 5–6 years of age with sudden onset of diplopia and esotropia.
- Treatment – prisms, Botulinum toxin injection, or surgery.

4. Secondary (sensory) – unilateral reduction in visual acuity which interferes with or abolishes fusion, such as cataract, optic atrophy or hypoplasia, macular scarring or retinoblastoma.

5. Consecutive – follows surgical overcorrection of exotropia.

6. Cyclic – alternating manifest esotropia with suppression and BSV, each lasting 24 hours.

Exotropia

Constant (early onset) exotropia

1. Presentation – often at birth.

2. Signs
- Normal refraction.
- Large and constant angle.
- DVD may be present.

3. Neurological anomalies – common.

4. Treatment – lateral rectus recession and medial rectus resection.

Intermittent exotropia

1. Presentation – around 2 years with exophoria breaking down to exotropia.

2. Signs – eyes are straight with BSV at times (Fig. 20.12a) and divergent with suppression at other times (Fig. 20.12b).

3. Classification

a. *Distance* – angle is greater for distance.

b. *Non-specific* – angle is the same for distance and near.

c. *Near* – angle is greater for near.

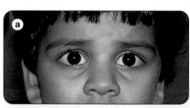
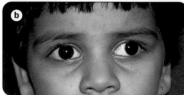

Fig. 20.12 Intermittent exotropia

4. Treatment options – correction of myopia, part-time occlusion, and surgery.

Sensory exotropia

Sensory (secondary) exotropia is the result of monocular or binocular visual impairment by acquired lesions, such as cataract (Fig. 20.13) or other opacities of the media.

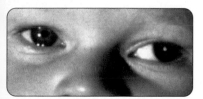

Fig. 20.13 Left sensory exotropia due to mature cataract

Consecutive exotropia

Consecutive exotropia develop spontaneously in an amblyopic cyc or more frequently following surgical correction of an esodeviation. Most cases present in adult life with concerns about cosmesis (*Fig. 20.14*) and social function, and can be greatly helped by surgery.

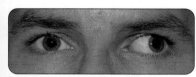

Fig. 20.14 Large left consecutive exotropia

Special syndromes

Duane retraction syndrome

1. Signs of left Duane
- BSV in the primary position (*Fig. 20.15a*).
- Limited left abduction (*Fig. 20.15b*).
- Limited left adduction accompanied by retraction of the globe and narrowing of the palpebral fissure (*Fig. 20.15c*).
- Upshoots or downshoots of the affected eye on adduction.
- Convergence deficiency.

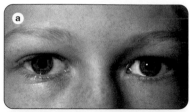

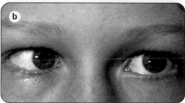

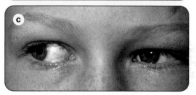

Fig. 20.15 Left Duane syndrome

2. Classification (Huber)
  a. *Type I*
- Primary position – straight or slight esotropia.
- Abduction – limited or absent.
- Adduction – normal or mildly limited.

  b. *Type II*
- Primary position – straight or slight exotropia.
- Adduction – limited.
- Abduction – normal or mildly limited.

  c. *Type III*
- Primary position – straight or slight esotropia.
- Adduction and abduction – both limited.

3. Treatment – not required if BSV is maintained; surgery if there is loss of binocular function.

Brown syndrome

1. Classification
  a. *Congenital*
- Idiopathic.
- Congenital click syndrome – impaired movement of the superior oblique tendon through the trochlea.

  b. *Acquired*
- Trauma to the trochlea or superior oblique tendon.
- Tendonitis associated with rheumatoid arthritis, pansinusitis, and scleritis.

2. Major signs of right Brown
- BSV in the primary position (*Fig. 20.16a*).
- Limited elevation in adduction (*Fig. 20.16b*).
- Limited elevation on up-gaze.
- Normal left elevation in abduction (*Fig. 20.16c*).
- Absence of left superior oblique overaction.

3. Variable signs
- Down shoot in adduction.
- Hypotropia in primary position.
- AHP with chin elevation and ipsilateral head tilt.

4. Treatment
  a. *Congenital* – not required as long as BSV is maintained with an acceptable AHP.
  b. *Acquired* – may benefit from steroids, either orally or by injection near the trochlea.

Monocular elevator deficit

1. Aetiology – tight or contracted inferior rectus, or hypoplastic or ineffective superior rectus.

2. Signs
- Profound inability to elevate one eye (*Fig. 20.17*).
- Straight in the primary position in about one-third of cases.
- Chin elevation to obtain fusion in down-gaze may be present.

3. Treatment – base-up prism over the involved eye or surgery.

Möbius syndrome

1. Ocular features
- Horizontal gaze palsy in 50% of cases.
- Bilateral 6th nerve palsy.

2. Systemic features
- Bilateral facial paresis.
- Paresis of the 9th and 12th cranial nerves; the latter results in atrophy of the tongue.
- Mild mental handicap.
- Limb anomalies.

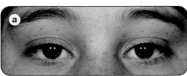

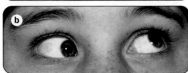

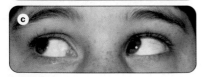

Fig. 20.16 Right Brown syndrome

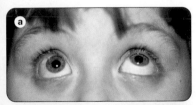

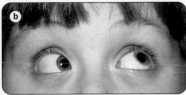

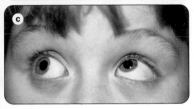

Fig. 20.17 Right monocular elevation deficit

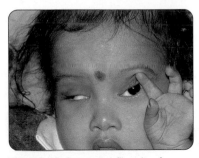

Fig. 20.18 Congenital fibrosis of extraocular muscles

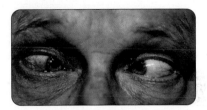

Fig. 20.19 Strabismus fixus

Congenital fibrosis of extraocular muscles

Congenital fibrosis of extraocular muscles syndrome is a rare non-progressive usually AD disorder characterized by bilateral ptosis and restrictive external ophthalmoplegia (*Fig. 20.18*).

Strabismus fixus

Strabismus fixus is a very rare condition, in which both eyes are fixed by fibrous tightening of the medial recti (convergent strabismus fixus – *Fig. 20.19*), or the lateral recti (divergent strabismus fixus).

Alphabet patterns

'V 'or 'A' patterns may occur when the relative contributions of the superior rectus and inferior oblique to elevation, or of the inferior rectus and superior oblique to depression are abnormal, resulting in abnormal balance of their horizontal vectors in up- and down-gaze.

1. **'V' pattern** – difference between up- and down-gaze is $\geq 15\ \Delta$, allowing for a small physiological variation between up- and down-gaze (*Figs 20.20 & 20.21*).
2. **'A' pattern** – difference between up- and down-gaze is $\geq 10\ \Delta$ (*Figs 20.22 & 20.23*).

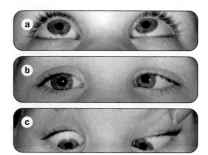

Fig. 20.20 V pattern esotropia

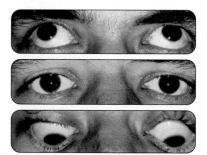

Fig. 20.21 V pattern exotropia

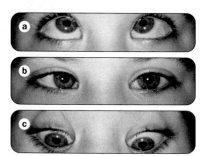

Fig. 20.22 A pattern esotropia

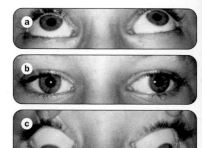

Fig. 20.23 A pattern exotropia

Surgery

The most common aims of surgery on the extraocular muscles are to correct misalignment to improve appearance and, if possible, restore BSV. Surgery can also be used to reduce an AHP and to expand or centralize a field of BSV.

Weakening procedures

1. **Recession** – slackens a muscle by moving it away from its insertion (*Fig. 20.24*).

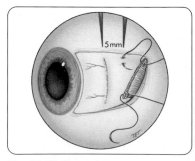

Fig. 20.24 Recession

2. **Disinsertion** – muscle is detached from its insertion without reattachment.
3. **Posterior fixation suture (Faden)** – muscle belly is sutured to the sclera posteriorly so as to decrease the pull of the muscle in its field of action without affecting the eye in the primary position.

Strengthening procedures

1. **Resection** – shortens a muscle to enhance its effective pull (*Fig. 20.25*).

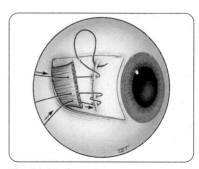

Fig. 20.25 Resection

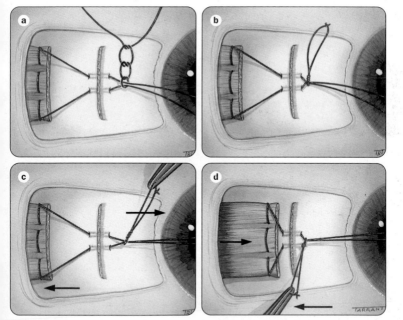

Fig. 20.26 Adjustable sutures. (a, b) Initial steps; (c, d) postoperative adjustment

2. Tucking – enhances the action of the superior oblique muscle in congenital 4th nerve palsy.

3. Advancement – nearer to the limbus can be used to enhance the action of a previously recessed rectus muscle.

Adjustable sutures

Results of strabismus surgery can be improved by the use of adjustable suture techniques on the rectus muscles (*Fig. 20.26*). These are particularly indicated when a precise outcome is essential and when the results with more conventional procedures are likely to be unpredictable.

Botulinum toxin chemodenervation

Temporary paralysis of an extraocular muscle can be created by an injection of Botulinum toxin under topical anaesthesia and EMG control (*Fig. 20.27*).

The effect takes several days to develop, is usually maximal at one to two weeks following injection and has generally worn off by 3 months.

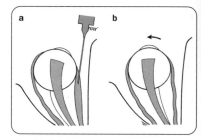

Fig. 20.27 Botulinum chemodenervation

Optic nerve disease

Signs of optic nerve dysfunction

1. **Reduced visual acuity.**
2. **Afferent pupillary defect.**
3. **Dyschromatopsia.**
4. **Diminished light brightness sensitivity.**
5. **Diminished contrast sensitivity.**
6. **Visual field defects.**

Primary optic atrophy

1. **Pathogenesis** – lesions affecting the visual pathways from the retrolaminar portion of the optic nerve to the lateral geniculate body, without antecedent swelling.
2. **Signs** (*Fig. 21.1*)
   - Pale, flat disc with clearly delineated margins, reduction in number of small vessels on the disc surface (Kestenbaum sign) and attenuation of peripapillary vessels.
   - Atrophy may be diffuse or sectoral depending on the cause and level of lesion.

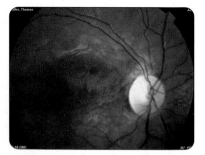

Fig. 21.1 Primary optic atrophy

3. **Causes**
   - Following retrobulbar neuritis.
   - Compression by tumours and aneurysms.
   - Hereditary optic neuropathies.
   - Toxic and nutritional optic neuropathies.

Secondary optic atrophy

Secondary optic atrophy is preceded by swelling of the optic nerve head.
1. **Signs** (*Fig. 21.2*)
   - White or dirty grey, slightly raised disc with poorly delineated margins.
   - Reduction in number of small vessels on the disc surface.

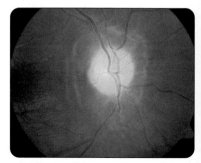

Fig. 21.2 Secondary optic atrophy

2. **Causes** – papilloedema, anterior ischaemic optic neuropathy, and papillitis.

Demyelinating optic neuritis

1. **Presentation** – 3rd–5th decade with subacute monocular visual impairment; discomfort around the eye frequently exacerbated by ocular movements.

2. Signs
- Disc is normal in the majority of cases (retrobulbar neuritis); the remainder show papillitis.
- Temporal disc pallor (*Fig. 21.3*) may indicate previous attacks.

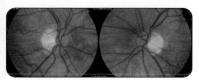

Fig. 21.3 Bilateral temporal pallor

3. Course – vision worsens over several days to 2 weeks and then begins to recover within 2–4 weeks.
4. Prognosis – visual acuity of 6/9 or better in 75%.
5. Treatment – speeds up recovery but does not influence the visual outcome. Where appropriate the treatment regimen is:
a. *Intravenous methylprednisolone sodium succinate* (1 g daily) for 3 days followed by oral prednisolone (1 mg/kg daily) for 11 days and then tapered for 3 days.
b. *Intramuscular interferon beta-1a* – reduces the risk of clinical MS over the following 3 years in patients at high risk of MS based on the presence of subclinical brain lesions on MR.

Parainfectious optic neuritis

1. Pathogenesis – viral infections such as measles, mumps, chickenpox, rubella, whooping cough, and glandular fever; may also follow immunization.

2. Presentation – in childhood with acute severe visual loss, which may be bilateral.
3. Signs – bilateral papillitis characterized by disc hyperaemia and oedema which may be associated with peripapillary flame-shaped haemorrhages (*Fig. 21.4*).

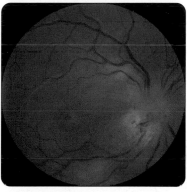

Fig. 21.4 Papillitis

4. Treatment – not required in most cases because the prognosis for spontaneous visual recovery is very good.

Infectious optic neuritis

1. Sinus-related – recurrent attacks associated with severe headache and spheno-ethmoidal sinusitis.
2. Cat-scratch fever – typically causes neuroretinitis.
3. Syphilis – acute papillitis or neuroretinitis during the primary or secondary stages.
4. Lyme disease – neuroretinitis and occasionally acute retrobulbar neuritis.

5. Cryptococcal meningitis in AIDS – acute optic neuritis.

6. Varicella zoster virus – papillitis by spread from contiguous retinitis.

Non-infectious optic neuritis

1. Sarcoidosis – optic neuritis affects 1–5% of patients with neurosarcoid and may be the presenting feature.

2. Autoimmune
- Retrobulbar neuritis or anterior ischaemic optic neuropathy.
- Some patients may have slowly progressive visual loss suggestive of optic nerve compression.

Neuroretinitis

1. Signs in chronological order:
- Papillitis.
- Macular star formation as the papillitis is gradually resolving (*Fig. 21.5*).
- Resolution of the macular star with improvement of vision within 6–12 months.

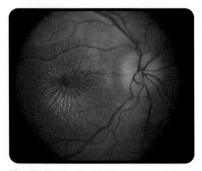

Fig. 21.5 Neuroretinitis

3. Systemic associations
- Idiopathic (Leber stellate neuroretinitis) – 25% of cases.
- Cat scratch fever – 60% of cases.
- Other causes – syphilis and Lyme disease.

4. Treatment – varies according to the underlying cause.

Non-arteritic anterior ischaemic optic neuropathy

1. Pathogenesis – infarction of the optic nerve head caused by occlusion of the short posterior ciliary arteries.

2. Predispositions – small or absent physiological cup, hypertension, diabetes mellitus, hypercholesterolaemia, collagen vascular disease, antiphospholipid antibody syndrome, hyperhomocysteinaemia, sudden hypotensive events, cataract surgery, sleep apnoea syndrome, and sildenafil citrate (Viagra).

3. Presentation – 6th–7th decade with sudden, painless, monocular visual loss not associated with premonitory visual obscurations.

4. Signs
- Hyperaemic disc swelling often with a few peripapillary splinter-shaped haemorrhages (*Fig. 21.6*).
- Swelling gradually resolves and pallor ensues after 3–6 weeks.
- Fellow eye involvement in 10% of patients after 2 years and 15% after 5 years.

5. Treatment – not available, although underlying systemic predispositions should be addressed.

6. Prognosis – guarded.

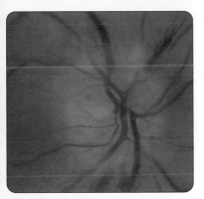

Fig. 21.6 Non-arteritic AION

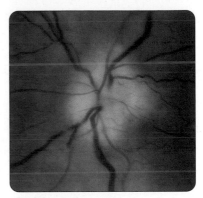

Fig. 21.7 Arteritic AION

Arteritic anterior ischaemic optic neuropathy

1. **Pathogenesis** – occlusion of the posterior ciliary arteries due to giant cell arteritis (GCA).
2. **Presentation** – 8th–9th decade with sudden, profound unilateral visual loss which may be preceded by transient visual obscurations and flashing lights; bilateral simultaneous involvement is rare.
3. **Signs**
   - Strikingly pale ('chalky white') oedematous disc (*Fig. 21.7*).
   - Occasionally combined with cilioretinal artery occlusion (see *Fig. 16.31*).
   - Swelling gradually resolves and severe optic atrophy ensues after 1–2 months.
4. **ESR** and **CRP** are usually raised.
5. **Treatment** is aimed at preventing blindness of the fellow eye.
   a. *Intravenous methylprednisolone sodium succinate* 1 g/day for 3 days then oral prednisolone 80 mg daily.

- After 3 days the oral dose is reduced to 60 mg and then 50 mg for 1 week each.
- Daily dose is then reduced by 5 mg weekly; headache, ESR and CRP permitting, until a maintenance dose of 10 mg is reached.
   b. *Oral prednisolone* (80–120 mg daily) alone if intravenous therapy is inappropriate.
6. **Prognosis** – very poor.

Posterior ischaemic optic neuropathy

1. **Pathogenesis** – ischaemia to the retrolaminar portion of the optic nerve which is supplied by the surrounding pial capillary plexus.
2. **Diagnosis** – after other causes of retrobulbar optic neuropathy, such as compression or inflammation, have been excluded.
3. **Classification**
   a. *Operative* – follows a variety of surgical procedures, most notably involving the spine.
   b. *Arteritic* – GCA.
   c. *Non-arteritic* – same systemic risk factors as AION.

Diabetic papillopathy

1. **Definition** – transient visual dysfunction associated with optic disc swelling which may occur in both type 1 and type 2 diabetics.
2. **Signs**
   - VA is usually 6/12 or better.
   - Unilateral or bilateral, mild disc swelling and hyperaemia, that may be associated with surface telangiectasia (*Fig. 21.8*).

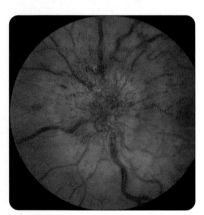

Fig. 21.8 Diabetic papillopathy

3. **Course** – improvement occurs after several months.
4. **Treatment** – posterior sub-Tenon steroid injections.

Leber hereditary optic neuropathy

1. **Pathogenesis** – maternally inherited mitochondrial DNA mutations, most notably 11778, that affect males.
2. **Presentation** – 2nd–4th decade with:

   - Unilateral, acute or subacute, severe, painless loss of central vision.
   - Fellow eye becomes similarly affected within weeks or months.
3. **Signs**
   - Disc hyperaemia with dilated surface capillaries and swelling of the peripapillary nerve fibre layer (*Fig. 21.9a*).
   - Resolution is followed by severe optic atrophy (*Fig. 21.9b*).

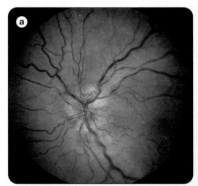

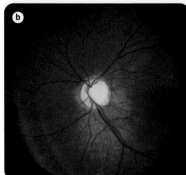

Fig. 21.9 Leber optic neuropathy.
(a) Acute stage; (b) severe optic atrophy

4. Treatment – not possible.
5. Prognosis – poor.

Hereditary optic atrophy

The hereditary optic atrophies (neuropathies) are a very rare group of disorders that are primarily characterized by bilateral optic atrophy.

Kjer syndrome

1. Inheritance – AD.
2. Presentation – 1st–2nd decade with insidious visual loss.
3. Optic atrophy – subtle temporal or diffuse.
4. Prognosis – variable.
5. Systemic abnormalities – few cases develop sensorineural hearing loss.

Behr syndrome

1. Inheritance – AR.
2. Presentation – 1st decade with progressive visual loss which stabilizes after a variable period.
3. Optic atrophy – diffuse.
4. Prognosis – fair to poor.
5. Systemic abnormalities – spastic gait, ataxia, and mental handicap.

Wolfram syndrome

Also referred to as DIDMOAD = Diabetes Insipidus, Diabetes Mellitus, Optic Atrophy and Deafness.
1. Inheritance – AR.
2. Presentation – 1st–2nd decade.
3. Optic atrophy – diffuse and severe.
4. Prognosis – very poor.
5. Systemic abnormalities (apart from DIDMOAD) – anosmia, ataxia, seizures, mental handicap, short stature, endocrine abnormalities, and elevated CSF protein.

Nutritional optic neuropathy

1. Pathogenesis – dietary deficiency of proteins and B-complex vitamins, often associated with alcoholism and smoking cigars or pipes.
2. Presentation – insidious onset of progressive, bilateral, symmetrical visual impairment associated with dyschromatopsia.
3. Signs – usually normal optic discs at presentation.
4. Visual field defects – bilateral centrocaecal scotomas (*Fig. 21.10*).

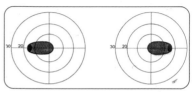

Fig. 21.10 Centrocaecal scotomas

5. Treatment – weekly injections of 1000 units of hydroxocobalamin for 10 weeks.
6. Prognosis – good if treated early.

Papilloedema

1. Definition – swelling of the optic nerve head, secondary to raised intracranial pressure; nearly always bilateral although may be asymmetrical.
2. Early papilloedema (*Fig. 21.11*)
   • Disc hyperaemia, mild elevation, and slightly indistinct margins.
   • Loss of previous spontaneous venous pulsation.
3. Established (acute) papilloedema (*Fig. 21.12*)
   • Severe disc hyperaemia with indistinct margins and obscuration of small surface vessels.

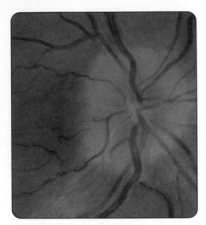

Fig. 21.11 Early papilloedema

- Venous engorgement, peripapillary flame-shaped haemorrhages, and frequently cotton-wool spots.
- Hard exudates forming an incomplete macular star ('macular fan').

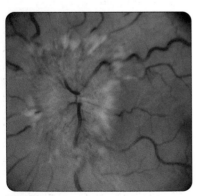

Fig. 21.12 Acute papilloedema

4. Chronic papilloedema (*Fig. 21.13*)
- Severe disc elevation with a 'champagne cork' appearance.
- Cotton-wool spots and haemorrhages are absent.

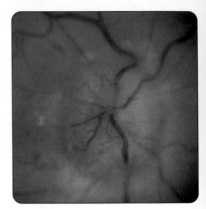

Fig. 21.13 Chronic papilloedema

- Opto-ciliary shunts and drusen-like crystalline deposits (corpora amylacea) may be present on the disc surface.

5. Atrophic papilloedema (secondary optic atrophy)
- VA is severely impaired.
- Greyish disc elevation with indistinct margins and few crossing blood vessels (*Fig. 21.14*).

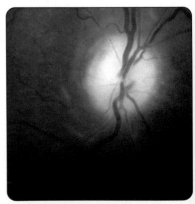

Fig. 21.14 Atrophic papilloedema

Pupillary reactions

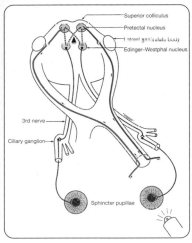

Fig. 21.15 Anatomic pathway of the light reflex

Afferent pupillary defects

1. **Absolute afferent pupillary defect** (amaurotic pupil) – caused by a complete optic nerve lesion; characterized by:
   - Eye is completely blind (i.e. no PL).
   - Both pupils are equal in size.
   - When the affected eye is stimulated by light neither pupil reacts (*Fig. 21.16a*).
   - When the normal eye is stimulated both pupils react normally (*Fig. 21.16b*).
   - Near reflex is normal in both eyes.
2. **Relative pupillary defect** (Marcus Gunn pupil) – caused by an incomplete optic nerve lesion or severe retinal disease.

- Signs are those of an amaurotic pupil but more subtle.
- Pupils respond weakly to stimulation of the diseased eye and briskly to that of the normal eye as demonstrated by the 'swinging flashlight' test.

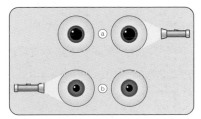

Fig. 21.16 Left afferent defect

Light-near dissociation

The light reflex is absent or sluggish but the near response is normal. The causes are listed in *Table 21.1*.

Table 21.1 **Causes of light-near dissociation**
1. *Unilateral*
· Afferent conduction defect
· Adie pupil
· Herpes zoster ophthalmicus
· Aberrant regeneration of the 3rd nerve
2. *Bilateral*
· Neurosyphilis
· Type 1 diabetes
· Myotonic dystrophy
· Parinaud dorsal midbrain syndrome
· Familial amyloidosis
· Encephalitis
· Chronic alcoholism

Adie pupil

1. **Pathogenesis** – denervation of the postganglionic supply to the sphincter pupillae and the ciliary muscle which may follow a viral illness.
2. **Signs of right Adie**
   - Large and regular pupil (*Fig. 21.17a*).

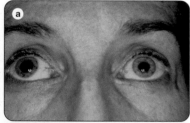

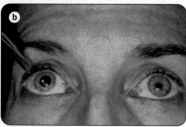

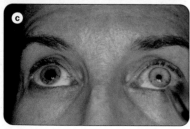

Fig. 21.17 Right Holmes–Adie pupil

- Direct light reflex – absent or sluggish (*Fig. 21.17b*) and associated with vermiform movements of the pupillary border.
- Consensual light reflex – absent or sluggish (*Fig. 21.17c*).
- Near reflex – slow constriction and re-dilatation.
- Accommodation – may manifest similar tonicity.
- In longstanding cases the pupil may become small ('little old Adie').
3. **Associations** – diminished deep tendon reflexes (Holmes–Adie syndrome) and autonomic nerve dysfunction.
4. **Pharmacological testing** – if 2.5% methacholine or 0.125% pilocarpine is instilled into both eyes, the normal pupil will not constrict but the abnormal one will because of denervation hypersensitivity.

Oculosympathetic palsy (Horner syndrome)

1. **Anatomical pathway** (*Fig. 21.18*).
2. **Signs** – usually unilateral (*Figs 21.19 & 21.20*).
   - Mild ptosis and miosis.
   - Slight elevation of the lower lid.
   - Normal reactions to light and near.
   - Hypochromic heterochromia may be seen if congenital or longstanding.
   - Reduced ipsilateral sweating if the lesion is below the superior cervical ganglion.
3. **Pharmacological tests**
   a. *Cocaine 4%* – confirms the diagnosis; normal pupil dilates but Horner pupil does not.

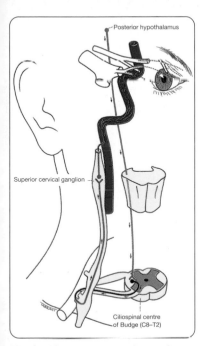

Fig. 21.18 Anatomical pathway of sympathetic supply

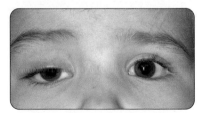

Fig. 21.20 More obvious right congenital Horner

Table 21.2 **Causes of Horner syndrome**

1. *Central (first-order neurone)*
   - Brain stem disease (tumour, vascular, demyelination)
   - Syringomyelia
   - Lateral medullary (Wallenberg) syndrome
   - Spinal cord tumour
   - Diabetic autonomic neuropathy
2. *Preganglionic (second-order neurone)*
   - Pancoast tumour
   - Carotid and aortic aneurysm and dissection
   - Neck lesions – glands, trauma, postsurgical
3. *Postganglionic (third-order neurone)*
   - Cluster headaches (migrainous neuralgia)
   - Internal carotid artery dissection
   - Nasopharyngeal tumour
   - Otitis media
   - Cavernous sinus mass

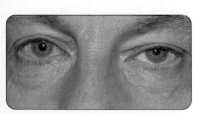

Fig. 21.19 Subtle left acquired Horner

b. Hydroxyamphetamine 1% – differentiates a preganglionic (both pupils will dilate) from a postganglionic lesion (Horner pupil will not dilate).

c. *Adrenaline 1:1000* – demonstrates denervation supersensitivity and a preganglionic (neither pupil dilates) from a postganglionic lesion (Horner pupil dilates and ptosis may improve).

4. Causes (*Table 21.2*).

Chiasm

Causes of chiasmal disease

1. **Tumours** – pituitary adenoma, craniopharyngioma, meningioma, glioma, chordoma, dysgerminoma, nasopharyngeal tumours, and metastases.
2. **Non-neoplastic masses** – aneurysms, Rathke pouch cysts, fibrous dysplasia, sphenoidal sinus mucoceles, and arachnoid cysts.
3. **Miscellaneous** – demyelination, inflammation, trauma, radiation-induced necrosis, and vasculitis.

Pituitary adenoma

1. **Definition** – anterior pituitary tumour that may or may not secrete specific hormones; most common is a chromophobe adenoma.
2. **Presentation** – 3rd–5th decade with headache, visual field defects, or endocrine disturbance.
3. **Visual field defects** – initially superotemporal with subsequent inferior spread (*Fig. 21.21*).

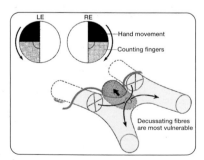

Fig. 21.21 Visual field defects caused by pituitary adenoma

4. **Colour desaturation** – across the vertical midline of the uniocular visual field is an early sign (*Fig. 21.22*).

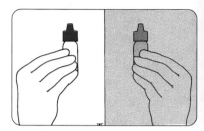

Fig. 21.22 Demonstration of colour desaturation

5. **Optic atrophy** – in 50% of cases with field defects.
6. **Miscellaneous** – diplopia and see-saw nystagmus of Maddox.
7. **MR** – hypointense on T1-weighted images; hyperintense on T2-weighed images and strong enhancement with gadolinium (*Fig. 21.23*).

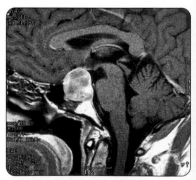

Fig. 21.23 Sagittal T1-weighted MR of a gadolinium enhanced pituitary adenoma

8. Treatment.
   a. *Observation* – if clinically silent.
   b. *Medical* – with dopamine agonists to shrink a prolactin-secreting tumour.
   c. *Surgery* – for severe compressive problems or failure to respond to medical therapy or radiotherapy.
   d. *Radiotherapy* – adjunct following incomplete removal and can also be used as primary treatment.
   e. *Gamma knife stereotactic radiotherapy.*

Craniopharyngioma

1. **Definition** – slow-growing tumour arising from vestigial remnants of Rathke pouch along the pituitary stalk.
2. **Presentation**
   - In children – dwarfism, delayed sexual development and obesity.
   - In adults – visual impairment and field defects.
3. **Visual field defects** – initially inferotemporal with subsequent superior spread (Fig. 21.24).

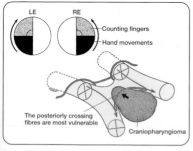

Fig. 21.24 Visual field defects caused by craniopharyngioma

4. MR – on T1-weighted images the solid component is isointense and the cystic hyperintense (Fig. 21.25).

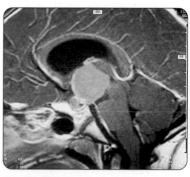

Fig. 21.25 Sagittal T1-weighted MR of craniopharyngioma with secondary hydrocephalus

5. Treatment – surgical.

Meningioma

Visual field defects and clinical signs depend on the location of the tumour (Fig. 21.26).

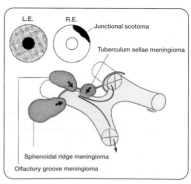

Fig. 21.26 Compression of anterior visual pathways by meningioma

1. **Tuberculum sellae** – compresses the junction of the chiasm with the optic nerve, resulting in an ipsilateral central scotoma and contralateral upper temporal defect (junctional scotoma) due to damage to the anterior knee of Wilbrand.
2. **Olfactory groove** – anosmia and optic nerve compression.
3. **Sphenoidal ridge** – compresses the optic nerve early if the tumour is located medially, and late if it involves the lateral aspect of the sphenoid bone and middle cranial fossa.
4. **Treatment** – surgery.

Retrochiasmal lesions

Optic tract

1. **Incongruous homonymous hemianopia** – mismatch between the two hemifields.
2. **Wernicke hemianopic pupil**
   - Light reflex – normal when the unaffected hemiretina is stimulated.
   - Light reflex – absent when the involved hemiretina is stimulated (i.e. light is shone from the hemianopic side).
3. **Optic atrophy**
   - Ipsilateral disc shows atrophy of the superior and inferior aspects of the neuroretinal rim.
   - Contralateral disc shows 'bow tie' pattern of atrophy.
4. **Contralateral pyramidal signs** – damage to ipsilateral cerebral peduncle.

Temporal optic radiations

1. **Visual field defect** – contralateral, homonymous, superior quadrant-anopia ('pie in the sky' – *Fig. 21.27a*).

2. **Associated features** – contralateral hemisensory disturbance, mild hemiparesis, paroxysmal olfactory and gustatory hallucinations (uncinate fits), formed visual hallucinations, seizures, and receptive dysphasia if the dominant hemisphere is involved.

Anterior parietal radiations

1. **Visual field defect** – incongruous, contralateral, homonymous, inferior quadrantanopia ('pie on the floor' – *Fig. 21.27b*).
2. **Associated features**
   - Of dominant parietal lobe disease – acalculia, agraphia, left–right disorientation and finger agnosia.
   - Of non-dominant lobe disease – dressing and constitutional apraxia and spatial neglect.

Main radiations

1. **Visual field defects** – complete homonymous hemianopia (*Fig. 21.27c*).
2. **Optokinetic nystagmus** (OKN) may be useful in localizing a lesion causing an isolated homonymous hemianopia that does not conform to any set pattern in a patient without associated neurological deficits.
   - Incongruous homonymous hemianopia with asymmetrical OKN indicates a parietal lesion.
   - Congruous hemianopia with symmetrical OKN indicates occipital lobe disease.

Striate cortex

1. **Visual field defects**
   - Occlusion of the posterior cerebral artery produces a macular sparing congruous homonymous hemianopia (*Fig. 21.27d*).

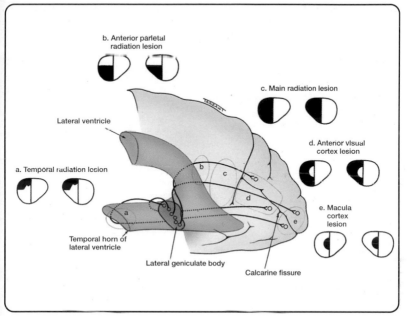

Fig. 21.27 Field defects caused by lesions of the optic radiations and visual cortex

- Damage to the tip of the occipital cortex, as might occur from a head injury, gives rise to congruous, homonymous, macular defects (*Fig. 21.27e*).
2. **Associated features** of visual cortex disease (cortical blindness):
   - Formed visual hallucinations, particularly involving the hemianopic field.
   - Denial of blindness (Anton syndrome).
   - Riddoch phenomenon.
3. **Causes** – vascular disease, migraine, trauma, and tumours.

Higher visual function

From the striate cortex (area 17), visual information is relayed to the visual association areas (18 and 19) of the cerebral cortex, where it is processed, analysed and interpreted. Lesions of various areas of the cerebral cortex produce characteristic clinical pictures.

1. **Alexia** – inability to read, commonly accompanied by agraphia, may be produced by lesions of the angulate gyrus of the dominant hemisphere.
2. **Visual agnosia** – inability to recognize objects by sight, whilst the

ability to recognize by touch is retained may be caused by bilateral disease of the inferior occipito-temporal area.

3. **Visual hallucinations.**

Third nerve

Applied anatomy

1. **Nuclear complex** – in the midbrain at the level of the superior colliculus, ventral to the Sylvian aqueduct (*Fig. 21.28*) is composed of the following paired and unpaired subnuclei.

   a. *Levator subnucleus* – unpaired caudal midline structure which innervates both levator muscles.

   b. *Superior rectus subnuclei* – paired, each innervates the respective contralateral superior rectus.

   c. *Medial rectus, inferior rectus* and *inferior oblique subnuclei* – paired and innervate corresponding ipsilateral muscles.

2. **Fasciculus** – efferent fibres pass through the red nucleus and the medial aspect of the cerebral peduncle.

   a. *Benedikt syndrome* – ipsilateral 3rd and contralateral extrapyramidal signs.

   b. *Weber syndrome* – ipsilateral 3rd and contralateral hemiparesis.

   c. *Nothnagel syndrome* – ipsilateral 3rd and cerebellar ataxia.

   d. *Claude syndrome* – combination of Benedikt and Nothnagel syndromes.

3. **Basilar**

   • Starts as a series of 'rootlets' which leave the midbrain on the medial aspect of the cerebral peduncle before coalescing to form the main trunk.

   • Runs lateral to and parallel with the posterior communicating artery and traverses the base of the skull along its subarachnoid course (*Fig. 21.29*).

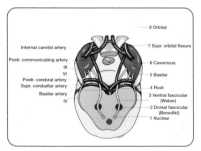

Fig. 21.28 Dorsal view of the course of the 3rd nerve

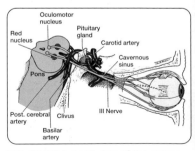

Fig. 21.29 Lateral view of the course of the 3rd nerve

• Causes of isolated basilar palsies – posterior communication aneurysm, and subdural or extradural haematoma (*Fig. 21.30*).

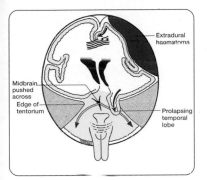

Fig. 21.30 3rd nerve palsy due to extradural haematoma

- superficially and derive their blood supply from the pial blood vessels.
- The main trunk of the 3rd nerve is supplied by the vasa nervorum.
- Pupillary involvement indicates a 'surgical' (e.g. aneurysm) cause whereas sparing indicates a 'medical' (e.g. hypertension) cause.

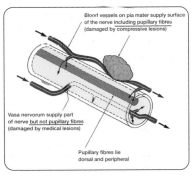

Fig. 21.31 Location of pupillomotor fibres within the trunk of the 3rd nerve

4. Intracavernous

- Runs in the lateral wall above the 4th nerve and divides into superior and inferior branches which enter the orbit through the superior orbital fissure within the annulus of Zinn.
- Causes of intracavernous palsies – diabetes, pituitary apoplexy, and intracavernous pathology such as aneurysm, meningiomas, and carotid-cavernous fistula.

5. Intraorbital

- Superior division innervates the levator and superior rectus muscles.
- Inferior division innervates the medial rectus, the inferior rectus and the inferior oblique muscles.
- The branch to the inferior oblique contains pre-ganglionic parasympathetic fibres from the Edinger–Westphal subnucleus, which innervate the sphincter pupillae and the ciliary muscle.

6. Pupillomotor fibres (Fig. 21.31)

- Between the brain stem and the cavernous sinus, pupillomotor parasympathetic fibres are located

Diagnosis

Signs of right 3rd nerve palsy:
- Profound ptosis (Fig. 21.32a).
- Abducted eye in the primary position (Fig. 21.32b).
- Normal abduction (Fig. 21.32c).
- Limited adduction (Fig. 21.32d).
- Limited depression (Fig. 21.32e) and elevation (Fig. 21.32f).
- Intact superior oblique muscle causes intorsion of the eye at rest which increases on attempted down-gaze.
- Parasympathetic involvement causing mydriasis and cycloplegia.

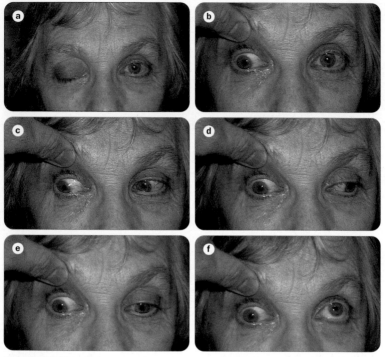

Fig. 21.32 Right 3rd nerve palsy

Causes of isolated third nerve palsy

1. **Idiopathic** – about 25%.
2. **Vascular** – hypertension and diabetes.
3. **Aneurysm** – of posterior communicating artery at its junction with the internal carotid.
4. **Trauma** – both direct and secondary to subdural haematoma with uncal herniation.
5. **Miscellaneous** – tumours, syphilis, giant cell arteritis, and other collagen vascular disorders.

Fourth nerve

Applied anatomy

1. **Important features**
   - Only cranial nerve to emerge from the dorsal aspect of the brain.
   - Crossed cranial nerve – i.e. 4th nerve nucleus innervates the contralateral superior oblique muscle.
   - Very long and slender.
2. **Nucleus** – at the level of the inferior colliculi ventral to the Sylvian aqueduct (*Fig. 21.33*).

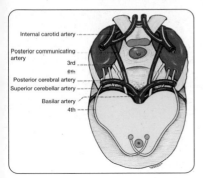

Internal carotid artery
Posterior communicating artery
3rd
6th
Posterior cerebral artery
Superior cerebellar artery
Basilar artery
4th

Fig. 21.33 Dorsal view of the course of the 4th nerve

3. Fasciculus – axons curve posteriorly around the aqueduct and decussate in the anterior medullary velum.

4. Trunk
- Leaves the brain stem on the dorsal surface and curves laterally around the brain stem.
- Runs forwards beneath the free edge of the tentorium and passes between the posterior cerebral artery and the superior cerebellar artery.
- Pierces the dura and enters the cavernous sinus.

5. Intracavernous
- Runs in the lateral wall of the sinus, inferiorly to the 3rd nerve and above the 1st division of the 5th.
- In the anterior part of the cavernous sinus it rises and passes through the superior orbital fissure above and lateral to the annulus of Zinn.

6. Intraorbital – innervates the superior oblique muscle.

Diagnosis

1. Signs of left 4th nerve palsy:
- Left hypertropia ('left over right') in the primary position when uninvolved right eye is fixating (*Fig. 21.34a*).
- Left hypertropia increased on right gaze due to inferior oblique overaction (*Fig. 21.34b*).
- Left limitation of depression in adduction (*Fig. 21.34c*).
- Normal – left abduction (*Fig. 21.34d*), depression (*Fig. 21.34e*), and elevation (*Fig. 21.34f*).
- Excyclotorsion.
- Diplopia is vertical, torsional, and worse on looking down.

2. Abnormal head posture (*Fig. 21.35*).
- Contralateral head tilt.
- Contralateral face turn.
- Chin depressed.

3. Bilateral involvement – always suspect until proved otherwise.
- Right hypertropia in left gaze, left hypertropia in right gaze.
- Greater than 10° of cyclodeviation on double Maddox rod test (see below).
- V pattern esotropia.
- Bilaterally positive Bielschowsky test (see below).

Special tests

1. Parks three step test
   a. *First step* – which eye is hypertropic in the primary position?
   - Left hypertropia may be caused by weakness of one of the following four muscles: one of the depressors of the left eye (superior oblique or inferior rectus) or one of the elevators of the right eye (superior rectus or inferior oblique).

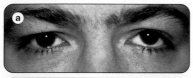

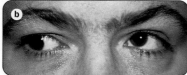

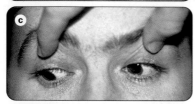

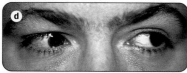

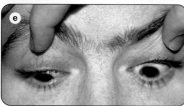

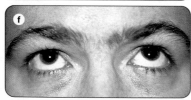

Fig. 21.34 Left 4th nerve palsy

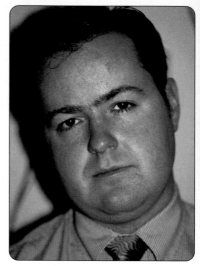

Fig. 21.35 Abnormal head posture

- In 4th nerve palsy the involved eye is higher.
- **b.** *Step two* – is left hypertropia is greater in right gaze or left gaze?
- Increase on right gaze implicates either the right superior rectus or left superior oblique.
- Increase on left gaze implicates either the right inferior oblique or left inferior rectus (in 4th nerve palsy the deviation is **W**orse **O**n **O**pposite **G**aze – **WOOG**).
- **c.** *Step three* – Bielschowsky head tilt test.
- The head is tilted to the right and then to the left (*Fig. 21.36*).
- Increase of left hypertropia on left head tilt (*Fig. 21.3*) implicates the left superior oblique.
- Increase of right hypertropia on left head tilt implicates the right inferior rectus (in 4th nerve palsy the deviation is **B**etter **O**n **O**pposite **T**ilt – **BOOT**).

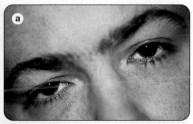

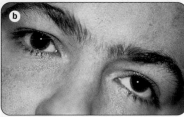

Fig. 21.36 Positive Bielschowsky test in left 4th nerve palsy

Causes of isolated fourth nerve palsy

1. **Congenital** – frequent, although symptoms may not develop until decompensation occurs in adult life.
2. **Trauma** – frequently causes bilateral paresis.
3. **Vascular**.

Sixth nerve

Applied anatomy

1. **Nucleus** – in the pons ventral to the floor of the 4th ventricle (*Fig. 21.37*).
2. **Fasciculus** – passes ventrally and leaves the brain stem at the pontomedullary junction, just lateral to the pyramidal prominence.

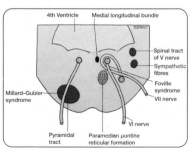

Fig. 21.37 Pons at the level of the 6th nerve nucleus

- **a.** Foville syndrome
  - 5th nerve palsy – facial analgesia.
  - 6th nerve palsy combined with gaze palsy (PPRF).
  - 7th nerve (nuclear or fascicular damage) – facial weakness.
  - 8th nerve damage – deafness.
  - Central Horner syndrome.
- **b.** Millard–Gubler syndrome
  - Ipsilateral 6th nerve palsy
  - Contralateral hemiplegia.
  - Variable number of signs of a dorsal pontine lesion.

3. **Basilar**
   - Enters prepontine basilar cistern, passes upwards close to the base of the skull and is crossed by the anterior inferior cerebellar artery (*Fig. 21.38*).
   - Pierces the dura and angles forwards over the tip of the petrous bone, passing through Dorello canal to enter the cavernous sinus.
   - Causes of basilar palsies – acoustic neuroma, nasopharyngeal tumours, raised intracranial pressure, basal skull fracture, and Gradenigo syndrome.

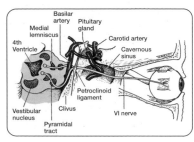

Fig. 21.38 Lateral view of the course of the 6th nerve

4. **Intracavernous** – runs forwards below the 3rd and 4th nerves, and the first division of the 5th.
5. **Intraorbital** – enters the orbit through the superior orbital fissure within the annulus of Zinn to innervate the lateral rectus muscle.

Diagnosis

1. **Signs** of a left 6th nerve palsy.
   - Primary position – left esotropia if recent, straight if longstanding (*Fig. 21.39a*).
   - Limited left abduction (*Fig. 21.39b*).
   - Normal left adduction (*Fig. 21.39c*).
2. **Compensatory face turn** – into the field of action of the paralysed muscle (i.e. to the right) to minimize diplopia.
3. **Causes** – already mentioned; aneurysms are rare but vascular causes (especially diabetes and hypertension) are common.

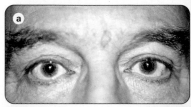

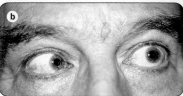

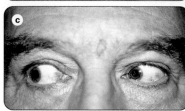

Fig. 21.39 Left 6th nerve palsy

Horizontal gaze palsy

Applied anatomy

- Horizontal movements are generated from the horizontal gaze centre in the PPRF (*Fig. 21.40*).
- From here motor neurones connect to the ipsilateral 6th nerve nucleus which innervates the lateral rectus.
- From the 6th nerve nucleus internuclear neurones cross the midline at the level of the pons and pass up the contralateral medial longitudinal fasciculus (MLF) to synapse with motor neurones in the

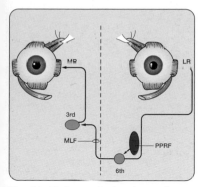

Fig. 21.40 Anatomical pathways for horizontal eye movements (PPRF = pontine paramedian reticular formation; MLF = medial longitudinal fasciculus; MR = medial rectus; LR = lateral rectus)

medial rectus subnucleus in the 3rd nerve complex which innervates the medial rectus.

- Stimulation of the PPRF on one side causes a conjugate movement of the eyes to the same side.
- Loss of normal horizontal eye movements occurs when these pathways are disrupted; causes are shown in *Table 21.3*.

Table 21.3 **Causes of internuclear ophthalmoplegia**

- Demyelination
- Vascular disease
- Tumours of the brain stem and 4th ventricle
- Trauma
- Encephalitis
- Hydrocephalus
- Progressive supranuclear palsy
- Drug-induced
- Remote effects of carcinoma

Diagnosis

1. **PPRF** – ipsilateral horizontal gaze palsy with inability to look in the direction of the lesion.
2. **MLF** – signs of left internuclear ophthalmoplegia (INO).
   - Primary position – straight.
   - Right gaze – limited left adduction and ataxic nystagmus of the right eye (*Fig. 21.41a*).
   - Left gaze – normal (*Fig. 21.41b*).
   - Convergence – intact with discrete lesions (21.41c).
   - Vertical nystagmus on attempted up-gaze.

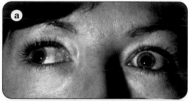

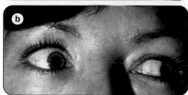

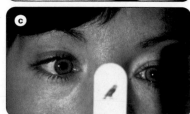

Fig. 21.41 Left INO

3. Bilateral INO
- Left gaze – limitation of right adduction and ataxic nystagmus of the left eye (*Fig. 21.42a*).
- Right gaze – limitation of left adduction and ataxic nystagmus of the right eye (*Fig. 21.42b*).
- Convergence – absent with extensive lesions (*Fig. 21.42c*).

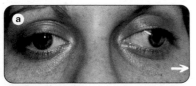

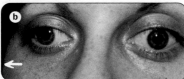

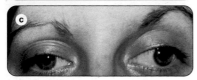

Fig. 21.42 Bilateral INO

4. PPRF and **MLF** combined lesions on the same side give rise to the 'one-and-a-half syndrome' which is characterized by a combination of ipsilateral gaze palsy and INO.

Vertical gaze palsy

Anatomy
- Vertical movements are generated from the vertical gaze centre (rostral interstitial nucleus of the MLF).

- From the vertical gaze centre, impulses pass to the subnuclei of the eye muscles controlling vertical gaze in both eyes.
- Cells mediating upward and downward eye movements are intermingled in the vertical gaze centre.

Parinaud dorsal midbrain syndrome

1. Signs
- Primary position – straight.
- Supranuclear up-gaze palsy.
- Convergence – limited.
- Pupils – large with light-near dissociation.
- Lid retraction (Collier sign).
- Convergence–retraction nystagmus.

2. Causes
a. *In children* – aqueduct stenosis, meningitis, and pinealoma (*Fig. 21.43*).

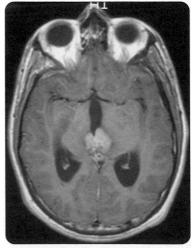

Fig. 21.43 T1-weighted axial MR of pinealoma with secondary ventricular enlargement

b. *In young adults* – demyelination, trauma and arteriovenous malformations.

c. *In the elderly* – midbrain vascular accidents, mass lesions involving the periaqueductal grey matter, and posterior fossa aneurysms.

Progressive supranuclear palsy (Steele–Richardson–Olszewski syndrome)

1. **Definition** – severe degenerative disease which presents in old age.
2. **Signs**
   - Supranuclear gaze palsy.
   - Horizontal movements subsequently become impaired and eventually global gaze palsy develops.
   - Pseudobulbar palsy.
   - Extrapyramidal rigidity, gait ataxia and dementia.
   - Paralysis of convergence.

Chronic progressive external ophthalmoplegia

1. **Definition** – group of disorders characterized by ptosis and slowly progressive bilateral ocular immobility.
2. **Classification** – isolated, Kearns–Sayre syndrome, and oculopharyngeal dystrophy.
3. **Signs**
   a. *Bilateral ptosis* – usually the first sign (Fig. 21.44a).
   b. *Progressive external ophthalmoplegia* – initially involving up-gaze and subsequently lateral gaze (Fig. 21.44b,c) so that the eyes may become virtually fixed.

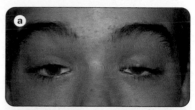
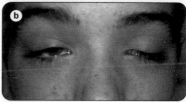
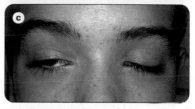

Fig. 21.44 CPEO. (a) Primary position; (b) left gaze; (c) right gaze

Intracranial aneurysm

Neurological considerations

Most (85%) intracranial aneurysms arise from the anterior half of the circle of Willis. The majority remain asymptomatic during life although occasionally they may cause the following life-threatening complications:

1. **Subarachnoid haemorrhage** (*Fig. 21.45*) – presents with sudden onset of severe headache, photophobia, clouding consciousness, vomiting and signs of meningeal irritation – including neck stiffness and positive Kernig sign.

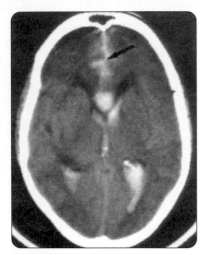

Fig. 21.45 Axial CT showing blood in the ventricles due to subarachnoid haemorrhage

2. Pressure effects – associated with 'giant' aneurysms (>25 mm).
3. Treatment – clipping the neck of the aneurysm or less frequently inserting metallic coils into the lumen.

Ophthalmic considerations

1. **Isolated 3rd nerve palsy** – compression by an aneurysm of the posterior communicating artery at its junction with the internal carotid artery in the subarachnoid space.
2. **Isolated 6th nerve palsy** – aneurysms of the intracavernous part of the internal carotid artery.
3. **Combined palsies** – 3rd and 6th with intracavernous carotid aneurysms and other cavernous sinus lesions.
4. **Monocular visual loss** – compression of the intracranial part of the optic nerve by an aneurysm arising

from the internal carotid artery near the origin of the ophthalmic artery, at its terminal bifurcation.
5. **Visual field defects** – involving the nasal field may be caused by a giant aneurysm at or near the origin of the ophthalmic artery.
6. **Terson syndrome** – combination of frequently bilateral and intraretinal and subhyaloid haemorrhage (*Fig. 21.46*) and subarachnoid haemorrhage secondary to aneurysmal rupture, most commonly arising from the anterior communicating artery.

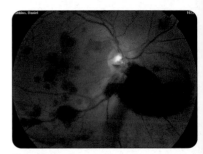

Fig. 21.46 Intraocular haemorrhage in Terson syndrome

Nystagmus

Definition

Nystagmus is a repetitive, involuntary, to-and-fro eye oscillation of the eyes, which may be physiological or pathological. In pathological nystagmus, each cycle of movement is usually initiated by an involuntary, defoveating drift of the eye away from the object of interest, followed by a returning refixation saccadic movement.

1. **Plane** – horizontal, vertical, torsional or non-specific.
2. **Amplitude** – fine or coarse.
3. **Frequency** – high, moderate or low.

Classification

1. **Jerk** – saccadic with a slow defoveating 'drift' movement and a fast corrective refoveating saccadic movement. The direction of nystagmus is described in terms of the direction of the fast component.
2. **Pendular** – velocity is equal in both directions. It may be congenital or acquired.
3. **Mixed** – pendular nystagmus in the primary position and jerk nystagmus on lateral gaze.

The characteristics of any form of nystagmus can be documented using the scheme shown in *Figure 21.47*.

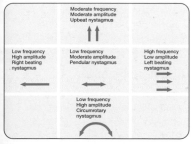

Fig. 21.47 Schematic for documenting nystagmus

Physiological nystagmus

1. **End-point** – fine jerk nystagmus of moderate frequency found when the eyes are in extreme positions of gaze. The fast phase is in the direction of gaze.
2. **Optokinetic** – jerk nystagmus induced by moving repetitive targets across the visual field. The slow phase is a pursuit movement in which the eyes follow the target; the fast phase is a saccadic movement in the opposite direction as the eyes fixate on the next target.
3. **Vestibular** – jerk nystagmus caused by altered input from the vestibular nuclei to the horizontal gaze centres. It may be elicited by caloric stimulation as follows:
   - When cold water is poured into the right ear the patient will develop left jerk nystagmus (i.e. fast phase to the left).
   - When warm water is poured into the right ear the patient will develop right jerk nystagmus (i.e. fast phase to the right).
   - A useful mnemonic is 'COWS' (cold–opposite, warm–same) indicating the direction of the nystagmus.

Primary congenital nystagmus

1. **Inheritance** – X-LR or AD.
2. **Presentation** – 2–3 months after birth and persists throughout life.
3. **Signs**
   - Uniplanar horizontal jerk nystagmus that may be dampened by convergence and is not present during sleep.
   - There is usually a null point in which nystagmus is minimal.
   - An abnormal head posture may be adopted to move the eye into the null point.

Spasmas nutans

1. **Presentation** – 3–18 months after birth.
2. **Signs** – unilateral or bilateral, small-amplitude, high-frequency horizontal nystagmus associated with head nodding.

3. Causes
- Idiopathic; spontaneously resolves by age 3 years.
- Glioma of anterior visual pathway, empty sella syndrome and porencephalic cyst.

Latent nystagmus

1. Association – infantile esotropia and DVD.

2. Signs
- With both eyes open there is no nystagmus.
- Horizontal nystagmus becomes apparent on covering one eye or reducing the amount of light reaching the eye.
- Fast phase is in the direction of the uncovered fixating eye.
- Occasionally, an element of latency may be superimposed on a manifest nystagmus so that when one eye is covered the amplitude of nystagmus increases (latent-manifest nystagmus).

Periodic alternating nystagmus

1. Signs – conjugate horizontal jerk nystagmus that periodically reverses its direction.

2. Causes – congenital, cerebellar disease, ataxia telangiectasia (Louis–Bar syndrome) and drugs such as phenytoin.

Convergence–retraction nystagmus

Convergence–retraction nystagmus is caused by co-contraction of the extraocular muscles, particularly the medial recti.

1. Signs
- Jerk nystagmus induced by passing an OKN tape downwards.
- The upward refixation saccade brings the two eyes towards each other in a convergence movement.
- Associated retraction of the globe.

2. Causes – lesions of the pre-tectal area such as pinealoma and vascular accidents (dorsal midbrain syndrome).

Downbeat nystagmus

1. Signs – vertical nystagmus with the fast phase beating downwards, which is more easily elicited in lateral gaze and downgaze.

2. Causes – Arnold–Chiari malformation, syringobulbia, drugs (e.g. phenytoin, barbiturates), Wernicke encephalopathy, demyelination and hydrocephalus.

Upbeat nystagmus

1. Signs – vertical nystagmus with the fast phase beating upwards.

2. Causes – posterior fossa lesions, drugs and Wernicke encephalopathy.

See-saw nystagmus of Maddox

1. Signs – pendular nystagmus, in which one eye elevates and intorts while the other depresses and extorts; the eyes then reverse direction.

2. Causes – parasellar tumours often producing bitemporal hemianopia, syringobulbia and brain stem stroke.

Ataxic nystagmus

Horizontal jerk nystagmus of the abducting eye in INO (see above).

Sensory deprivation nystagmus

1. **Signs** – horizontal pendular nystagmus that can often be dampened by convergence.
2. **Cause** – severe visual impairment before the age of 2 years.

Nystagmoid movements

Ocular flutter and opsoclonus

1. **Signs**
   - Saccadic oscillations with no intersaccadic interval.
   - In ocular flutter they are purely horizontal and in opsoclonus they are multiplanar.
2. **Causes** – viral encephalitis, infantile myoclonic encephalopathy, drug-induced, and idiopathic in healthy infants.

Ocular bobbing

1. **Signs** – rapid, conjugate, downward eye movements with a slow drift up to the primary position.
2. **Causes** – pontine haemorrhage, cerebellar lesions, and metabolic encephalopathy.

Migraine

Clinical features

1. **Common migraine** (migraine without aura) – headache with autonomic nervous system dysfunction without stereotypical neurological or ophthalmic features.
2. **Classical migraine** (migraine with aura)
   - Expanding scintillation scotoma that resolves after about 30 minutes (*Fig. 21.48*).
   - Supervening headache is hemicranial and associated with nausea and photophobia.

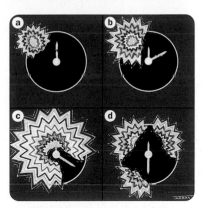

Fig. 21.48 Progression of scintillating scotoma

3. **Cluster headache** (migrainous neuralgia) – oculotemporal, excruciating headache accompanied by various autonomic phenomena such as lacrimation and rhinorrhoea, occurring almost every day for a period of some weeks.
4. **Focal migraine** – transient dysphasia, hemisensory symptoms or even focal weakness in addition to other symptoms of migraine.
5. **Migraine sine migraine** – episodic visual disturbances without headache.
6. **Retinal migraine** – acute, transient unilateral visual loss.
7. **Ophthalmoplegic migraine** – recurrent transient 3rd nerve palsy which begins after the headache.
8. **Familial hemiplegic migraine** – failure of full recovery of focal neurological features after an attack of migraine subsides.
9. **Basilar migraine** – in children, characterized by a typical migrainous aura associated with numbness and tingling of the lips and extremities.

Treatment

1. **General measures** – elimination of conditions and agents that may precipitate an attack of migraine.
2. **Prophylaxis** – beta-blockers, calcium channel blockers, amitriptyline, clonidine, pizotifen, and low-dose aspirin.
3. **Treatment of acute attack** – simple analgesics and, if appropriate, an anti-emetic such as metoclopramide.

Facial spasm

Essential blepharospasm

1. **Definition** – uncommon but distressing, idiopathic disorder which presents in the 6th decade and affects women more commonly than men by a 3:1 ratio. It is characterized by progressive bilateral involuntary spasm of the orbicularis oculi and upper facial muscles.
2. **Meige syndrome** – combination of blepharospasm and involvement of the lower facial and neck muscles.
3. **Brueghel syndrome** – associated with severe mandibular and cervical muscle involvement.
4. **Treatment** – Botulinum toxin injection along the upper and lower eyelid and eyebrow affords temporary relief in most patients.

Facial hemispasm

1. **Presentation** – 5th–6th decade of life with brief spasm of the orbicularis oculi which later spreads along the distribution of the facial nerve.
2. **Treatment** – similar to essential blepharospasm.

Cornea

Vortex keratopathy

1. **Signs** – whorl-like pattern of epithelial deposits which originate from a point below the pupil and swirl outwards, sparing the limbus (*Fig. 22.1*).

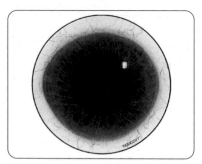

Fig. 22.1 Vortex keratopathy

2. **Causes**
   a. *Antimalarials* (chloroquine and hydroxychloroquine) – unrelated to the dose or duration of administration and may clear despite continued administration.
   b. *Amiodarone* – universal and reversible on discontinuation of medication.

Chlorpromazine

Some patients on long-term therapy may develop innocuous, subtle, diffuse, yellowish-brown granular deposits in the endothelium and deep stroma. Other toxic effects are anterior lens capsule deposits and retinopathy.

Argyrosis

Argyrosis is a discoloration of ocular tissues secondary to silver deposits which may be iatrogenic or from occupational exposure. Greyish-brown, granular deposits in Descemet membrane (*Fig. 22.2a*) that may also involve the conjunctiva (*Fig. 22.2b*).

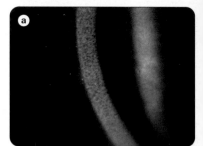

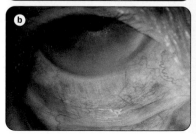

Fig. 22.2 Argyrosis

Chrysiasis

Virtually all patients on continuous gold therapy for rheumatoid arthritis, who have received a total dose of gold compound exceeding 1000 mg, develop innocuous dust-like or glittering purple stromal granules (*Fig. 22.3a*); marginal keratitis is uncommon (*Fig. 22.3b*).

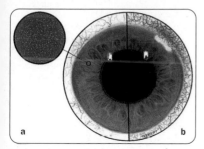

Fig. 22.3 Chrysiasis

Lens

1. **Steroids** – posterior subcapsular opacities (*Fig. 22.4*) may be caused by topical and systemic steroids.

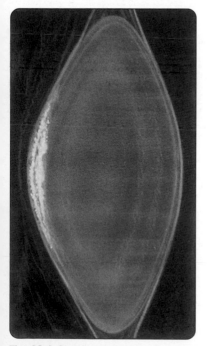

Fig. 22.4 Steroid cataract

2. **Chlorpromazine** – innocuous, fine, stellate, yellowish-brown granules on the anterior lens capsule within the pupillary area (*Fig. 22.5*).

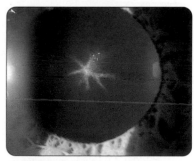

Fig. 22.5 Chlorpromazine deposits

3. **Busulphan** – occasionally causes lens opacities.
4. **Gold** – innocuous anterior capsular deposits in about 50% of patients on treatment for longer than 3 years.
5. **Allopurinol** – increases the risk of cataract formation in elderly patients, if the cumulative dose exceeds 400 g or duration of administration exceeds 3 years.

Uveitis

Rifabutin

Rifabutin is used mainly in *Mycobacterium avium* complex infections in AIDS patients with low CD4 counts.
1. **AAU** – unilateral and frequently associated with hypopyon.
2. **Treatment** – withdrawal of the drug or reduction of dose.

Cidofovir

Cidofovir is used in CMV retinitis.
1. **AAU** – few cells but a marked fibrinous exudate may develop following several intravenous infusions.
2. **Treatment** – topical steroids.

Retina

Antimalarials

Drugs

1. **Risks**
   - Normal dose of chloroquine is 250 mg.
   - Cumulative dose of less than 100 g or duration under one year is rarely associated with retinal damage.
   - The risk increases significantly when the cumulative dose exceeds 300 g (i.e. 250 mg daily for 3 years).
   - Risk of retinopathy from hydroxy-chloroquine is negligible if the daily dose does not exceed 400 mg.
2. **Stages**
   a. *Premaculopathy* – normal visual acuity and a scotoma to a red target 4–9° from fixation; reversible if the drug is discontinued.
   b. *Early maculopathy* – visual acuity is 6/9–6/12 and a subtle 'bull's eye' macular lesion (*Fig. 22.6a*) which may progress even if the drug is stopped.
   c. *Moderate maculopathy* – visual acuity is 6/18–6/24 and an obvious 'bull's eye' macular lesion (*Fig. 22.6b*); irreversible.
   d. *Severe maculopathy* – visual acuity is (6/36–6/60) with widespread RPE atrophy surrounding the fovea (*Fig. 22.6c*).
   e. *End-stage* – atrophy of the RPE and choriocapillaris, arteriolar attenuation, and peripheral pigment clumping (*Fig. 22.6d*).

Screening

1. **Hydroxychloroquine** – unnecessary although some authorities have recommended annual screening if the patient has been on medication for over 6 years.
2. **Chloroquine**
   - Recording of visual acuity and ophthalmoscopy by the prescribing doctor is all that is required.
   - The patient can be given an Amsler grid to use once a week. If symptoms occur or an abnormality is found, then an ophthalmic opinion should be sought.

Phenothiazines

1. **Thioridazine** (Melleril) – normal dose is 150–600 mg.
   - Doses which exceed 800 mg/day may be retinotoxic.
   - Salt-and-pepper pigmentary disturbance involving the mid-periphery and posterior pole.
   - Plaque-like pigmentation and focal loss of the RPE and choriocapil-laris (*Fig. 22.7*).
   - Diffuse loss of the RPE and choriocapillaris.
2. **Chlorpromazine** – normal dose is 75–300 mg; retinotoxicity character-ized by non-specific pigmentary granularity and clumping may occur if very much larger doses are used over a prolonged period.

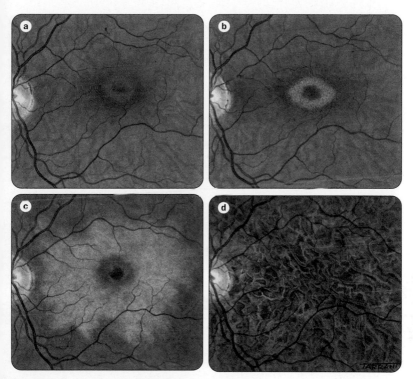

Fig. 22.6 Progression of chloroquine maculopathy

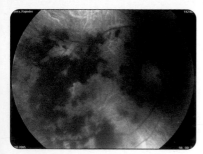

Fig. 22.7 Thioridazine retinopathy

Crystalline maculopathies

1. **Tamoxifen** – normal dose is 20–40 mg.
   - Toxicity may develop with higher doses and rarely on normal doses.
   - Retinopathy – bilateral, fine, superficial, yellow, crystalline deposits in the inner layers of the retina and punctate grey lesions in the outer retina and RPE (*Fig. 22.8*).

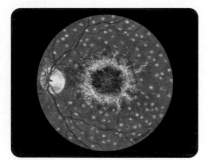

Fig. 22.8 Tamoxifen retinopathy

2. **Canthaxanthin** – prolonged use may cause the deposition of innocuous, inner retinal, tiny, glistening, yellow deposits, arranged symmetrically in a doughnut shape at the posterior poles (*Fig. 22.9*).

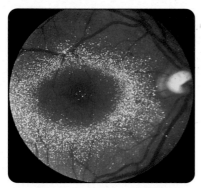

Fig. 22.9 Canthaxanthin retinopathy

3. **Methoxyflurane** – prolonged administration may lead to renal failure and secondary hyperoxalosis, with deposition of calcium oxalate crystals in the retina and a black macular lesion (*Fig. 22.10*).

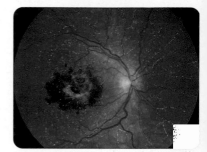

Fig. 22.10 Oxalosis

4. **Nitrofurantoin** – superficial and deep intraretinal glistening deposits distributed in a circinate pattern throughout the posterior pole.

Miscellaneous agents

1. **Interferon alpha** – cotton-wool spots and intraretinal haemorrhages may develop (*Fig. 22.11*), particularly with high doses. Other ocular side-effects include CMO, oculomotor nerve palsy, disc oedema, and retinal vein occlusion.

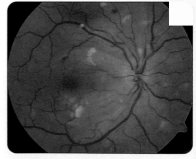

Fig. 22.11 Interferon retinopathy

2. **Desferrioxamine mesylate** – macular and/or equatorial pigmentary degeneration associated with reduced ERG amplitudes and reduced EOG light-peak to dark-trough ratios.

3. **Nicotinic acid** – reversible CMO without leakage on fluorescein angiography when doses greater than 1.5 g daily are used.

4. **Gentamicin** – severe retinal ischaemia when injected intravitreally for the treatment of bacterial endophthalmitis; rarely retinal toxicity may result from periocular injection.

Optic nerve

1. **Ethambutol** – may cause optic neuritis, colour vision abnormalities and visual field defects. Toxicity is dose and duration dependent, the incidence is up to 6% at a daily dose of 25 mg/kg and rare with a daily dose not exceeding 15 mg/kg.

2. **Amiodarone** – optic neuropathy occurs in 1–2% of patients and is not dose-related.

3. **Vigabatrin** – bilateral concentric or binasal visual field defects, often asymptomatic, months or years after starting treatment.

Eyelid trauma

Haematoma

A haematoma (black eye – *Fig. 23.1*) is the most common result of blunt injury and is generally innocuous, although it is important to exclude associated trauma to the globe or orbit, and basal skull fracture.

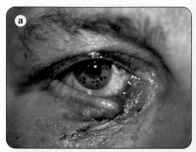

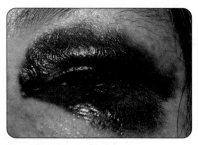

Fig. 23.1 Black eye

Fig. 23.2 (a) Laceration; (b) after treatment

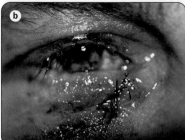

Laceration

1. **Eyelid laceration** – should be repaired by direct closure (*Fig. 23.2*) whenever possible, even under tension, since this affords the best functional and cosmetic results.
2. **Canalicular laceration** – repaired by bridging with silicone tubing threaded down the lacrimal system and tied in the nose, and suturing of the laceration.

Orbital fractures

Blow-out orbital floor fracture

1. **Pathogenesis** – sudden increase in the orbital pressure by a striking object greater than 5 cm in diameter (*Fig. 23.3*).
2. **Periocular signs** – ecchymosis, oedema, and subcutaneous emphysema.

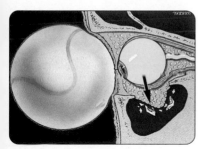

Fig. 23.3 Mechanism of blow-out orbital floor fracture

3. **Infraorbital nerve anaesthesia** – lower lid, cheek, side of nose, upper lip, upper teeth and gums.
4. **Diplopia** – limitation of elevation (*Fig. 23.4a*) and depression due to entrapment of the inferior rectus and inferior oblique.
5. **Enophthalmos** – in severe fractures.

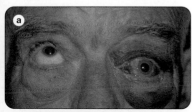

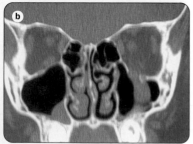

Fig. 23.4 (a) Defective left elevation; (b) CT coronal section shows the fracture and antral opacification

6. **CT** – to assess the severity of the fracture and maxillary antral opacities (*Fig. 23.4b*).
7. **Treatment** – release of entrapped tissue and repair of the bony defect with synthetic material (*Fig. 23.5*).

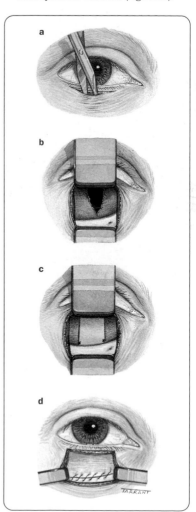

Fig. 23.5 Repair of blow-out fracture

Blow-out medial wall fracture

Most medial wall orbital fractures are usually associated with floor fractures.

1. Signs
- Periorbital haematoma and subcutaneous emphysema on blowing the nose.
- Defective adduction (*Fig. 23.6a*) and abduction due to entrapment of the medial rectus.

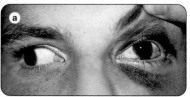

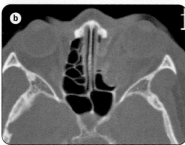

Fig. 23.6 (a) Defective left adduction; (b) axial CT shows the fracture

2. CT – shows the bony defect (*Fig. 23.6b*).

3. Treatment – release of the entrapped tissue and repair of the bony defect.

Roof fracture

Isolated roof fractures may be caused by falling on a sharp object or a blow to the brow or forehead.

1. Presentation – haematoma of the upper eyelid and periocular ecchymosis.

2. Signs
- Inferior or axial globe displacement.
- Pulsation of the globe unassociated with a bruit in a large fracture.

3. Treatment – small fractures may not require treatment but sizeable defects with downwardly displaced fragments usually require reconstructive surgery.

Lateral wall fracture

Acute lateral wall fractures (*Fig. 23.7a*) are rarely encountered by ophthalmologists. Because the lateral wall of the orbit is more solid than the other walls, a fracture is usually associated with extensive facial damage so that residual deformity following treatment is common (*Fig. 23.7b*).

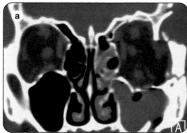

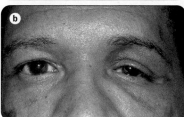

Fig. 23.7 (a) Coronal CT of a left lateral wall fracture; (b) residual deformity following repair

Trauma to the globe

Definitions

1. **Closed injury** – corneo-scleral wall of the globe is intact but intraocular damage is present.
2. **Open injury** – full-thickness wound of the corneo-scleral wall.
3. **Contusion** – closed injury resulting from blunt trauma.
4. **Rupture** – full-thickness wound caused by blunt trauma.
5. **Laceration** – full-thickness wound caused by a sharp object at the site of impact.
6. **Lamellar laceration** – partial-thickness wound caused by a sharp object.
7. **Penetration** – single full-thickness wound, usually caused by a sharp object, without an exit wound.
8. **Perforation** – two full-thickness wounds, one entry and one exit, usually caused by a missile.

Principles of management

1. **Initial assessment**
   - Determination of the nature and extent of any life-threatening problems.
   - History of the injury.
   - Examination of both eyes and orbits.
2. **Special investigations**
   a. *CT* – for detection and localization of intraocular foreign bodies.
   b. *US* – for intraocular foreign bodies, globe rupture, suprachoroidal haemorrhage, and RD.
   c. *ERG* – to assess the integrity of the optic nerve and retina.

Blunt trauma

Cornea

1. **Corneal abrasion** – stains with fluorescein (*Fig. 23.8*); treatment involves topical cycloplegia and antibiotic ointment; the epithelium heals faster without patching.

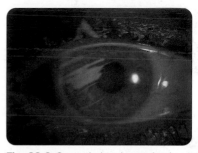

Fig. 23.8 Corneal abrasion stained with fluorescein

2. **Acute corneal oedema** – may be associated with folds in Descemet membrane and stromal thickening.
3. **Tears in Descemet membrane** – usually vertical and may be associated with birth trauma (*Fig. 23.9*).

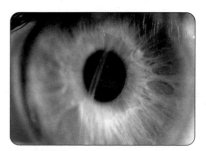

Fig. 23.9 Vertical tears in Descemet membrane

Hyphaema

1. Signs – red cell floating in the aqueous with or without an inferior fluid level (*Fig. 23.10a*).

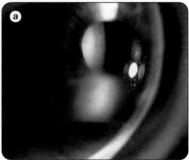

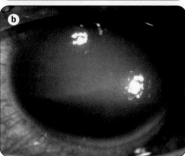

Fig. 23.10 (a) Hyphaema; (b) secondary haemorrhage

2. Observation
- Most are innocuous and transient.
- The immediate risk is that of secondary haemorrhage, often larger than the original bleed (*Fig. 23.10b*).

3. Treatment
- Oral tranexamic acid 25 mg/kg t.i.d. to prevention secondary haemorrhage.
- Atropine with or without topical steroids.

Anterior uvea

1. Pupil – pigment imprinting on the anterior lens capsule (Vossius ring – *Fig. 23.11*), mydriasis, and radial pupillary margin tears.

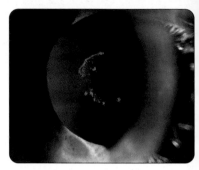

Fig. 23.11 Vossius ring

2. Iridodialysis – D-shaped pupil and a dark bi-convex area near the limbus (*Fig. 23.12*).

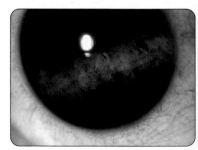

Fig. 23.12 Large iridodialysis

3. Ciliary body – temporary cessation of aqueous secretion (ciliary shock) resulting in ocular hypotony.

Lens

1. Cataract – flower-shaped ('rosette') opacity (*Fig. 23.13*).

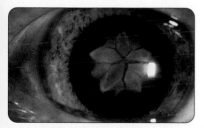

Fig. 23.13 Rosette cataract

2. **Subluxation** – lens tends to deviate towards the meridian of intact zonule (*Fig. 23.14*).

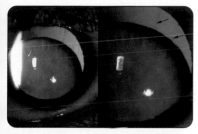

Fig. 23.14 Lens subluxation (arrows indicate ruptured zonule)

3. **Dislocation** – due to 360° zonular rupture may be into the vitreous (*Fig. 23.15*) or anterior chamber (*Fig. 23.16*).

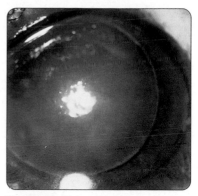

Fig. 23.16 Dislocation into anterior chamber

Globe rupture

Rupture is usually in the vicinity of Schlemm canal, and may be associated with prolapse of intraocular structures. Occasionally, the rupture is posterior (occult) with little visible anterior segment damage.

Retina and choroid

1. **Commotio retinae** – grey appearance most frequently involves the temporal fundus (*Fig. 23.17*).

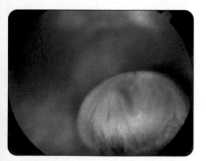

Fig. 23.15 Dislocation into vitreous

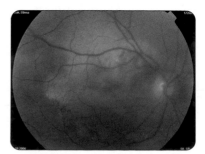

Fig. 23.17 Commotio retinae

2. **Choroidal rupture** – white crescent-shaped, vertical streak of exposed underlying sclera concentric with the optic disc (*Fig. 23.18*).

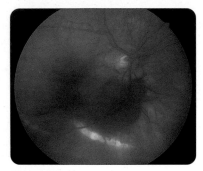

Fig. 23.18 Choroidal rupture

3. **Retinal breaks and RD** (see Chapter 19).

Optic nerve

1. **Optic neuropathy** – fundus examination is initially normal and then optic atrophy ensues; treatment is unsatisfactory.
2. **Optic nerve avulsion** – striking cavity where the optic nerve head has retracted from the dural sheath.

Non-accidental injury (shaken baby syndrome)

1. **Definition** – physical abuse in children usually under the age of 2 years; suspected whenever characteristic ophthalmic features are identified in the absence of a convincing alternative explanation.
2. **Presentation** – irritability, lethargy, and vomiting.

3. **Systemic features** – subdural haematoma and impact injuries to the head.
4. **Ocular features** – periorbital bruising and subconjunctival haemorrhages, retinal haemorrhages typically involving different retinal layers, poor visual responses, and APD.

Penetrating corneal trauma

The technique of primary repair depends on the extent of the wound and associated complications such as iris incarceration, flat anterior chamber and damage to intraocular contents.

1. **Small shelving** – often heal spontaneously or with the aid of a soft bandage contact lens.
2. **Medium-sized** – usually require suturing, especially if the anterior chamber is shallow or flat.
3. **With iris involvement** (*Fig. 23.19*) – requires iris abscission and suturing.

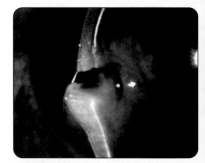

Fig. 23.19 Penetrating wound with iris incarceration

4. **With lens damage** – requires suturing and lens removal.

Penetrating scleral trauma

1. **Anterior** – may be associated with uveal prolapse (*Fig. 23.20*) and vitreous incarceration which must be managed appropriately to prevent subsequent fibrous proliferation and tractional RD.

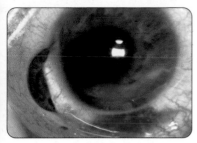

Fig. 23.20 Scleral laceration with iris prolapse

2. **Posterior** – frequently associated with retinal breaks that require prophylactic treatment after the wound has been sutured.

Superficial foreign bodies

1. **Subtarsal** – pathognomonic pattern of linear corneal abrasions; lid is everted and the foreign body removed.
2. **Corneal** – easy to remove with a hypodermic needle; ferrous foreign bodies often result in rust staining of the bed of the abrasion (rust ring) which must also be removed.

Intraocular foreign bodies

Technique of removal

1. **Magnet** – of ferrous foreign bodies involves a sclerotomy adjacent to the foreign body, application of a magnet followed by cryotherapy to the retinal break.
2. **Forceps** – of non-magnetic foreign bodies and magnetic foreign bodies that cannot be removed with a magnet involves pars plana vitrectomy and removal of the foreign body with forceps either through the pars plana or limbus depending on its size.

Siderosis

1. **Definition** – intraocular ferrous foreign body undergoes dissociation that results in the deposition of iron in the intraocular epithelial structures – notably the lens epithelium, iris and ciliary body epithelium (*Fig. 23.21*), and sensory retina where it exerts a toxic effect.

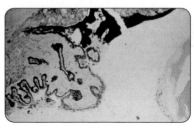

Fig. 23.21 Iron deposits in the anterior uvea stained black

2. **Signs** – radial iron deposits on the anterior lens capsule and reddish brown staining of the iris (*Fig. 23.22*).
3. **Complications** – secondary glaucoma and pigmentary retinopathy.
4. **ERG** – progressive attenuation of the b-wave.

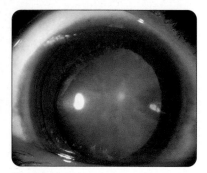

Fig. 23.22 Siderosis caused by an iron foreign body in the lens

Chalcosis

- The ocular reaction to an intraocular foreign body with a high copper content involves a violent endophthalmitis-like picture.
- An alloy such as brass or bronze, with a relatively low copper content, results in chalcosis, a picture similar to that of Wilson disease with a Kayser–Fleischer ring, anterior 'sunflower' cataract, and golden retinal plaques.

Enucleation

1. Primary – performed only for very severe injuries with no prospect of retention of vision (*Fig. 23.23*).

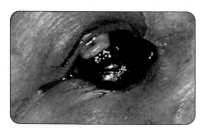

Fig. 23.23 Eye suitable for primary enucleation

2. Secondary – may be considered following primary repair if the eye is severely and irreversibly damaged, particularly if it is also unsightly and uncomfortable (*Fig. 23.24*).

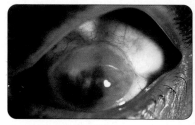

Fig. 23.24 Eye suitable for secondary enucleation

Sympathetic ophthalmitis

1. Definition
- Bilateral granulomatous panuveitis occurring after penetrating trauma often associated with uveal prolapse or intraocular surgery.
- The traumatized eye is referred to as the *exciting* eye and the fellow eye, which also develops uveitis, is the *sympathizing* eye.

2. Presentation – in 65% of cases is between 2 weeks and 3 months after initial injury; 90% of all cases occur within the first year.

3. Signs in chronological order:
- Exciting eye – evidence of the initial trauma and is red and irritable.
- Sympathizing – photophobic and irritable.
- Both eyes – granulomatous anterior uveitis (*Fig. 23.25*).
- Multifocal mid-peripheral choroidal infiltrates (*Fig. 23.26*).

- Exudative RD in severe cases.
- 'Sunset-glow' appearance as in VKH (see Fig. 14.28).

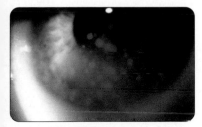

Fig. 23.25 Mutton fat keratic precipitates

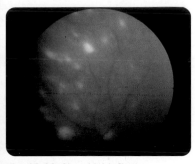

Fig. 23.26 Choroidal infiltrates

4. **Systemic manifestations** – same as in VKH but less common.
5. **Treatment**
   a. *Enucleation* – within first 10 days following trauma only if the visual prognosis is hopeless (see Fig. 23.23).
   b. *Topical* – steroids and mydriatics.
   c. *Systemic* – steroids and occasionally ciclosporin or azathioprine.

Bacterial endophthalmitis

- Endophthalmitis develops in about 8% of cases of penetrating trauma with retained foreign body. *Staphylococcus* spp. and *Bacillus* spp. are isolated from about 90% of culture positive cases.
- Risk factors – delay in primary repair, retained intraocular foreign body, and the position and extent of the laceration.
- Clinical signs and treatment – same in acute postoperative endophthalmitis.
- Prophylactic ciprofloxacin 750 mg b.d. in open globe injuries.

Chemical injuries

Emergency treatment

1. **Copious irrigation** – normal saline (or equivalent) should be used to irrigate the eye for 15–30 minutes or until pH is normalized.
2. **Double-eversion of the eyelids** – to remove any retained particulate matter trapped in the fornices.
3. **Debridement of necrotic epithelium** – to allow for proper re-epithelialization.

Grading of severity

Grading is performed on the basis of corneal clarity and severity of limbal ischaemia.
1. **Grade 1** – clear cornea and no limbal ischaemia (excellent prognosis).
2. **Grade 2** – hazy cornea but with visible iris details and less than

one-third of limbal ischaemia (good prognosis – *Fig. 23.27*).

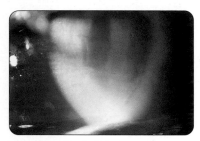

Fig. 23.27 Grade 2 burn

3. **Grade 3** – total loss of corneal epithelium, stromal haze obscuring iris details and between one-third and half of limbal ischaemia (guarded prognosis – *Fig. 23.28*).

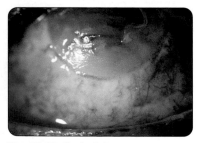

Fig. 23.28 Grade 3 burn

4. **Grade 4** – opaque cornea and more than half of limbal ischaemia (very poor prognosis – *Fig. 23.29*).

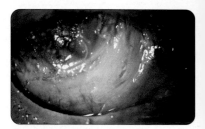

Fig. 23.29 Grade 4 burn

Treatment

1. **Mild (grade 1 and 2) burns** – short course of topical steroids, cycloplegics and prophylactic antibiotics for about 7 days.
2. **Severe burns**
   a. *Topical steroids* – used initially but must be tailed off after 7–10 days and replaced by topical NSAIDs.
   b. *Topical sodium ascorbate 10%* – 2-hourly in addition to a systemic dose of 2 g q.i.d.
   c. *Topical sodium citrate 10%* – 2-hourly for about 10 days.
   d. *Tetracyclines* – topical and systemically (doxycycline 100 mg b.d.).
   e. *Other* – limbal cell transplantation and amniotic membrane grafting.

Chapter 24

Systemic Disease

Connective tissue disease

Rheumatoid arthritis

1. Systemic
- Female preponderance.
- Symmetrical, destructive, deforming, inflammatory polyarthropathy.
- Associations – rheumatoid nodules (*Fig. 24.1*), pulmonary fibrosis, peripheral neuropathy, and cutaneous vasculitis.

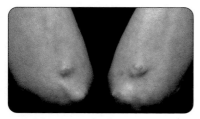

Fig. 24.1 Rheumatoid nodules

2. Ophthalmic – KCS, scleritis, ulcerative keratitis, and acquired superior oblique tendon sheath syndrome.

Juvenile idiopathic arthritis

1. Systemic – inflammatory arthritis of at least 6 weeks duration occurring before the age of 16 years; three types of presentation:
   a. Pauciarticular (<5 joints).
   b. Polyarticular (>4 joints – *Fig. 24.2*).
   c. Systemic (variable number of joints).
2. Ophthalmic – CAU.

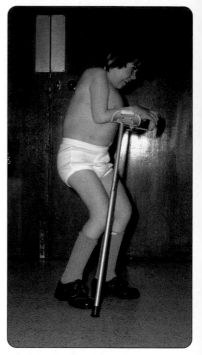

Fig. 24.2 Polyarticular JIA

Systemic lupus erythematosus

1. Systemic
- Predominantly affects young females.
- Non-organ specific disease characterized by widespread vasculitis and tissue damage; butterfly facial rash (*Fig. 24.3*), arthritis, renal and cardiovascular disease, and anaemia.

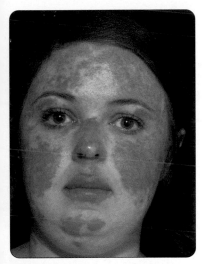

Fig. 24.3 Butterfly rash in SLE

2. Ophthalmic – madarosis, KCS, scleritis, peripheral ulcerative keratitis, retinal vasculitis, and optic neuropathy.

Wegener granulomatosis

1. Systemic – Idiopathic, multisystem granulomatous disorder affecting predominantly the respiratory tract (Fig. 24.4) and kidneys.

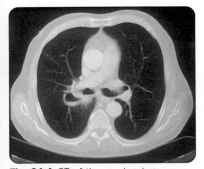

Fig. 24.4 CT of thorax showing pulmonary cavitation

2. Ophthalmic – necrotizing scleritis, peripheral ulcerative keratitis, orbital inflammatory disease, nasolacrimal obstruction, dacryocystitis, tarsal-conjunctival disease, and occlusive retinal periarteritis.

Polyarteritis nodosa

1. Systemic – idiopathic, potentially lethal, vasculitis; purpura (Fig. 24.5), livedo reticularis, dermal infarcts, muscular weakness, renal disease, and cardiovascular disease; ocular involvement may precede the systemic manifestations by several years.

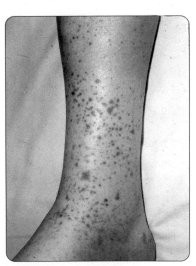

Fig. 24.5 Purpura in PAN

2. Ophthalmic – necrotizing scleritis, peripheral ulcerative keratitis, orbital inflammatory disease, and occlusive retinal periarteritis.

Relapsing polychondritis

1. **Systemic** – small vessel vasculitis primarily involving cartilage; swelling of the pinnae, hoarse voice, cardiac valve defects, arthritis, and saddle-shaped nasal deformity (*Fig. 24.6*).

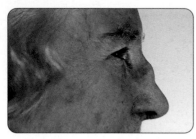

Fig. 24.6 Saddle-shaped nose in relapsing polychondritis

2. **Ophthalmic** – scleritis and anterior uveitis.

Sjögren syndrome

1. **Systemic** – autoimmune inflammation and destruction of lacrimal and salivary glands; enlargement of salivary glands, xerostomia that may result in dental caries (*Fig. 24.7*), dry nasal passages and vagina, and Raynaud phenomenon.
   a. *Primary* – exists in isolation.
   b. *Secondary* – associated with other diseases such as rheumatoid arthritis, SLE, systemic sclerosis, primary biliary cirrhosis, chronic active hepatitis and myasthenia gravis.
2. **Ophthalmic** – KCS and Adie pupil (rare).

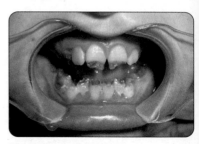

Fig. 24.7 Dental caries in severe Sjögren syndrome

Systemic sclerosis

1. **Systemic**
   - Female preponderance.
   - Chronic disease affecting the skin and internal organs.
   - Fixed facial expression, sclerodactyly (*Fig. 24.8*), subcutaneous calcification, oesophageal dysmobility, and cardiac, pulmonary are renal disease.

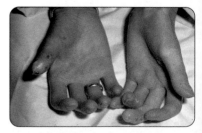

Fig. 24.8 Sclerodactyly

2. **Ophthalmic** – eyelid tightening and telangiectasia, KCS, conjunctival forniceal shortening, nodular episcleritis, and retinal cotton-wool spots.

Giant cell arteritis

1. **Systemic** – granulomatous necrotizing arteritis with a predilection for large and medium-size arteries, particularly the superficial temporal (*Fig. 24.9*), ophthalmic, posterior ciliary and proximal vertebral.

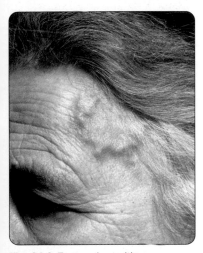

Fig. 24.9 Temporal arteritis

2. **Ophthalmic** – AION, cilioretinal artery occlusion (may be combined with optic neuropathy), central retinal artery occlusion, transient ischaemic attacks, cotton-wool spots, ocular ischaemic syndrome, and ophthalmoplegia.

Dermatomyositis – polymyositis

1. **Systemic** – autoimmune degenerative and inflammatory changes in skeletal muscle; widespread erythematous rash (not in polymyositis), muscular pain and weakness, ulceration over bony prominences (*Fig. 24.10*), and high incidence of systemic malignancy.

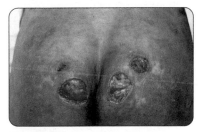

Fig. 24.10 Ulceration in dermatomyositis

2. **Ophthalmic** – eyelid heliotrope rash, periorbital erythema and oedema, KCS, scleritis, cotton-wool spots, and retinal periarteritis.

Mixed connective tissue disease

1. **Systemic** – combination of SLE, systemic sclerosis, and polymyositis.
2. **Ophthalmic** – KCS.

Ehlers–Danlos syndrome type 6

1. **Inheritance** – AR.
2. **Error** – deficiency of procollagen lysyl hydroxylase.
3. **Systemic** – fragile hyperelastic skin (*Fig. 24.11*), joint hypermobility, bleeding diathesis, and cardiovascular disease.

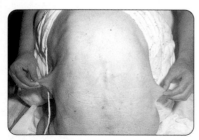

Fig. 24.11 Hyperelastic skin

4. **Ophthalmic** – ocular fragility, keratoconus, ectopia lentis, blue sclera, high myopia and RD, microcornea, angioid streaks, and epicanthic folds.

Marfan syndrome

1. **Inheritance** – AD.
2. **Systemic** – tall, thin, stature, high-arched palate, arachnodactyly (*Fig. 24.12*), and cardiovascular disease.

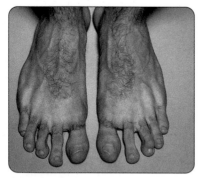

Fig. 24.12 Arachnodactyly

3. **Ophthalmic** – ectopia lentis, hypoplasia of dilator pupillae, angle anomaly, glaucoma, keratoconus, cornea plana, microspherophakia, myopia and RD.

Weill–Marchesani syndrome

1. **Inheritance** – AR.
2. **Systemic** – short stature, brachydactyly, and mental handicap.
3. **Ophthalmic** – microspherophakia, ectopia lentis, and glaucoma.

Stickler syndrome (hereditary arthro-ophthalmopathy)

1. **Inheritance** – AD.
2. **Systemic** – flat nasal bridge and maxillary hypoplasia (*Fig. 24.13*), deafness, and arthropathy.

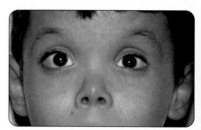

Fig. 24.13 Stickler syndrome

3. **Ophthalmic** – empty vitreous, myopia, lens subluxation, atypical lattice degeneration and RD.

Pseudoxanthoma elasticum

1. **Inheritance** – AR or AD.
2. **Systemic**
   - Calcification, fragmentation and degeneration of elastic fibres in the skin (*Fig. 24.14*), eyes, and cardiovascular system.
   - Loss of peripheral pulses, coronary artery disease, hypertension, and mitral valve prolapse.

- Inflammation, calcification and ossification of ligaments and capsules of joints with resultant bony ankylosis of the axial skeleton; calcification of spinal ligaments gives rise to a 'bamboo' appearance on x-ray (*Fig. 24.15*).
- Association – inflammatory bowel disease.

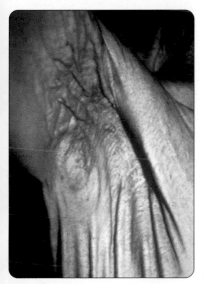

Fig. 24.14 Loose skin in pseudo-xanthoma elasticum

3. Ophthalmic – angioid streaks (Groenblad–Strandberg syndrome) and blue sclera.

Takayasu disease

1. Systemic – progressive obliterative arteritis of the aorta and its main branches.
2. Ophthalmic – slow-flow retinopathy, amaurosis fugax, and ocular ischaemic syndrome.

Spondyloarthropathies

Ankylosing spondylitis

1. Systemic
- Affects young males, 90% of whom are HLA-B27 positive.

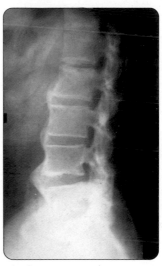

Fig. 24.15 Bamboo spine

2. Ophthalmic – AAU and rarely conjunctivitis.

Reiter syndrome (reactive arthritis)

1. Systemic
- Affects young males, 85% of whom are HLA-B27 positive; 30% develop spondyloarthropathy.
- Triad of non-specific (non-gonococcal) urethritis, conjunctivitis, and arthritis.

- Associations – oral ulceration, circinate balanitis, keratoderma blenorrhagica (*Fig. 24.16*), and cardiac disease.

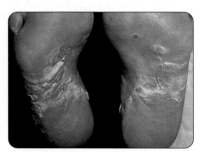

Fig. 24.16 Keratoderma blenorrhagica

2. Ophthalmic – conjunctivitis, AAU, nummular keratitis, episcleritis, and scleritis.

Psoriatic arthritis

1. Systemic
- Increased prevalence of HLA-B27 and HLA-B17.
- Nail dystrophy and peripheral arthritis (*Fig. 24.17*), and occasionally spondyloarthropathy.

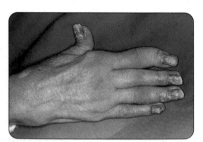

Fig. 24.17 Nail dystrophy and arthritis

2. Ophthalmic – AAU, conjunctivitis, KCS, and marginal corneal infiltrates.

Skeletal disease

Paget disease

1. Systemic
- Chronic, progressive disease characterized by excessive and disorganized resorption and formation of bone.
- Enlargement and deformity of bone (*Fig. 24.18*), compressive phenomena, deafness, heart failure and predisposition to osteosarcoma.

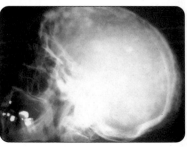

Fig. 24.18 Enlarged skull

2. Ophthalmic – optic atrophy, proptosis, ocular motor nerve palsies, and angioid streaks.

Osteogenesis imperfecta

Type 1
1. Inheritance – AD.
2. Systemic – deafness; few fractures with little or no deformity.
3. Ophthalmic – blue sclera, megalocornea, and corneal arcus.

Type 2

1. **Inheritance** – AR or sporadic.
2. **Systemic** – severe deafness, dental anomalies, multiple fractures and short limbs; uniformly lethal.
3. **Ophthalmic** – blue sclera.

Type 3

1. **Inheritance** – heterogenous.
2. **Systemic** – dental anomalies, triangular face, and bony deformity (*Fig. 24.19*)

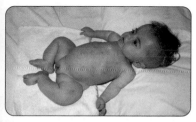

Fig. 24.19 Osteogenesis imperfecta type 3

3. **Ophthalmic** – blue sclera.

Type 4

1. **Inheritance** – heterogenous.
2. **Systemic** – variable deafness and skeletal anomalies.
3. **Ophthalmic** – blue sclera is uncommon.

Parry–Romberg syndrome

1. **Systemic** – idiopathic progressive hemifacial atrophy (*Fig. 24.20*).
2. **Ophthalmic** – enophthalmos, restrictive strabismus, congenital iris hypochromia, and Horner syndrome.

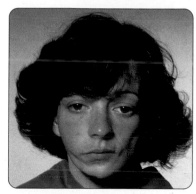

Fig. 24.20 Parry–Romberg syndrome

Gastrointestinal disease

Ulcerative colitis

1. **Systemic**
   - Chronic, relapsing inflammatory disease, involving the rectum and extending proximally to involve part or all of the large intestine.
   - Associations – spondyloarthropathy, pyoderma gangrenosum (*Fig. 24.21*), hepatic disease, and thrombosis; predisposition to colonic carcinoma.

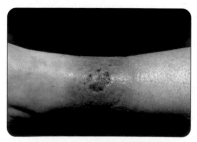

Fig. 24.21 Pyoderma gangrenosum

2. **Ophthalmic** – AAU, peripheral corneal infiltrates, conjunctivitis, episcleritis, scleritis, and retinal vasculitis.

Crohn disease (regional ileitis)

1. **Systemic**
   - Chronic, relapsing disease characterized by multifocal, full-thickness, non-caseating granulomatous inflammation of the intestinal wall that may cause strictures.
   - Associations – peripheral arthritis or spondyloarthropathy, finger clubbing, and perianal abscess and fistula (*Fig. 24.22*).

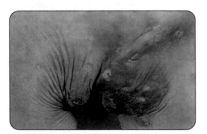

Fig. 24.22 Perianal abscess and fistula

2. **Ophthalmic** – AAU, conjunctivitis, episcleritis, peripheral corneal infiltrates, and retinal periphlebitis.

Cirrhosis – primary biliary

1. **Systemic** – autoimmune, cholestatic disease which typically affects women; fatigue, hepatomegaly, jaundice, spider naevi (*Fig. 24.23*), white nails, and palmar erythema; predisposition to liver carcinoma.
2. **Ophthalmic** – KCS.

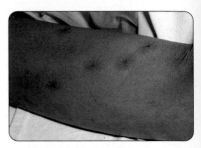

Fig. 24.23 Spider naevi

Pancreatitis – acute

1. **Systemic** – acute abdomen, often associated with biliary disease and alcoholism.
2. **Ophthalmic** – cotton-wool spots (Purtscher-like retinopathy).

Alagille syndrome (arteriohepatic dysplasia)

1. **Inheritance** – AD.
2. **Systemic** – neonatal jaundice due to absence or paucity of intrahepatic bile ducts, cardiopulmonary malformations, peculiar facies, and vertebral and CNS abnormalities.
3. **Ophthalmic** – posterior embryotoxon, optic disc drusen, and pigmentary retinopathy.

Hirschsprung disease

1. **Systemic** – congenital absence of intestinal ganglion cells, resulting in constipation and abdominal distension (congenital megacolon).
2. **Ophthalmic** – bilateral sectoral iris hypochromia (*Fig. 24.24*).

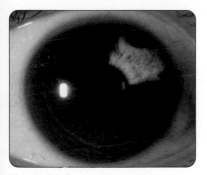

Fig. 24.24 Sectoral iris hypochromia

Turgot syndrome

1. **Inheritance** – AD.
2. **Systemic** – intestinal adenomatous polyposis predisposing to carcinoma, and CNS tumours.
3. **Ophthalmic** – atypical CHRPE.

Acquired non-infectious multisystem disease

Sarcoidosis

1. **Systemic**
   - Non-caseating granulomatous disorder with a clinical spectrum of disease varying from mild single-organ involvement to potentially fatal multisystem disease.
   - Tissues most commonly involved – mediastinal (*Fig. 24.25*) and superficial lymph nodes, lungs, liver, spleen, skin, parotid glands, phalangeal bones, and the eye.
2. **Ophthalmic** – anterior uveitis (acute or chronic) intermediate uveitis, posterior uveitis, KCS, and conjunctival nodules.

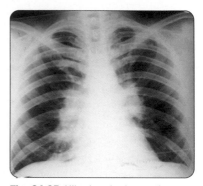

Fig. 24.25 Hilar lymphadenopathy

Behçet syndrome

1. **Systemic**
   - Idiopathic disease that presents in the 3rd decade with a masculine preponderance.
   - Typically affects patients from the eastern Mediterranean region and Japan and is strongly associated with HLA-B51.
   - Recurrent orogenital ulceration (*Fig. 24.26*), and vasculitis.
   - Associations – cardiovascular disease, venous thrombosis, skin hypersensitivity, and arthritis.
2. **Ophthalmic** – panuveitis, occlusive vasculitis, conjunctivitis, conjunctival ulceration, episcleritis, and scleritis.

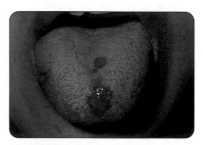

Fig. 24.26 Aphthous ulceration

Vogt–Koyanagi–Harada syndrome

1. Systemic
- Autoimmune disease against melanocytes causing inflammation of melanocyte-containing tissues such as the uvea, ear and meninges.
- Predominantly affects Hispanics, Japanese and pigmented individuals, and is associated with HLA-DR1 and HLA-DR4.

2. Subdivision
- **a.** *Vogt–Koyanagi* – skin changes (vitiligo and poliosis – *Fig. 24.27*) and anterior uveitis.
- **b.** *Harada* – neurological features and exudative RD predominate.

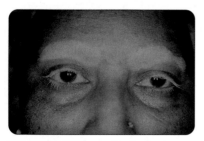

Fig. 24.27 Vitiligo and poliosis

3. Ophthalmic – bilateral granulomatous anterior or multifocal posterior uveitis and exudative RD.

Goodpasture syndrome

1. Systemic – rapidly progressive disease involving the lungs and kidneys caused by a linear deposition of anti-basement membrane antibodies.

2. Ophthalmic – retinal haemorrhages, cotton-wool spots, and exudative RD.

Churg–Strauss syndrome (allergic granulomatosis)

1. Systemic – allergic disease characterized by granulomatous inflammation involving the respiratory tract and necrotizing vasculitis; pulmonary hilar adenopathy and infiltrates (Löffler syndrome), cutaneous vasculitis, heart disease and hypertension, arthralgia, and renal disease.

2. Ophthalmic – conjunctival granuloma, scleritis, orbital inflammation, and retinal periarteritis.

Kawasaki disease (mucocutaneous lymph node syndrome)

1. Systemic – idiopathic, vasculitis-like illness affecting young children; lymphadenopathy, strawberry tongue, rash, indurated oedema of extremities (*Fig. 24.28*), and arthropathy; later cardiac disease.

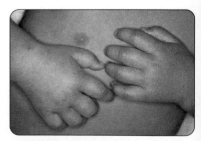

Fig. 24.28 Oedema in Kawasaki syndrome

2. Ophthalmic – acute bilateral conjunctivitis, superficial punctate keratitis, AAU, and retinal vasculitis.

Familial juvenile systemic granulomatosis syndrome (Blau syndrome, Jabs disease)

1. Inheritance – AD.
2. Systemic – childhood onset of involvement of skin, eyes, and joints; painful cystic joint swelling and contractures and intermittent perioral rash.
3. Ophthalmic – panuveitis and multifocal choroiditis.

Neonatal-onset multisystem inflammatory disease

1. Systemic – idiopathic, chronic relapsing disease that involves skin, joints, and the CNS.
2. Ophthalmic – anterior uveitis.

Viral infection

Acquired immunodeficiency syndrome (AIDS)

1. Systemic – HIV acquired by homosexual contact and occasionally by contaminated blood or needles; opportunistic infections, tumours (notably Kaposi sarcoma – *Fig. 24.29*), wasting syndrome, and encephalopathy.
2. Ophthalmic
   a. *Eyelids* – blepharitis, Kaposi sarcoma, multiple molluscum lesions, and severe HZO.
   b. *Orbit* – cellulitis and B-cell lymphoma.

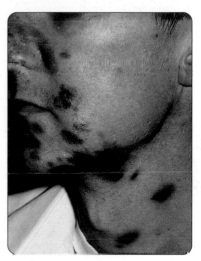

Fig. 24.29 Kaposi sarcoma

   c. *Anterior segment*
   • Conjunctiva – Kaposi sarcoma, squamous cell carcinoma and microangiopathy.
   • Keratitis – microsporidial, herpes simplex and herpes zoster.
   • KCS.
   d. *Posterior segment* – HIV retinopathy, CMV retinitis, PORN, toxoplasma retinitis, choroidal cryptococcosis, choroidal pneumocystosis, and B-cell intraocular lymphoma.

Bacterial infection

Tuberculosis

1. Systemic – *M. tuberculosis* which primarily affects the lungs but it may spread by the blood stream to other sites to form a generalized (miliary) infection involving many organs and bone; scrofula describes lymph node

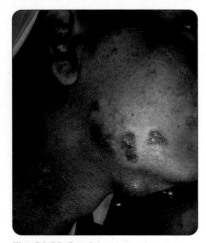

Fig. 24.30 Scrofula

enlargement with discharging
sinuses (*Fig. 24.30*).

2. Ophthalmic – Parinaud oculoglandular syndrome, phlyctenulosis, IK,
granulomatous anterior uveitis,
scleritis, focal or multifocal
choroiditis, serpiginous-like choroiditis, occlusive retinal periphlebitis,
and Eales disease.

Acquired syphilis

1. Systemic – *Treponema pallidum*
sexually acquired; divided into the
following stages:
   a. *Primary* – chancre.
   b. *Secondary* – lymphadenopathy,
   maculopapular rash (*Fig. 24.31*),
   mucous patches, and condylo-
   mata lata.
   c. *Latent* – may last for years.
   d. *Tertiary* – gummatous infiltration,
   aortitis, tabes dorsalis, and
   general paralysis of the insane.

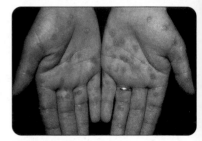

Fig. 24.31 Syphilitic rash

2. Ophthalmic – AAU, granulomatous
anterior uveitis, IK, scleritis,
madarosis, optic neuritis, Argyll–
Robertson pupils, and ocular motor
nerve palsies.

Lyme disease (borreliosis)

1. Systemic – *Borrelia burgdorferi*
transmitted through the bite of a
hard-shelled tick of the genus *Ixodes*
which feeds on deer.
   • Early stage – annular expanding
   skin lesion (erythema chronicum
   migrans – *Fig. 24.32*), lymphadenopathy, and constitutional
   features.
   • Late complications – chronic
   arthritis, polyneuropathy, and
   encephalopathy.

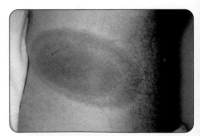

Fig. 24.32 Erythema chronica migrans

2. Ophthalmic – transient follicular conjunctivitis, keratitis, episcleritis, scleritis, uveitis, orbital myositis, optic neuritis, neuroretinitis, ocular motor nerve palsies, and reversible Horner syndrome.

Leprosy (Hansen disease)

1. Systemic – *M. leprae* that has an affinity for skin, peripheral nerves, and the eye
   a. *Lepromatous* – leonine facies, neuropathy that may result in shortening of digits (*Fig. 24.33*), cutaneous nodules, and saddle-shaped nose.
   b. *Tuberculoid* – hypopigmented skin patches and thickened cutaneous nerves.

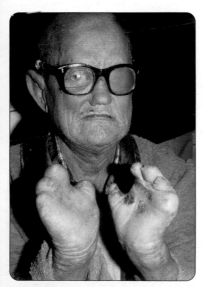

Fig. 24.33 Shortening of digits in leprosy

2. Ophthalmic – madarosis, trichiasis, conjunctivitis, episcleritis, scleritis, and CAU.

Cat-scratch disease (benign lymphoreticulosis)

1. Systemic – *Bartonella henselae* transmitted by the scratch or bite of a cat; constitutional features, pustule at the site of inoculation and regional lymphadenopathy.
2. Ophthalmic – neuroretinitis, Parinaud oculoglandular syndrome, focal choroiditis, intermediate uveitis, exudative maculopathy, retinal vascular occlusion and panuveitis.

Chlamydial genital infection

1. Systemic – *Chlamydia trachomatis* transmitted sexually or occasionally acquired by transmission from an infected mother to baby during delivery.
   a. *In males* – urethritis, epididymitis, and may act as a trigger for Reiter disease.
   b. *In females* – cervicitis, chronic salpingitis, peritonitis and perihepatitis (Fitz-Hugh–Curtis syndrome).
2. Ophthalmic – chronic conjunctivitis in adults and neonatal conjunctivitis.

Gonorrhoea

1. Systemic – *Neisseria gonorrhoeae* transmitted sexually; urethral discharge in males (*Fig. 24.34*) and vaginal discharge in females.
2. Ophthalmic – purulent conjunctivitis and secondary keratitis.

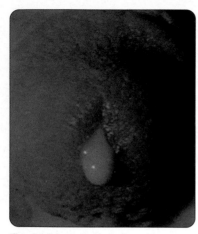

Fig. 24.34 Urethral discharge in gonorrhoea

Nocardia

1. **Systemic** – *Nocardia asteroides,* opportunistic infection in immuno-compromised patients acquired by inhalation; suppurative necrosis and abscess formation in the lungs, brain, and skin.
2. **Ocular disease** – intraocular suppuration.

Bacterial endocarditis

1. **Systemic** – *S. aureus* infection in patients with pre-existing cardiac abnormalities; fever, heart murmurs, finger clubbing, splenomegaly, petechial skin haemorrhages, finger clubbing, Osler nodes (tender lesions on finger tips), and subungual splinter haemorrhages (*Fig. 24.35*)
2. **Ophthalmic** – subconjunctival haemorrhage, Roth spots, endogenous endophthalmitis, and retinal artery occlusion.

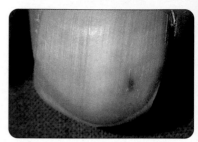

Fig. 24.35 Subungual haemorrhage

Whipple disease (intestinal lipodystrophy)

1. **Systemic** – *Tropheryma whipplei* infection that presents with weight loss, diarrhoea, and abdominal pain; later involvement of the CNS, lungs, and joints may occur.
2. **Ophthalmic** – secondary to CNS involvement or various types of intraocular inflammation.

Lymphogranuloma venereum

1. **Systemic** – strain of *Chlamydia trachomatis* transmitted sexually; painless genital ulceration and painful inguinal lymphadenopathy (*Fig. 24.36*).

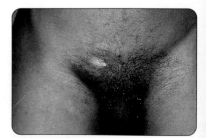

Fig. 24.36 Lymphogranuloma venereum

2. Ophthalmic – Parinaud oculoglandular syndrome and IK.

Chancroid

1. Systemic – *Haemophilus ducreyi* transmitted sexually; painful genital ulceration and inguinal lymphadenopathy that may suppurate.
2. Ophthalmic – Parinaud oculoglandular fever.

Leptospirosis

1. Systemic – *Leptospira interrogans* acquired by the bite of a rat; subsequent renal, liver, meningeal and brain disease.
2. Ophthalmic – subconjunctival haemorrhage, anterior uveitis, retinal haemorrhages and cotton-wool spots, choroiditis, and papilloedema.

Tularaemia

1. Systemic – *Francisella tularensis*; transmitted from an infected animal, by a tick bite, by ingestion of infected meat, or by inhalation; cutaneous ulceration and regional lymphadenopathy, and pneumonia.
2. Ophthalmic – Parinaud oculoglandular syndrome.

Fungal infection

Cryptococcosis

1. Systemic – *Cryptococcus neoformans* acquired through inhalation and primarily affects immunocompromised patients; meningitis, mucocutaneous lesions, and multiple organ involvement.
2. Ophthalmic – choroiditis.

Candidiasis – systemic

1. Systemic – *C. albicans* acquired by intravenous drug abuse, long-term indwelling catheters, and affects severely immunocompromised patients causing multiple organ involvement.
2. Ophthalmic – multifocal choroiditis, vitreous 'cotton' ball colonies, retinal haemorrhages, endophthalmitis and retinal necrosis.

Parasitic infestation

Toxoplasmosis

1. Systemic – *Toxoplasma gondii* acquired transplacentally, by ingestion of uncooked meat, or ingestion of cysts following accidental contamination of hands when disposing of cat litter trays and then subsequent transfer on to food (see *Fig. 14.30*).
2. Ophthalmic – congenital macular scars or retinitis in later life.

Toxocariasis

1. Systemic – *Toxocara canis* acquired by accidental ingestion of soil or food contaminated with ova shed in dog faeces; very young children who eat dirt (pica) or are in close contact with puppies are at particular risk of acquiring the disease.
2. Ophthalmic – posterior pole granuloma, peripheral granuloma, or chronic endophthalmitis.

Onchocerciasis (river blindness)

1. Systemic – *Onchocerca volvulus* transmitted by the bite of the black fly; microfilariae cause cutaneous lesions, subcutaneous nodules

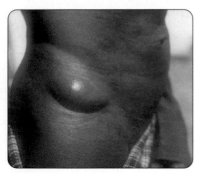

Fig. 24.37 Onchocercoma

(onchocercomas – *Fig. 24.37*), and lymphoedema.
2. **Ophthalmic** – microfilariae in the aqueous, CAU, keratitis, and chorioretinitis.

Cysticercosis

1. **Systemic** – *Cysticercus cellulosae* acquired by ingesting contaminated pork, vegetables or water; involvement of the lungs, muscle, and brain
2. **Ophthalmic** – involvement of the orbit, vitreous, and retina.

Coccidioidomycosis

1. **Systemic** – *Coccidioides immitis* acquired by inhalation; pulmonary infection, erythema nodosum, arthropathy, and meningitis.
2. **Ophthalmic** – multifocal choroiditis, phlyctenulosis, and anterior uveitis.

Histoplasmosis

1. **Systemic** – *Histoplasma capsulatum* acquired by inhalation; usually asymptomatic occasionally pulmonary involvement, or disseminated disease in AIDS.

2. **Ophthalmic** – wet maculopathy, and multifocal choroiditis associated with peripapillary atrophy.

Rhinosporidiosis

1. **Systemic** – *Rhinosporidium seeberi*; warts and polyps in the nasal mucosa.
2. **Ophthalmic** – polyp-like conjunctival lesions (*Fig. 24.38*).

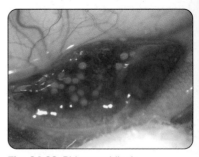

Fig. 24.38 Rhinosporidiosis

Sporotrichosis

1. **Systemic** – *Sporothrix schenckii*; warts and ulcers, and occasionally dissemination to the lungs, bone, and brain.
2. **Ophthalmic** – Parinaud oculoglandular syndrome and chronic endophthalmitis.

Intrauterine infections (embryopathies)

Rubella

1. **Systemic** – deafness, cardiac malformation, and mental handicap.
2. **Ophthalmic** – microphthalmos, cataract, keratitis, glaucoma, and retinopathy.

Toxoplasmosis

1. **Systemic** – seizures, hydrocephalus, intracranial calcification (Fig. 24.39), and deafness.

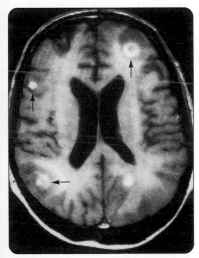

Fig. 24.39 Axial CT shows intracranial calcification

2. **Ophthalmic** – chorioretinitis, microphthalmos, cataract, and optic atrophy.

Cytomegalovirus

1. **Systemic** – jaundice, hepatospleno-megaly and intracranial calcification.
2. **Ophthalmic** – chorioretinitis, microphthalmos, keratitis, cataract, and optic atrophy.

Varicella

1. **Systemic** – mental handicap, cutaneous scarring and limb deformities.

2. **Ophthalmic** – microphthalmos, Horner syndrome, cataract, chorioretinitis, optic disc hypoplasia, and optic atrophy.

Syphilis

1. **Systemic** – deafness, malformed incisors, saddle-shaped nose, and osteopathy.
2. **Ophthalmic** – IK, anterior uveitis, retinopathy, and optic atrophy.

Mucocutaneous disease

Mucous membrane pemphigoid

1. **Systemic** – autoimmune blistering disease that most frequently involves mucous membranes, particularly the mouth (Fig. 24.40), and less commonly the skin.

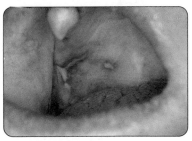

Fig. 24.40 Oral blisters

2. **Ophthalmic** – cicatrizing conjunctivitis in 75% of cases with oral involvement but only 25% of those with skin lesions; occasionally it occurs in isolation.

Stevens–Johnson syndrome

1. **Systemic** – delayed hypersensitivity response to drugs or a response to epithelial cell antigens modified by drug exposure; oral involvement and haemorrhagic crusting of the lips (*Fig. 24.41*), genital involvement, and 'target' skin lesions.

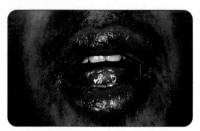

Fig. 24.41 Stevens–Johnson syndrome

2. **Ophthalmic** – self-limiting papillary conjunctivitis, pseudo-membranous or membranous conjunctivitis, and cicatrizing conjunctivitis.

Atopic eczema (dermatitis)

1. **Systemic** – idiopathic, often familial, disease, often associated with asthma and hay fever; two types are facial and flexural (*Fig. 24.42*).

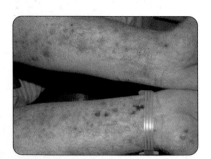

Fig. 24.42 Flexural eczema

2. **Ophthalmic** – madarosis, staphylo-coccal blepharitis, chronic keratocon-junctivitis, vernal disease, keratoconus, early-onset cataract, and RD.

Acne rosacea

1. **Systemic** – common, idiopathic, chronic dermatosis involving the sun-exposed skin of the face and upper neck; erythema, telangiectasia, papules, pustules, sebaceous gland hypertrophy (*Fig. 24.43*), and rhinophyma.

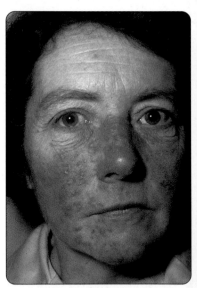

Fig. 24.43 Acne rosacea

2. **Ophthalmic** – conjunctival hyper-aemia, marginal keratitis, corneal thinning, and phlyctenulosis.

Dermatitis herpetiformis

1. **Systemic** – chronic disease associated with gluten enteropathy; groups of small, symmetrical itching blisters on extensor surfaces (*Fig. 24.44*), scalp and buttocks.

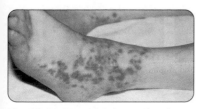

Fig. 24.44 Dermatitis herpetiformis

2. **Ophthalmic** – cicatrizing conjunctivitis.

Pemphigus vulgaris

1. **Systemic** – severe and potentially fatal autoimmune disease; widespread flaccid thin-walled blisters that initially involve the oral mucosa and then the skin (*Fig. 24.45*).

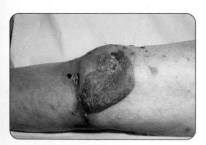

Fig. 24.45 Pemphigus vulgaris

2. **Ophthalmic** – conjunctivitis without scarring.

Epidermolysis bullosa

1. **Inheritance** – AD or AR.
2. **Systemic** – chronic blistering and sloughing following minor trauma (*Fig. 24.46*), mucosal involvement, nail dystrophy, and partial syndactyly of hands and feet.
3. **Ophthalmic** – eyelid scarring, corneal erosions, and cicatrizing conjunctivitis.

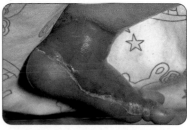

Fig. 24.46 Epidermolysis bullosa

Ichthyosis – congenital

1. **Inheritance** – AR.
2. **Systemic** – dry scaly, tight and shiny skin (collodion baby – *Fig. 24.47*).

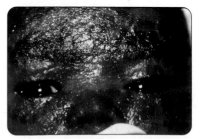

Fig. 24.47 Collodion baby

3. **Ophthalmic** – ectropion and congenital cataract.

Linear naevus sebaceus of Jadassohn

1. **Systemic** – warty or scaly lesion often on the scalp, forehead (*Fig. 24.48*) or face; infantile spasms, CNS anomalies, and developmental delay.
2. **Ophthalmic** – ptosis, epibulbar dermoids, cloudy cornea, lid colobomas, fundus colobomas, and microphthalmos.

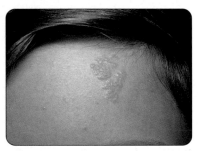

Fig. 24.48 Linear naevus sebaceus of Jadassohn

Menke disease

1. **Inheritance** – X-LR.
2. **Systemic** – abnormal hair (like wire wool), cutaneous hypopigmentation, developmental retardation, and seizures.
3. **Ophthalmic** – pigmentary retinopathy, tortuous retinal vessels, and optic atrophy.

Rothmund–Thomson syndrome

1. **Inheritance** – AR.
2. **Systemic** – poikiloderma, sparse hair, short stature, hypodontia, and nail dystrophy.
3. **Ophthalmic** – congenital cataract.

Sjögren–Larsson syndrome

1. **Inheritance** – AR.
2. **Systemic** – congenital ichthyosis, spastic diplegia or tetraplegia, and mental handicap.
3. **Ophthalmic** – macular crystals, cataract, colobomatous microphthalmos, and pigmentary retinopathy.

Waardenburg syndrome

1. **Inheritance** – AD.
2. **Systemic** – AD; partial albinism, deafness, poliosis, white hair forelock, poliosis, and synophrys (*Fig. 24.49*) or an unusual facial hair distribution.

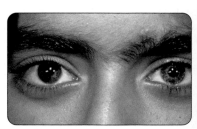

Fig. 24.49 Waardenburg syndrome

3. **Ophthalmic** – telecanthus and short palpebral fissure, heterochromia iridis, fundus hypopigmentation, microcornea, and glaucoma.

Naevus of Ota (oculodermal melanocytosis)

1. **Systemic** – unilateral facial skin hyperpigmentation (*Fig. 24.50*).
2. **Ophthalmic** – episcleral pigmentation, iris heterochromia and mammillations, glaucoma, fundus

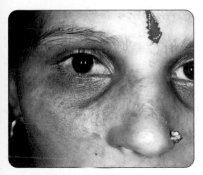

Fig. 24.50 Naevus of Ota

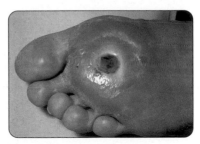

Fig. 24.51 Neuropathic ulcer

hyperpigmentation in Caucasians, and increased risk of uveal melanoma.

Acquired metabolic and endocrine disease

Diabetes mellitus

1. **Defect** – sustained hyperglycaemia of varying severity secondary to lack or diminished efficacy of endogenous insulin.
2. **Systemic** – nephropathy, accelerated atherosclerosis, peripheral vascular disease, neuropathic ulceration (*Fig. 24.51*), cranial nerve palsies, and skin infections.
3. **Ophthalmic**
   a. *Common* – retinopathy, iridopathy, and unstable refraction.
   b. *Uncommon* – papillopathy, accelerated senile cataract, rubeosis iridis, ocular motor nerve palsies, and reduced corneal sensation.
   c. *Rare* – pupillary light-near dissociation, Wolfram syndrome, acute-onset cataract, and rhino-orbital mucormycosis.

Thyrotoxicosis (hyperthyroidism)

1. **Defect** – excessive secretion of thyroid hormones.
2. **Systemic** – goitre (*Fig. 24.52*), fine hand tremor, intolerance to warmth,

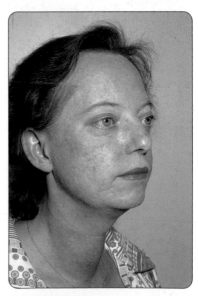

Fig. 24.52 Goitre

diarrhoea, weight loss, vitiligo, tachycardia, and acropachy.
3. **Ophthalmic** – lid retraction, chemosis, proptosis, superior limbic keratoconjunctivitis, KCS, diplopia, compressive optic neuropathy, and choroidal folds.

Myxoedema

1. **Defect** – thyroid hormone deficiency.
2. **Systemic** – cold intolerance, husky voice, alopecia, puffy face (*Fig. 24.53*) and hands, bradycardia, and dry skin.

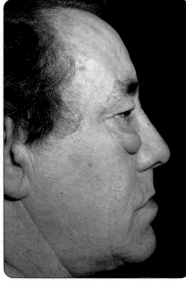

Fig. 24.53 Myxoedema

3. **Ophthalmic** – madarosis, periorbital and eyelid puffiness, and corneal arcus.

Hyperlipoproteinaemia

1. **Defect** – increased levels of circulating lipoprotein that may be primary or secondary.
2. **Systemic** – tendon xanthomata; atherosclerosis and coronary heart disease.

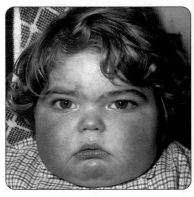

Fig. 24.54 Cushing syndrome

3. **Ophthalmic** – eyelid xanthelasma, corneal arcus, retinal vein occlusion, and lipaemia retinalis.

Cushing syndrome

1. **Defect** – prolonged elevation of free plasma glucocorticoid levels.
2. **Systemic** – obesity, moon face (*Fig. 24.54*), cutaneous striae, hirsutism in females, diabetes, and hypertension.
3. **Ophthalmic** – steroid-induced cataracts and ocular hypertension in iatrogenic Cushing syndrome, and chiasmal compression by a pituitary adenoma.

Acromegaly

1. **Defect** – hypersecretion of growth hormone by an acidophilic pituitary adenoma.
2. **Systemic** – facial coarseness, enlargement of nose, jaws, fingers, toes, tongue (macroglossia – Fig. 24.55) and internal organs, osteoarthrosis, hypertension, diabetes, and cardiomyopathy.

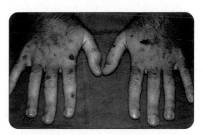

Fig. 24.56 Porphyria cutanea tarda

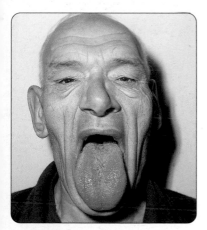

Fig. 24.55 Macroglossia

3. **Ophthalmic** – chiasmal compression and angioid streaks.

Porphyria cutanea tarda (cutaneous hepatic porphyria)

1. **Inheritance** – AD.
2. **Defect** – deficiency of uroporphyrinogen decarboxylate.
3. **Systemic** – cutaneous fragility, eruptions on exposure to sunlight, scarring and hyperpigmentation (Fig. 24.56); hepatomegaly, and hirsutism in females.

4. **Ophthalmic** – cicatricial ectropion, cicatrizing conjunctivitis, and scleritis.

Gout

1. **Systemic** – hyperuricaemia with deposition of monosodium urate in tissues; presents with acute monoarticular arthritis; later chronic arthritis (Fig. 24.57), tophi, renal disease, and hypertension.

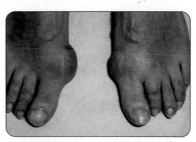

Fig. 24.57 Arthritis in gout

2. **Ophthalmic** – corneal crystals, band keratopathy, and scleritis.

Hyperparathyroidism – primary

1. **Systemic** – hypercalcaemia due to hypersecretion of parathyroid

hormone; renal calculi, bone disease, hypotonicity, and neurological problems.

2. **Ophthalmic** – band keratopathy.

Haemochromatosis – primary

1. **Systemic** – AR; increased iron absorption with subsequent deposition in various organs, resulting in hepatomegaly, arthropathy, diabetes and cardiomyopathy.
2. **Ophthalmic** – KCS.

Meretoja syndrome

1. **Inheritance** – AD.
2. **Systemic** – amyloidosis, mask-like facies and protruding lip, cranial nerve palsies, particularly facial, and skin laxity.
3. **Ophthalmic** – lattice dystrophy type 2.

Cardiovascular disease

Systemic hypertension

1. **Systemic** – blood pressure >140/90 mmHg that is most commonly idiopathic (essential) and occasionally secondary to a renal or metabolic disorder; may cause heart failure, coronary artery disease, renal disease, and stroke.
2. **Ophthalmic** – retinal arteriolosclerosis, branch retinal vein occlusion, retinopathy, choroidopathy, retinal artery occlusion, retinal artery macroaneurysm, AION, exudative RD, and ocular motor nerve palsies.

Carotid stenosis

1. **Systemic** – atheromatous narrowing often associated with ulceration, at the bifurcation of the common carotid artery; embolic stroke.
2. **Ophthalmic** – transient retinal ischaemic attacks (amaurosis fugax), retinal artery occlusion, and ocular ischaemic syndrome.

Myopathies

Myasthenia gravis

1. **Systemic** – impairment of neuromuscular conduction causes weakness and fatiguability of skeletal musculature; presents in the 3rd decade and may be ocular (*Fig. 24.58*), bulbar or generalized; thymoma in 10%.

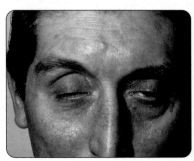

Fig. 24.58 Ocular myasthenia

2. **Ophthalmic** – ptosis, diplopia, and nystagmoid movements.

Myotonic dystrophy (dystrophia myotonica, Steinert disease)

1. **Inheritance** – AD.
2. **Defect** – delayed muscular relaxation after cessation of voluntary effort (myotonia).
3. **Systemic** – mournful facial expression, frontal baldness (*Fig. 24.59*), and slurred speech.

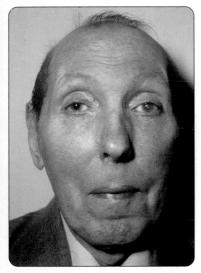

Fig. 24.59 Myotonic facies

4. **Ophthalmic** – early-onset cataract, ptosis, ophthalmoplegia, pupillary light-near dissociation, mild pigmentary retinopathy, bilateral optic atrophy, and low intraocular pressure.

Kearns–Sayre syndrome

1. **Defect** – mitochondrial cytopathy associated with mitochondrial DNA deletions.

2. **Systemic** – ataxia, cardiac conduction defects, deafness, short stature, and diabetes.
3. **Ophthalmic** – bilateral ptosis and limitation of ocular movements in all directions of gaze (progressive external ophthalmoplegia), and pigmentary retinopathy.

Oculopharyngeal dystrophy

1. **Inheritance** – AD.
2. **Systemic** – weakness of pharyngeal muscles and wasting of temporalis.
3. **Ophthalmic** – bilateral ptosis and progressive external ophthalmoplegia.

Neurological disease

Multiple sclerosis

1. **Systemic**
   - Idiopathic demyelinating disease involving white matter within the CNS that presents in the 3rd–4th decade either with relapsing–remitting disease or progressive involvement without remissions.
   - MR shows ovoid periventricular and corpus callosum plaques with their long axes perpendicular to the ventricular margins (*Fig. 24.60*).

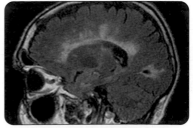

Fig. 24.60 MR sagittal FLAIR image shows plaques of demyelination

2. Ophthalmic – optic neuritis (usually retrobulbar), internuclear ophthalmoplegia, nystagmus, skew deviation, ocular motor nerve palsies, intermediate uveitis, and retinal periphlebitis.

Wernicke encephalopathy (Wernicke–Korsakoff syndrome)

1. Systemic – neuropathy associated with thiamine deficiency, most commonly secondary to chronic alcohol abuse.
2. Ophthalmic – nystagmus, unreactive pupils, gaze palsy, and bilateral 6th nerve palsies.

Syringomyelia

1. Systemic – cavitation surrounded by gliosis involving the crossing spinothalamic tracts in the spinal cord and medulla (syringobulbia); loss of pain and temperature but preservation of touch and wasting of the small muscles of the hands.
2. Ophthalmic – Horner syndrome.

Cogan syndrome

1. Systemic – acute onset of tinnitus, vertigo and deafness in a young adult. Some patients may develop necrotizing vasculitis and aortitis.
2. Ophthalmic – IK, uveitis, scleritis, and retinal vasculitis.

Devic disease (neuromyelitis optica)

1. Systemic – transverse myelitis of the spinal cord.
2. Ophthalmic – bilateral retrobulbar neuritis.

Steele–Richardson–Olszewski syndrome

1. Systemic – idiopathic condition characterized by neurological and mental deterioration in old age.
2. Ophthalmic – progressive supranuclear palsy.

Louis–Bar syndrome (ataxia telangiectasia)

1. Inheritance – AR.
2. Systemic – ataxia, slurred speech, skin telangiectasis, lymphopenia, growth retardation, and mental handicap.
3. Ophthalmic – bulbar conjunctival telangiectasia (*Fig. 24.61*) and disorders of ocular movements.

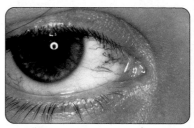

Fig. 24.61 Conjunctival telangiectasia in Louis–Bar syndrome

Cerebellar ataxia type 1

1. Inheritance – AD.
2. Systemic – progressive ataxia and dysarthria with reduced life span.
3. Ophthalmic – nystagmus, strabismus, lid retraction, supranuclear ophthalmoplegia, and optic atrophy.

Friedreich ataxia

1. **Inheritance** – AR.
2. **Systemic** – ataxia, dysarthria, scoliosis, diabetes, and cardiac disease.
3. **Ophthalmic** – pigmentary retinopathy, nystagmus, and optic atrophy.

Olivopontocerebellar atrophy type III

1. **Inheritance** – AD.
2. **Systemic** – ataxia, tremor and involuntary movements.
3. **Ophthalmic** – bull's-eye maculopathy.

Frontonasal dysplasia (medial clefting syndrome)

1. **Systemic** – midfacial anomalies, basal skull defect (Fig. 24.62) and encephalocele, absent corpus callosum (Fig. 24.63), and pituitary deficiency.

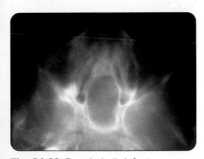

Fig. 24.62 Basal skull defect

2. **Ophthalmic** – hypertelorism, morning glory anomaly, disc coloboma, and microphthalmos.

de Morsier syndrome (septo-optic dysplasia)

1. **Systemic** – absence of the septum pellucidum, thinning or absence of the corpus callosum (see Fig. 24.63), and hypopituitarism.

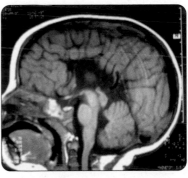

Fig. 24.63 MR sagittal image shows absence of corpus callosum

2. **Ophthalmic** – bilateral optic disc hypoplasia.

Gillespie syndrome

1. **Inheritance** – AR.
2. **Systemic** – cerebellar ataxia and mental handicap.
3. **Ophthalmic** – aniridia.

Hallervorden–Spatz syndrome

1. **Inheritance** – AR.
2. **Systemic** – progressive psychomotor deterioration.
3. **Ophthalmic** – retinal flecks and bull's-eye maculopathy.

Kjellin syndrome

1. **Inheritance** – AR.
2. **Systemic** – spastic paresis and dementia.
3. **Ophthalmic** – pattern retinal dystrophy.

Norrie disease

1. **Inheritance** – X-LR.
2. **Systemic** – psychomotor degeneration and deafness.
3. **Ophthalmic** – vitreoretinal dysplasia and retrolental mass, retinal folds, RD, cloudy cornea, cataract, and iris atrophy.

Riley–Day syndrome (familial dysautonomia)

1. **Inheritance** – AR.
2. **Systemic** – congenital aplasia of peripheral autonomic neurones.
3. **Ophthalmic** – KCS, corneal ulceration, and retinal vascular tortuosity.

Usher syndrome

1. **Inheritance** – AR.
2. **Systemic** – deafness.
3. **Ophthalmic** – pigmentary retinopathy.

Walker–Warburg syndrome

1. **Inheritance** – AR.
2. **Systemic** – hydrocephalus, cerebral malformation, epilepsy, muscular dystrophy, and early demise.
3. **Ophthalmic** – retinal dysplasia, Peters anomaly, cataract, uveal coloboma, microphthalmos, and optic nerve hypoplasia.

Phacomatoses

Neurofibromatosis 1 (von Recklinghausen disease)

1. **Inheritance** – AD.
2. **Systemic** – café-au-lait spots, axillary freckles, neurofibromas (*Fig. 24.64*), and bony abnormalities.

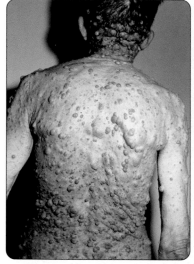

Fig. 24.64 Neurofibromas

3. **Ophthalmic** – eyelid neurofibromas, neural orbital tumours, optic nerve glioma, spheno-orbital encephalocele, Lisch iris nodules, iris mammillations, congenital ectropion uveae, glaucoma, prominent corneal nerves, choroidal naevi, retinal astrocytomas.

Neurofibromatosis 2

1. Inheritance – AD.
2. Systemic – bilateral acoustic neuromas (*Fig. 24.65*).

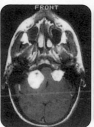 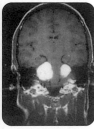

Fig. 24.65 MR with enhancement shows bilateral acoustic neuromas

3. Ophthalmic – early-onset cataract, combined hamartoma of the RPE and retina, and ophthalmoplegia.

Tuberous sclerosis (Bourneville disease)

1. Inheritance – AD in 60%.
2. Systemic
- Classic triad of (a) *epilepsy*, (b) *mental retardation* and (c) *adenoma sebaceum* (*Fig. 24.66*) is present in a minority of patients, but is diagnostic when present.
- Other manifestations – subungual hamartomas, ash-leaf spots, shagreen patches, intracranial astrocytomas, and visceral tumours.
3. Ophthalmic – fundus astrocytomas, patchy iris hypopigmentation, and atypical iris colobomas.

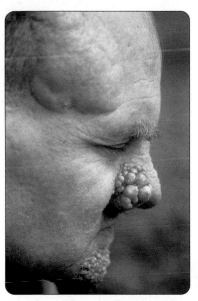

Fig. 24.66 Adenoma sebaceum and fibrous plaque on the forehead

Von Hippel–Lindau syndrome

1. Inheritance – AD.
2. Systemic – CNS haemangioblastoma involving the cerebellum (*Fig. 24.67*), spinal cord, medulla or pons, phaeochromocytoma, and tumours or cysts of other organs.
3. Ophthalmic – retinal haemangioblastoma, which may be multiple and bilateral.

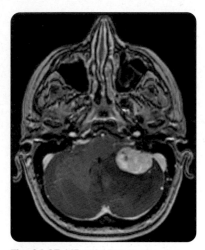

Fig. 24.67 MR axial image shows a cerebellar haemangioblastoma

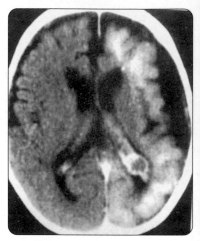

Fig. 24.68 CT axial image shows meningeal haemangioma and cerebral atrophy

Sturge–Weber syndrome (encephalotrigeminal angiomatosis)

1. **Systemic** – sporadic; facial port-wine stain and leptomeningeal haemangioma (*Fig. 24.68*) that may cause seizures, hemiparesis or hemianopia.
2. **Ophthalmic** – glaucoma, episcleral haemangioma, diffuse choroidal haemangioma, and heterochromia iridis.

Klippel–Treunaunay–Weber syndrome

1. **Systemic** – sporadic; facial naevus flammeus (port-wine stain), cutaneous haemangiomas, hypertrophy of one limb, soft tissue hypertrophy, and varicose veins or venous malformations.

2. **Ophthalmic** – ocular haemangiomas, orbital varices, and glaucoma.

Blood disease

Leukaemia

1. **Systemic**
   - Malignancies of the haematopoietic stem cells that may be acute or chronic and myelocytic or lymphocytic.
   - Fatigue, recurrent infections, easy bruising and bleeding (*Fig. 24.69*), lymphadenopathy and hepatosplenomegaly.
2. **Ophthalmic** – direct leukaemic infiltration may involve the uvea and orbit, and indirect involvement as a result of anaemia, thrombocytopenia and hyperviscosity resulting in intraocular bleeding, infection and vascular occlusion.

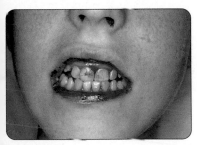

Fig. 24.69 Bleeding in acute leukaemia

Anaemia

1. Systemic
- Decrease in circulating erythrocytes or in amount of haemoglobin in each cell, or both, that occurs when the equilibrium between blood loss and production is disturbed.
- Pallor and atrophic glossitis (*Fig. 24.70*), koilonychia, and angular stomatitis.

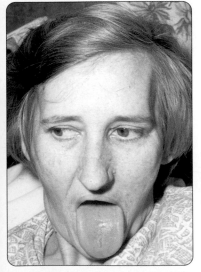

Fig. 24.70 Pallor and atrophic glossitis in anaemia

2. Ophthalmic – sickle cell retinopathy, optic neuropathy in pernicious anaemia, retinal flame-shaped haemorrhages, cotton-wool spots, Roth spots, and venous tortuosity.

Antiphospholipid antibody syndrome – primary

1. Systemic
- Prethrombotic autoimmune disease occurring in patients who do not have SLE but who are positive for antiphospholipid antibody.
- Presents in young adults with venous and arterial occlusion, and recurrent spontaneous abortion; also heart valve abnormalities, renal disease, and livedo reticularis.

2. Ophthalmic – retinal vascular occlusion, cotton-wool spots and venous dilatation; anterior ischaemic optic neuropathy, amaurosis fugax, and conjunctival telangiectasia.

Polycythaemia rubra vera

1. Systemic – neoplastic proliferation of erythrocytes; plethora (*Fig. 24.71*), splenomegaly, pruritus, and stroke.

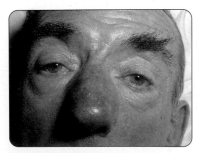

Fig. 24.71 Plethora

2. Ophthalmic – slow-flow retinopathy, conjunctival telangiectasia, and retinal vein occlusion.

Waldenström macroglobulinaemia

1. Systemic
- Malignant lymphoproliferative disorder with monoclonal IgM production.
- Fatigue, mucosal bleeding, lymphadenopathy, hepatospleno-megaly, Raynaud phenomenon, and peripheral vascular disease

2. Ophthalmic – slow-flow retinopathy, proptosis, corneal crystals, interme-diate uveitis, and cotton-wool spots.

Kasabach–Merrit syndrome

1. Systemic – thrombocytopenia and intravascular coagulation associated with rapidly expanding haemangio-mas of trunk, extremities and abdominal viscera.

2. Ophthalmic – eyelid and orbital haemangiomas.

Hermansky–Pudlak syndrome

1. Inheritance – AR.
2. Systemic – albinism, early bruising due to platelet dysfunction, and pulmonary fibrosis.
3. Ophthalmic – ocular albinism.

Rendu–Osler–Weber syndrome (hereditary haemorrhagic telangiectasia)

1. Inheritance – AD.
2. Systemic – telangiectasia of skin, lips, tongue (*Fig. 24.72*) and mouth;

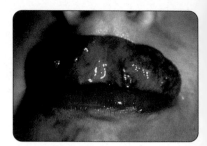

Fig. 24.72 Telangiectasia of the tongue

epistaxis, and bleeding from the gut and lungs.
3. Ophthalmic – conjunctival telangiec-tasis and retinal haemorrhages.

Neoplastic conditions

Lymphoma

1. Systemic – group of conditions characterized by neoplastic proliferation of cells of the immune system characterized by lymphade-nopathy, constitutional symptoms, and occasionally CNS involvement.

2. Ophthalmic
   a. *Hodgkin disease* – anterior uveitis, vitritis, and multifocal fundus lesions resembling chorioretinitis.
   b. *Non-Hodgkin lymphoma* – conjunctival involvement, orbital involvement, Mikulicz syndrome, and uveal infiltration.
   c. *CNS B-cell lymphoma* – intermedi-ate uveitis, sub-RPE infiltrates, and geographic encircling choroidal infiltration.

Multiple myeloma (myelomatosis)

1. **Systemic** – malignant proliferation of plasma cells; lytic bony lesions (*Fig. 24.73*), renal disease, anaemia, and increased blood viscosity.

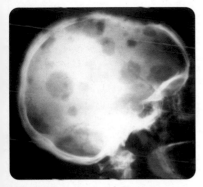

Fig. 24.73 Lytic skull lesions in myeloma

2. **Ophthalmic** – slow-flow retinopathy, proptosis, corneal crystals, pars plana cysts, and retinal vein occlusion.

Xeroderma pigmentosum

1. **Inheritance** – AR.
2. **Systemic** – skin dystrophy and multiple malignancies, bird-like facies (*Fig. 24.74*), ataxia and mental handicap.
3. **Ophthalmic** – eyelid malignancies, conjunctival scarring, conjunctival squamous cell carcinoma, and keratitis.

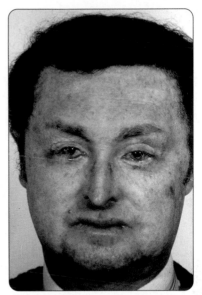

Fig. 24.74 Xeroderma pigmentosum

Eaton–Lambert myasthenic syndrome

1. **Systemic**
   - Autoimmune disorder of the neuromuscular junction often associated with underlying small cell bronchial carcinoma.
   - Gradual difficulty in walking that may precede the clinical manifestation of the associated carcinoma by up to two years.
2. **Ophthalmic** – ptosis and diplopia.

Histiocytosis X (Langerhans cell histiocytosis)

1. **Systemic** – three clinically different conditions in which multiple infiltrative foci of histiocytes occur that bear features of Langerhans cells.

2. Ophthalmic – incidence of ocular manifestations varies according to the subgroup:

   a. *Eosinophilic granuloma* – occasionally associated with proptosis.

   b. *Letterer–Siwe disease* – no ocular manifestations.

   c. *Hand–Schüller–Christian disease* – frequently associated with proptosis.

Muir–Torre syndrome

Cutaneous sebaceous gland tumours that may be single or multiple, benign or malignant, associated with visceral malignancies – most frequently colonic carcinoma.

Bazex syndrome

1. Inheritance – AD.

2. Systemic – eczematous and psoriasiform lesions associated with carcinomas of the upper respiratory and digestive tracts.

3. Ophthalmic – eyelid basal cell carcinoma.

Gardner syndrome

1. Inheritance – AD.

2. Systemic – adenomatous polyposis of the colon (*Fig. 24.75*) that

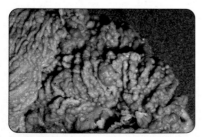

Fig. 24.75 Adenomatous polyposis

predisposes to carcinoma, supernumerary teeth, fibrous skull dysplasia, osteomas, fibromas, and epithelial cysts.

3. Ophthalmic – atypical CHRPE.

Gorlin–Goltz (naevoid basal cell carcinoma) syndrome

1. Inheritance – AD.

2. Systemic – multiple basal cell carcinomas and other tumours, broad facies (*Fig. 24.76*), macrocephaly, and rib anomalies.

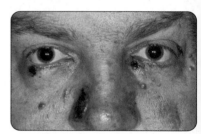

Fig. 24.76 Gorlin–Goltz syndrome

3. Ophthalmic – eyelid basal cell carcinoma, hypertelorism, cataract, iris coloboma, and microphthalmos.

Maffucci syndrome

1. Systemic – enchondromatosis associated with multiple cutaneous or visceral haemangiomas.

2. Ophthalmic – capillary haemangiomas of eyelids and orbit.

Multiple endocrine neoplasia type IIB (Sipple syndrome)

1. Inheritance – AD.

2. Systemic – multiple neuromas of tongue, lips (*Fig. 24.77*) and intestinal mucosa; Marfanoid

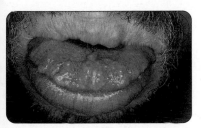

Fig. 24.77 Sipple syndrome

habitus, medullary thyroid carcinoma, phaeochromocytoma and hyperparathyroidism.
3. **Ophthalmic** – eyelid neurofibroma, conjunctival neuromas, prominent corneal nerves, and poor pupillary dilatation.

Renal disease

IgA nephropathy

1. **Systemic** – glomerulonephritis that principally affects young males and presents with haematuria, pharyngitis, lethargy and muscle pains.
2. **Ophthalmic** – anterior uveitis and scleritis.

Membranoproliferative glomerulonephritis type II

1. **Systemic** – idiopathic renal disorder with characteristic histological features that presents in childhood with nephritic syndrome or acute nephritis.
2. **Ophthalmic** – drusen-like deposits at the posterior pole.

Tubulointerstitial nephritis and uveitis (TINU)

1. **Systemic** – immune oculorenal disease that typically affects adolescent girls. Presentation is with constitutional symptoms, proteinuria, hypertension, and renal failure.
2. **Ophthalmic** – bilateral anterior uveitis follows renal manifestations.

Alport syndrome

1. **Inheritance** – AD or X-LR.
2. **Systemic** – progressive deafness and renal disease associated with abnormal glomerular basement membrane.
3. **Ophthalmic** – anterior lenticonus, fleck retinopathy, and posterior polymorphous corneal dystrophy.

Renal-coloboma syndrome (papillorenal syndrome)

1. **Inheritance** – AD.
2. **Systemic** – renal hypoplasia.
3. **Ophthalmic** – optic disc coloboma and microphthalmos.

Miscellaneous inborn errors of metabolism

Homocystinuria

1. **Inheritance** – AR.
2. **Defect** – deficiency of cystathionine-beta-synthetase results in accumulation of homocystine and methionine.
3. **Systemic** – fair complexion and malar flush (*Fig. 24.78*), Marfanoid habitus, failure to thrive, neurodevelopmental delay, osteoporosis, psychiatric problems, and thromboembolic phenomena.

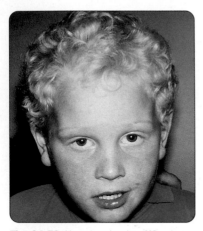

Fig. 24.78 Homocystinuria

4. **Ophthalmic** – ectopia lentis, myopia, and RD.

Alcaptonuria

1. **Inheritance** – AR.
2. **Defect** – in homogentistic acid oxidase results in accumulation of homogentistic acid in tissues.
3. **Systemic** – dark urine, dark sweat stains, greyish pigmentation of nasal cartilage and ear lobes (ochronosis), spinal disc degeneration (*Fig. 24.79*), and arthropathy.
4. **Ophthalmic** – ochronosis of sclera and tendons of horizontal recti, and oil-droplet corneal pigmentation just inside the limbus.

Wilson disease (hepatolenticular degeneration)

1. **Inheritance** – AR.
2. **Defect** – deficiency of caeruloplasmin results in the deposition of

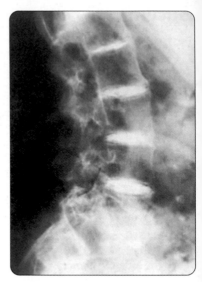

Fig. 24.79 Disc degeneration in alcaptonuria

copper in tissues, particularly the liver and brain.
3. **Systemic** – chronic liver disease, dysarthria, tremor, involuntary movements, and psychosis.
4. **Ophthalmic** – Kayser–Fleischer rings and sunflower cataract.

Refsum syndrome (heredopathic atactica polyneuritiformis)

1. **Inheritance** – AR.
2. **Defect** – deficiency in phytanoyl-CoA hydrolase results in accumulation of phytanic acid.
3. **Systemic** – cerebellar ataxia, peripheral neuropathy, ichthyosis (*Fig. 24.80*), deafness, anosmia, and cardiomyopathy.
4. **Ophthalmic** – pigmentary retinopathy, optic atrophy, cataract, and nystagmus.

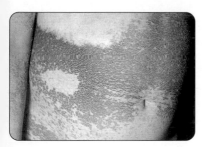

Fig. 24.80 Ichthyosis

Galactosaemia

1. **Inheritance** – AR.
2. **Defect** – absence of galactose-1-phosphate uridyl transferase results in impairment of galactose utilization.
3. **Systemic** – presents in infancy with failure to thrive, vomiting, hepatomegaly, and hypoglycaemia.
4. **Ophthalmic** – congenital 'oil droplet' cataract.

Bassen–Kornzweig syndrome (abetalipoproteiaemia)

1. **Inheritance** – AR.
2. **Defect** – deficiency of beta-lipoprotein results in malabsorption and vitamin A deficiency.
3. **Systemic** – spinocerebellar ataxia and acanthocytosis.
4. **Ophthalmic** – pigmentary retinopathy, ptosis and progressive external ophthalmoplegia, xanthelasma, and corneal arcus.

Tyrosinaemia type II (Richner–Hanhart syndrome)

1. **Inheritance** – AR.
2. **Defect** – deficiency of soluble tyrosine aminotransferase results in raised serum tyrosine.

3. **Systemic** – psychomotor retardation and palmar keratosis.
4. **Ophthalmic** – corneal pseudodendrites with crystalline edges, vortex keratopathy, and conjunctival thickening.

Hyperlysinaemia

1. **Inheritance** – AR.
2. **Defect** – deficiency of lysine alpha-ketoglutarate reductase.
3. **Systemic** – lax ligaments, muscular hypotonia, seizures, and mental handicap.
4. **Ophthalmic** – ectopia lentis.

Hyperornithinaemia

1. **Inheritance** – AR.
2. **Defect** – deficiency of ornithine aminotransferase.
3. **Systemic** – hyperornithinaemia and ornithinuria.
4. **Ophthalmic** – gyrate atrophy, myopia, and early-onset cataract.

Norum disease

1. **Inheritance** – AR.
2. **Defect** – deficiency of lecithin-cholesterol acyltransferase results in accumulation of unesterified cholesterol.
3. **Systemic** – early-onset atherosclerosis, renal disease, and anaemia.
4. **Ophthalmic** – progressive corneal opacification and arcus-like corneal clouding extending into the sclera.

Lowe syndrome (oculocerebrorenal syndrome)

1. **Inheritance** – X-LR.
2. **Defect** – amino acid metabolism.
3. **Systemic** – psychomotor retardation, muscular hypotonia, renal disease,

frontal prominence, sunken eyes, and chubby cheeks.
4. **Ophthalmic** – cataract, glaucoma, miosis and poor pupillary dilatation, and posterior lenticonus.

Mannosidosis

1. **Inheritance** – AR.
2. **Defect** – deficiency of alpha-mannosidase results in excretion of mannose-containing oligosaccharides in the urine.
3. **Systemic** – psychomotor retardation, hepatosplenomegaly, bone deformity, and deafness.
4. **Ophthalmic** – cataract, corneal clouding, abnormal eye movements, and optic atrophy.

Sulphite oxidase deficiency

1. **Inheritance** – AR.
2. **Systemic** – progressive psychomotor deterioration and early demise.
3. **Ophthalmic** – ectopia lentis.

Tangier disease

1. **Inheritance** – AR.
2. **Defect** – absence of high-density lipoprotein and accumulation of cholesterol esters in tissues.
3. **Systemic** – enlarged tonsil, facial diplegia, neuropathy, and spleno-megaly.
4. **Ophthalmic** – corneal crystals and vortex keratopathy.

Hyperoxaluria – primary

1. **Inheritance** – AR.
2. **Defect** – deficiency of glycoxylate metabolism results in excretion of large amounts of oxalate.

3. **Systemic** – renal disease and generalized deposition of calcium oxalate in other tissues (oxalosis).
4. **Ophthalmic** – retinal crystals and black macular lesions.

Mucopolysaccharidoses

Hurler syndrome (MPS IH)

1. **Inheritance** – AR.
2. **Systemic** – psychomotor retardation, stunted growth, large head, facial coarseness (*Fig. 24.81*), macro-glossia, stubby fingers and hepatosplenomegaly.

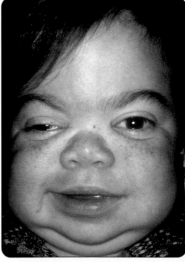

Fig. 24.81 Hurler syndrome

3. **Ophthalmic** – corneal clouding, glaucoma, pigmentary retinopathy, and optic atrophy.

Scheie syndrome (MPS IS)

1. **Inheritance** – AR.
2. **Systemic** – broad facies, macrostomia, short neck, truncal hirsutism, arthropathy, aortic valve disease and normal intellect.
3. **Ophthalmic** – pigmentary retinopathy, corneal clouding, and optic atrophy.

Hunter syndrome (MPS II)

1. **Inheritance** – X-LR.
2. **Systemic** – psychomotor retardation, stunted growth, large head, facial coarseness, kyphosis and hepatosplenomegaly.
3. **Ophthalmic** – pigmentary retinopathy and glaucoma.

Sanfilippo syndrome (MPS III A-D)

1. **Inheritance** – AR.
2. **Systemic** – moderate facial coarseness, hirsutism, hyperactivity and severe mental handicap.
3. **Ophthalmic** – pigmentary retinopathy and glaucoma.

Morquio syndrome (MPS IVA)

1. **Inheritance** – AR.
2. **Systemic** – mild facial coarseness, dwarfism, skeletal anomalies (*Fig. 24.82*), and normal intellect.

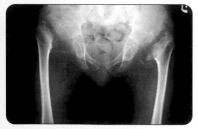

Fig. 24.82 Skeletal anomalies in Morquio syndrome

3. **Ophthalmic** – corneal clouding and glaucoma.

Maroteaux–Lamy syndrome (MPS VI)

1. **Inheritance** – AR.
2. **Systemic** – similar to Hurler syndrome but normal intellect.
3. **Ophthalmic** – corneal clouding, glaucoma, retinal vessel dilatation and tortuosity, and optic atrophy.

Sly syndrome (MPS VII)

1. **Inheritance** – AR.
2. **Systemic** – facial coarseness, macrocephaly, dysostosis multiplex, hepatosplenomegaly, and mental handicap.
3. **Ophthalmic** – corneal clouding, pigmentary retinopathy, and glaucoma.

Sphingolipidoses

Tay–Sachs disease (Gm2 gangliosidosis type I)

1. **Inheritance** – AR.
2. **Systemic** – progressive deafness, spasticity, and convulsions.
3. **Ophthalmic** – cherry-red spot at macula.

Sandhoff syndrome (Gm2 gangliosidosis type II)

1. **Inheritance** – AR.
2. **Systemic** – neurological degeneration similar to Tay–Sachs disease.
3. **Ophthalmic** – cherry-red spot at macula.

Niemann–Pick disease

Type A (acute neuronopathic)

1. **Systemic** – psychomotor deterioration and early demise.
2. **Ophthalmic** – cherry-red spot at macula and mild corneal clouding.

Type B (chronic non-neuronopathic)

1. **Systemic** – survival into adulthood.
2. **Ophthalmic** – bull's-eye maculopathy.

Type C (chronic neuronopathic)

1. **Systemic** – variable CNS involvement with death from 5 years to adulthood).
2. **Ophthalmic** – gaze palsy and abnormal eye movements.

Types D and E

1. **Systemic** – ataxia and athetosis.
2. **Ophthalmic** – gaze palsy.

Mucolipidoses

Type I (Goldberg syndrome – sialidosis)

1. **Inheritance** – AR.
2. **Systemic** – deafness, hypotonia, short trunk, cerebellar ataxia, Hurler-like features, and myoclonic seizures.
3. **Ophthalmic** – cataract and cherry-red spot at macula.

Type II (Leroy I-cell disease)

1. **Inheritance** – AR.
2. **Systemic** – psychomotor retardation, macroglossia, restricted joint mobility, and hip dislocation.
4. **Ophthalmic** – corneal clouding and glaucoma.

Type III (pseudo-Hurler polydystrophy syndrome)

1. **Inheritance** – AR.
2. **Systemic** – milder form of type II.
3. **Ophthalmic** – corneal clouding.

Type IV

1. **Inheritance** – AR.
2. **Systemic** – psychomotor retardation and organomegaly.
3. **Ophthalmic** – corneal clouding, cataract, and pigmentary retinopathy.

Nephropathic cystinosis

1. **Inheritance** – AR.
2. **Defect** – of lysosomal cystine transport resulting in accumulation of cysteine in the kidneys (Fanconi syndrome).
3. **Systemic** – failure to thrive, small stature, blond hair, fair complexion, hypothyroidism, and renal disease.
4. **Ophthalmic** – corneal and crystals, cataract, pigmentary retinopathy.

Fabry disease

1. **Inheritance** – X-LR.
2. **Defect** – lysosomal storage disease caused by deficiency of alpha-galactosidase.
3. **Systemic** – attacks of periodic burning pain in extremities and abdomen, purple cutaneous telangiectasia (angiokeratoma diffusum – *Fig. 24.83*), renal and cardiopulmonary disease, osteoporosis, and retarded growth.

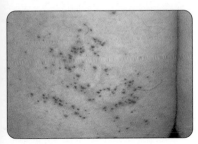

Fig. 24.83 Angiokeratoma diffusum

4. **Ophthalmic** – vortex keratopathy, wedge-shaped cataract, conjunctival telangiectasia, retinal vascular tortuosity, 3rd nerve palsy, and nystagmus.

Farber disease

1. **Inheritance** – AR.
2. **Defect** – lysosomal storage disease due to defective ceramidase.
3. **Systemic** – hoarseness, aphonia, dermatitis, lymphadenopathy, psychomotor retardation, and renal and cardiopulmonary disease.
4. **Ophthalmic** – cherry-red spot at macula, pinguecula-like conjunctival lesions, and nodular corneal opacity.

Jansky–Bielschowsky disease (CLN2)

1. **Systemic** – presentation is in early childhood with mental deterioration, ataxia, and epilepsy, with early demise.
2. **Ophthalmic** – retinal degeneration and optic atrophy.

Batten disease (neuronal ceroid lipofuscinosis – CLN3)

1. **Inheritance** – AR.
2. **Defect** – accumulation of lipopigments in tissues.
3. **Systemic** – psychomotor retardation, ataxia, hypotonia, and myoclonic jerks.
4. **Ophthalmic** – retinal dysplasia and leukocoria, bull's-eye maculopathy, pigmentary retinopathy, and optic atrophy.

Chromosomal defects

Down syndrome (mongolism)

1. **Defect** – trisomy 21.
2. **Systemic** – mental handicap, stunted growth, small antero-posteriorly flattened skull, flat nasal bridge, epicanthic folds and upslanting palpebral fissures (*Fig. 24.84*), excess skin on back of neck, short phalanges with a single transverse palmar (simian) crease, cardio-respiratory disease, and reduced life span.
3. **Ophthalmic** – epicanthic folds, iris Brushfield spots, myopia, blue dot cataract, strabismus, keratoconus, iris hypoplasia, and anomalous optic disc vasculature.

Turner syndrome

1. **Defect** – XO with 45 chromosomes.
2. **Systemic** – hypogonadism, hirsutism in females, webbed neck (*Fig. 24.85*), skeletal defects, and renal anomalies.

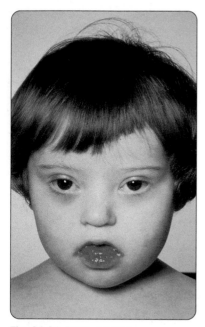

Fig. 24.84 Down syndrome

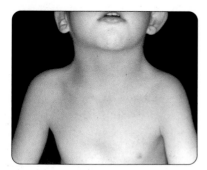

Fig. 24.85 Webbed neck in Turner syndrome

3. Ophthalmic – keratoconus, conjunctival telangiectasia, blue sclera, cataract, and Coats disease.

Edward syndrome

1. **Defect** – trisomy 18.
2. **Systemic** – skull abnormalities, micrognathia, webbed neck, short digits, low-set ears, deafness, cardiac anomalies, and mental handicap.
3. **Ophthalmic** – ptosis, microphthalmos, corneal opacity, cataract, uveal and disc coloboma, and vitreoretinal dysplasia.

Cat-eye syndrome

1. **Defect** – partial trisomy 22.
2. **Systemic** – anal atresia, cardiac defects, renal agenesis, preauricular anomalies and mental handicap.
3. **Ophthalmic** – uveal colobomas, microphthalmos, and morning glory anomaly.

Cri du chat syndrome

1. **Defect** – partial deletion of 5p.
2. **Systemic** – hypertelorism, microcephaly, growth retardation, low-set ears, cat-like cry, and mental handicap.
3. **Ophthalmic** – cataract and strabismus.

Patau syndrome

1. **Defect** – trisomy 13.
2. **Systemic** – forebrain defects, hare lip and cleft palate, polydactyly, cardiac defects and early demise.
3. **Ophthalmic** – cyclopia, anophthalmos, microphthalmos, cataract, uveal coloboma, retinal dysplasia, and optic nerve hypoplasia.

Prader–Willi syndrome

1. **Defect** – deletion of 15.
2. **Systemic** – obesity, short stature, hypogonadism, round face, CNS dysfunction, and mental handicap.
3. **Ophthalmic** – congenital ectropion uveae.

Craniosynostoses

Crouzon syndrome

1. **Inheritance** – AD.
2. **Systemic** – short anteroposterior head distance and wide cranium, midfacial hypoplasia, mandibular prognathism, inverted V-shaped palate, and acanthosis nigricans.
3. **Ophthalmic** – severe proptosis, hypertelorism, V pattern exotropia (Fig. 24.86), aniridia, blue sclera, cataract, ectopia lentis, glaucoma, coloboma, megalocornea, and optic nerve hypoplasia.

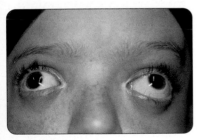

Fig. 24.86 Crouzon syndrome

Apert syndrome (acroceplalosyndactyly)

1. **Inheritance** – majority sporadic, remainder AD.
2. **Systemic** – oxycephaly, midfacial hypoplasia and beak-shaped nose (Fig. 24.87), low-set ears, high-arched cleft palate and a bifid uvula, syndactyly, anomalies of major organs, and occasional mental handicap.

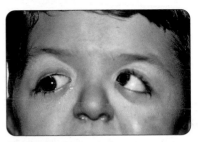

Fig. 24.87 Alpert syndrome

3. **Ophthalmic** – shallow orbits, mild proptosis, hypertelorism, exotropia, downward slanting palpebral apertures, keratoconus, ectopia lentis, and congenital glaucoma.

Mandibulofacial dysostoses

Treacher Collins syndrome

1. **Inheritance** – AD (40%), remainder sporadic.
2. **Systemic** – anomalies of pinnae, malar and mandibular hypoplasia (Fig. 24.88), cleft palate, and deafness.

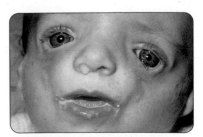

Fig. 24.88 Treacher Collins syndrome

3. Ophthalmic – downward slanting palpebral apertures, colobomas of the lateral lower eyelids, cataract, microphthalmos, epibulbar dermoids, and atresia of the lacrimal passages.

Goldenhar syndrome (oculo-auriculo-vertebral spectrum)

1. Systemic – mandibular hypoplasia (hemifacial microsomia – *Fig. 24.89*), microtia and preauricular appendages, and hemivertebrae.

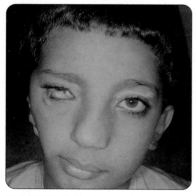

Fig. 24.89 Goldenhar syndrome

2. Ophthalmic – epibulbar dermoid, upper-lid notch or coloboma, microphthalmos, ptosis, nasolacrimal obstruction, and disc coloboma.

Hallermann–Streiff–François syndrome

1. Systemic – short stature, beak-shaped nose, micrognathia, sparse hair (hypotrichosis – *Fig. 24.90*), dental anomalies, and narrow upper respiratory airway.

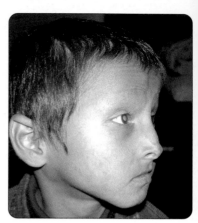

Fig. 24.90 Hallermann–Streiff–François syndrome

2. Ophthalmic – bilateral microphthalmos, cataract, nystagmus and strabismus, disc coloboma, and blue sclera.

Miscellaneous congenital syndromic conditions

Bardet–Biedl syndrome

1. Inheritance – AR.
2. Systemic – hypogonadism, polydactyly (*Fig. 24.91*), obesity, and mental handicap.
3. Ophthalmic – bull's-eye maculopathy, pigmentary retinopathy, cataract and myopia.

Laurence–Moon syndrome

1. Inheritance – AR.
2. Systemic – hypogonadism, spastic diplegia, and mental handicap.
3. Ophthalmic – pigmentary retinopathy and choroidal atrophy.

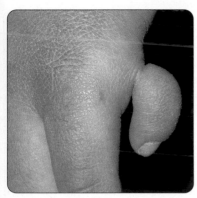

Fig. 24.91 Polydactyly

Bloch–Sulzberger syndrome (incontinentia pigmenti)

1. **Inheritance** – X-LD (lethal in males)
2. **Systemic** – initially vesciculobullous and later pigmentary (*Fig. 24.92*)

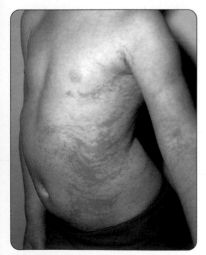

Fig. 24.92 Incontinentia pigmenti

skin changes, and anomalies of hair, bones, teeth and CNS.
3. **Ophthalmic** – cicatricial RD and leukocorea, and microphthalmos.

Chediak–Higashi syndrome

1. **Inheritance** – AR.
2. **Systemic** – albinism, pancytopenia, hepatosplenomegaly, recurrent or persistent bacterial infections, predisposition to lymphoma, and reduced life span.
3. **Ophthalmic** – ocular albinism.

Cockayne syndrome

1. **Inheritance** – AR.
2. **Systemic** – premature ageing, dwarfism, skeletal anomalies, deafness, progeria, photosensitivity, and mental handicap.
3. **Ophthalmic** – optic atrophy, pigmentary retinopathy, miosis, and cataract.

Cohen syndrome

1. **Inheritance** – AR.
2. **Systemic** – microcephaly, short stature, dysmorphic facies, hand anomalies, hypotonia, and mental handicap.
3. **Ophthalmic** – myopia, pigmentary retinopathy, and strabismus.

Cornelia de Lange syndrome

1. **Inheritance** – usually sporadic, occasionally AD.
2. **Systemic** – short stature, brachycephaly, low set ears, webbed neck, bushy eyebrows, synophrys, coarse hair, flared nostrils, depressed nasal bridge (*Fig. 24.93*), flat hands with short fingers, deafness, and severe mental handicap.

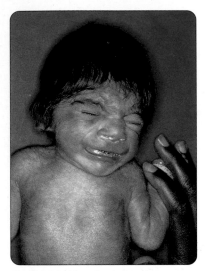

Fig. 24.93 Cornelia de Lange syndrome

3. **Ophthalmic** – microcornea, ptosis, nystagmus, myopia, and disc coloboma.

Goltz syndrome

1. **Inheritance** – X-LD.
2. **Systemic** – focal dermal hypoplasia and pigmentary changes, syndactyly, dental anomalies, facial hemihypertrophy, and nail dystrophy.
3. **Ophthalmic** – uveal and disc colobomas, microphthalmos, and anopthalmos.

Lenz microphthalmos syndrome

1. **Inheritance** – X-L.
2. **Systemic** – digital anomalies, narrow shoulders, bat ears, delayed development, congenital heart disease, and skeletal and urogenital defects.
3. **Ophthalmic** – bilateral or unilateral microphthalmos or anophthalmos, and ptosis.

Meckel–Gruber syndrome

1. **Inheritance** – AR.
2. **Systemic** – sloping forehead, posterior meningoencephalocele, polycystic disease of viscera, polydactyly, and early demise.
3. **Ophthalmic** – uveal colobomas, microphthalmos, and cataract.

Nance–Horan syndrome

1. **Inheritance** – X-LR.
2. **Systemic** – prominent ears and supernumerary abnormal teeth.
3. **Ophthalmic** – cataract, microcornea, and microphthalmos.

Pagon syndrome (CHARGE)

This is characterized by:
- **C**olobomas
- **H**eart defects
- **A**tresia of choanae
- **R**etarded growth
- **G**enital anomalies
- **E**ar anomalies – and/or deafness.

Pierre–Robin syndrome

1. **Inheritance** – AR.
2. **Systemic** – micrognathia and glossoptosis (*Fig. 24.94*), laryngeal displacement, and cleft palate.
3. **Ophthalmic** – uveal colobomas.

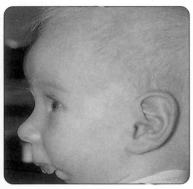

Fig. 24.94 Pierre–Robin syndrome

Rubinstein–Taybi syndrome

1. **Systemic** – psychomotor retardation, broad thumbs and great toes, dysmorphic facies (*Fig. 24.95*), short stature, large foramen magnum, and abnormalities of the vertebrae and sternum.

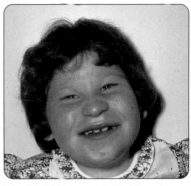

Fig. 24.95 Rubenstein–Taybi syndrome

2. **Ophthalmic** – hypertelorism, downslanting palpebral fissures, epicanthic folds, ptosis, long lashes, strabismus, congenital glaucoma, and uveal coloboma.

Index

Note: Page numbers in **bold** refer to figures.

O

S